HOME GYM TRAINING
with a personal trainer

First Printed 2001

Copyright © David and Melinda Obern, 2001-11-20

All rights reserved. No part of this publication may be reproduced, stored in a retrieval system, transmitted in any form or by any means, electronic, mechanical, photocopying, recording or otherwise without the prior written permission of the copyright owners.

National Library of Australia Cataloguing-in-Publication Entry

Obern, David, 1970-.
Home gym training with a personal trainer.

Bibliography.
Includes Index.
ISBN: 0 9580010 0 6

1. Exercise – Equipment and supplies. 2. Exercise. I. Obern, Melinda, 1968-. II. Title.

613.710284

Photolithography by:	Wakefields Digital Colour Solutions Limited, 102-108 Wakefield Street Wellington, New Zealand, Telephone: 04 473 3631, Fax: 04 473 3613
Printed by:	First printed in New Zealand by City Print Communications, 25 Bond Street, Wellington, Telephone: 04-473-8885, Fax: 04-473-8898
	Second edition printed in Taiwan by Pao Ying Printing CO., LTD. 366 Zi Jiang Road, Sha Lu Town, Taichung County, Taiwan, R.O.C., Telephone: +886-4-6314220-1, Fax: +886-4-6313515

Photography by: Adrian Obern and Paul Gosney • Book Design by: Sam Auger
• Project manager: Callum Calderwood

This book is intended to offer information and education on the topic of health and fitness. It is not intended to offer medical advice. Although the information contained in this book has been thoroughly researched, some material may not be suitable for every reader and may be affected by differences in a person's age, health, fitness level and other important factors. Please consult a medical or health professional before you begin any new exercise or nutritional program.

Warnings

1. Always consult your doctor before undertaking any exercise program.
2. Always wear suitable clothing and footwear eg tracksuit and training shoes.
3. Do not eat large meals two to three hours before exercising.
4. Remove jewellery, rings, chains and pins before exercising.
5. Where applicable make sure the weights and collars are secure.
6. Injuries to health may result from incorrect or excessive training.
7. Always warm up – cool down before and after exercising. This will help prevent straining muscles.
8. Start with a moderate weight so that you can perform the exercise correctly.
9. Breathing is very important. You should not hold your breath when exercising. The general rule is: inhale as you relax the muscles and exhale as you exert the muscles.
10. Keep yourself warm while exercising.

CONTENTS

SECTION ONE training at home   3
Motivation   4
Education   5
Commitment   6
Lets do it   6
Rest and recovery   8
Other benefits of exercise   12
Avoiding injury   12
Ten ways to stay motivated   14

SECTION TWO how to use this book   16
Using the forms at the back of the book   18
Our favourite exercises   18
Setting goals long term and short term   19
Tips on successfully setting
and achieving goals   23
Keeping a training diary   23
Rewarding yourself   25

**SECTION THREE
equipment for your home studio**   26
How much room do you have   26
A pleasant aspect   27
How much do you want to spend   28
What will you get for your money   29
The basics   32
Multi-gym   35
Advanced machines for advanced exercises   37
Cardio equipment   38
Boxing equipment   42
Accessories   43
Heart rate monitors   47

**SECTION FOUR
designing your home studio**   49
Layout   50
Section of an existing room   50
The spare room   52
The garage   54

SECTION FIVE strength training   57
Why lift weights   57
How long will it take   58
Advantages and disadvantages of machines   60
Advantages and disadvantages
of free weights   61
Reps and sets   62
How many reps should I do   62
How many sets should I do   63
How much rest do I take between sets   63
How do I know when I'm ready
for more weight   64
Fast reps/slow reps   64
Order of exercises   65
How many times per week should I train   66
How often should I change my routine   67
Dealing with muscle soreness   67

SECTION SIX exercise guide   69
Major muscles of the lower body   70
Major muscles of the upper body   71
Major muscles of the arms   73
Midsection exercise listing   74

SECTION SEVEN lower body — 75
- Front thigh quadriceps — 75
- Back thigh hamstring — 85
- Lower leg gastrocnemius — 90

SECTION EIGHT upper body — 95
- Back & upper back latissimus dorsi trapezius — 95
- Chest pectorals — 114
- Shoulders deltoids — 128

SECTION NINE arms — 141
- Front arms biceps — 141
- Back arms triceps — 152
- Wrists forearms — 164

SECTION TEN mid section — 167
- Torso abdominals — 167
- Torso lower back — 179

SECTION ELEVEN cardio training — 181
- Cardio for good health — 183
- Cardio for weight loss — 186
- Cardio for fitness — 191
- The four techniques in review — 195
- Target heart rates — 195
- Perceived rate of exertion — 197
- Cardio machines — 198

SECTION TWELVE getting started — 204
- What to wear — 204
- Choosing a program for you — 206
- Organising your twelve week planner — 207
- Filling in the forms — 207
- Choosing a start date — 208
- Your first training session — 209
- Lifestyle questionnaire — 211
- Medical questionnaire — 214
- Fitness assessment — 215

SECTION THIRTEEN programs — 220
- How to follow your 12-week program — 220
- Before you start — 220
- What are they for — 221
- Strength & muscle size – BEGINNERS — 224
- Strength & muscle size – INTERMEDIATE — 227
- Strength & muscle size – ADVANCED — 230
- Additional advanced strength training techniques — 233
- Fitness & fat loss - BEGINNERS — 235
- Fitness & fat loss – INTERMEDIATE — 238
- Fitness & fat loss – ADVANCED — 241
- The 30 minute express workout — 244
- Tips for writing your own program — 246
- Our ten favourite exercises — 252

SECTION FOURTEEN flexibility — 254
- Benefits of stretching — 255

SECTION FIFTEEN good nutrition — 268
- Where are you now — 269
- Popular myths — 270
- Starting the day — 271
- Eating on the run — 272
- Cooking dinner — 274
- Pantry survival list — 275
- The importance of drinking water — 276
- What about alcohol — 276
- Time out — 277
- Eating out — 278
- Good and bad fast foods — 279
- Fat grams in popular snack foods — 280
- Good fats bad fats — 280
- Healthy alternatives — 281
- What is a diet — 281
- Sample fitness/fat loss eating plan — 283
- Sample strength/muscle size eating plan — 285
- Sample eating for health plan — 287
- Glossary — 289
- Bibliography — 291
- Acknowledgments — 292
- Index — 293

SECTION ONE training at home

Training at home can be very time efficient and affective. Setting up a training area in your home means that you can exercise at the time of day or night that best suits your schedule and your body clock. 'Too busy' will never be a genuine excuse again!

Some people find exercising first thing in the morning a great start to the day, it can also be the time when they have the most energy. Having a home training studio means you can train with a bed-head, in your pyjama's if you want to, and get it done and out of the way for the day. No worrying about showering before and after a session, or the time involved in getting to and from the gym before work.

Others find mornings impossible and prefer to exercise in the evening, at the end of their day when work is finished and they can 'switch off'. Training in the evening suits those who can't shake off sleep easily or find it difficult to rouse the energy required for training early in the day. Put dinner in the oven and head off for a stress-busting workout in the next room ...can't do that in the gym can you?

Maybe you are a full-time parent who needs to exercise while the kids are asleep or at school. Do it while you catch up on a pre-recorded episode of your favourite show that you never get to watch anymore!

Both the purchase of a membership and the purchase of home equipment should be seen as a positive commitment towards better heath and greater achievements, a solid investment in your lifestyle.

Whatever your predicament, if you decide to set up a home training studio, there is no reason for you not to achieve the same or even greater results as committing to a gym membership. It doesn't take an expensive gym and fancy equipment to get results.

Home training is also cost-effective – you will probably only pay the equivalent of one or two years worth of gym memberships for some decent equipment, which is yours for life. What a great investment!

motivation

There is one downfall with home training – the absence of motivation and available information that will stop many people from committing to a regular training program and sticking to it.

The trouble with getting fit is that it isn't easy . It takes time and energy. Most people toy with the idea of committing, but few realise how much dedication is required. We will be straight with you right now, committing to a regular training program and achieving your goals is tough – but it really is worth it!

Unless you have a regular training partner, the only person that will hold you to your usual exercise session is yourself. When you decide you are too tired or busy to get through that session, there is no one else to kick you in the butt and say ' get on with it'. No commitment to a class booking or the thought of a lively and encouraging gym to get you going.

Motivation will be your toughest obstacle. Motivation is in fact most people's toughest obstacle. That's a big reason while personal trainers, fitness professional and sports coaches exist – to motivate and educate their clients.

There is no real trick to getting motivated or staying motivated. Our advice is to find out what works best or you and go with it. Try different approaches until you find something that hits the spot and once you start to see results you will be more motivated to carry on because you will know that you are capable of achieving what you want. Almost anything is possible, if you just put your mind to it and make a firm commitment.

- Forget quick fixes, they don't work, make a long term commitment and know that it will take time to achieve your goals and then perseverance to maintain them.

- Find a routine that suits you and stick with it. Choose days and times that don't interfere with what you would normally do. Getting our training sessions in should be as easy as possible, the harder it is to organise, the less likely you are to do it.

- Consider it an investment, in your life. We all know that regular exercise has endless advantages to our health and well-being.

- Set yourself realistic goals in an achievable period of time. Not reaching your goals is the biggest downer, so make sure you set out to achieve something realistic for your individual abilities without going too easy on yourself.

- Educate yourself. Learn as much as you can about the body you have been given and how it will respond to exercise. Knowing how your body benefits from exercise can be really motivating. Buy health and fitness magazines to get some ideas or a new perspective on your training. These magazines are full of great stuff, from the latest findings on exercise and equipment to good tasting healthy recipes (yes, they do exist!).

education

Once you have some knowledge of what you should be doing and for how long and how often, your sessions will be a little easier to get through. Knowing what you are doing and how to achieve your goals will see you getting results sooner, and once you start seeing some results you will feel better about your training. You will feel more in control because you will know how to look and feel your best.

You will look better because your body fat levels will have reduced and your lean muscle mass will have increased. This means that you will be stronger, leaner and healthier and more able to interpret the signals that your body sends you constantly, day and night. Healthy eating will also come easier as you will understand the difference between good food and bad food – the stuff you don't really need anyway but could have in small quantities occasionally so as not to deprive yourself of the things that you will always enjoy.

Read magazines and books on health and fitness and take note of articles in your newspaper on the subject. It's not hard to find constant sources of information on the subject these days, more and more people all over the world are becoming health conscious. Your nearest equipment specialist store can also be a good target for information. Speak to someone in the know, ask their opinion on your topic of interest and don't be afraid to ask them for suggestions.

commitment

Would you cook a meal and not eat it, or book a holiday and not go? Of course not, so why buy good quality home equipment and not use it? Training at home will require your initial commitment, and without that commitment, you won't achieve much at all. Initially it will not be easy, you are unlikely to see physical changes inside the first four to six weeks of an exercise and eating plan. You should feel healthier and more energetic almost immediately though, which is good because feeling better should be a large part of everyone's reason for starting an exercise regime.

Commitment is the most important word in the training vocabulary. But how do we achieve and maintain that elusive commitment to a healthier lifestyle? Good question. There is no sure-fire way or tried and tested method for it. You will have to want to get results, to achieve your goals, to be successful at something and feel good about it, even get recognition for it.

Your commitment will require strength, both mental and physical. But we believe that a commitment to something just about always ends in an achievement and that will make you a wiser, more competent person. So, expect to get results when you make that commitment and remember, making the decision to start is the hard part; exercising is easy.

lets do it!

OK, so you have made the commitment to look and feel better through an exercising and eating plan. Now lets talk more about the motivation you need to begin your journey. What is going to work for you? Music perhaps – it's a great motivator. Try a compilation of your favourite tracks; record them all on an audio tape and blast them out while you are training (be careful not to upset your neighbours).

Television is another great distraction, especially if there is a show on during the day or late in the evening that you usually miss. Record it on a tape and play it back while you are training. This will however, require you to set up a television and video in your training room. Be careful not to stop to watch it though, remember, it's only a distraction, not an excuse for extra long breaks between exercise sets!

A training partner is also an excellent idea. It can be someone who lives with you i.e. spouse or flatmate, a neighbour or a friend who lives nearby and can train at a mutually convenient time.

Having a training partner is a good idea because you will have someone to share goals and achievements with. Your partner will also provide a bit of healthy competition – you wouldn't want them to be fitter, stronger or leaner than you, would you?

Home training will require a good deal more motivation than training in a gym or working with a personal trainer. There are no obvious distractions like lots of other people all doing the same thing as you. Plenty of televisions, music and general commotion in a large gym all contribute to the motivation and distraction required, making your sessions easier to get through.

A personal trainer will provide you with the motivation you need to carry on, they will also tell what to do and when, so there is no thinking required on your part. Making an appointment to see a personal trainer at the same time each week is motivation in itself because they will waiting there for you to show up. They also tend to charge you for missed sessions, which is another incentive!

These extras are non-existent in your home training studio, so you will need to provide your own motivators. We suggest music as your first option, mostly because it is easy to organise and can be extremely influential on your moods. If you don't have a stereo to put in your training room, get yourself a mobile personal stereo. Set your music or pre-set radio station up before you begin exercising. If you intend on playing pre-recorded music, choose an upbeat style that will keep you moving at a steady pace while making you feel good. You will probably find yourself making the same choice in music every time. Try to change your music selections regularly to maintain a lively vibe while training.

The right kind of music creates a great atmosphere and before you know it, you will be halfway through your training program; and probably even enjoying it too!

Don't be discouraged by us coming on heavy in the motivation stakes, it really won't be easy initially, but you have already taken the first steps by buying this book. Let it become your complete companion, your own personal trainer and know that once you have begun your program, you will get results. Be assured also that it does get easier as time goes on, exercise should be enjoyable, and once you start to achieve some results and get a 'feel' for your training, there is no reason why you shouldn't look forward to doing it.

rest and recovery

No major project should involve constant hard work and discipline. Time out is really important. Like anything that requires commitment, your training regime will take a lot of energy and enthusiasm to maintain. And, like a job or full-time study, you will need a regular break from that regime, even a holiday every now and then.

No matter what kind of training you are doing, you should have at least one exercise-free day per week. This should be a day to relax and take it easy, not necessarily sit on the couch all day, but time to chill out and forget about exercise, training diaries and good or bad food.

Adequate recovery times between training sessions are also necessary if you want to remain injury free and maintain high energy levels. Forty-eight hours is about average for a medium to high intensity or advanced training program. Lighter programs which incorporate gentle weight training and cardio work may only require twenty four hours recovery time, and so could be performed most days of the week, depending upon your goals.

Recovery time with any program is essential to avoid burnout. Signs of burnout can include:

- Lethargy
- Tiredness
- Irritability
- Recurring colds and illness
- Persistent muscle soreness

Injuries are also more common if you are suffering from burnout.

If you do find that you are suffering from one or more of these symptoms, take a break. We recommend one to two weeks. If you find by the end of that period that your health has improved, you'll know that your program needs to include more rest time.

Don't be afraid to take regular breaks from your training or allow adequate recovery time between sessions. It won't reduce your level of results. In fact plenty of R&R will actually see you achieving greater results than running yourself into the ground training for two hours every day to get the perfect body.

Your body is a finely tuned machine; it will perform to its full capability when it is in good shape, healthy and happy and getting good quality fuel in the form of food to power it. If you are constantly sick you will suffer a lot of down time when you cant exercise at all – not great for achieving results. The other times when you are training, your sessions will be second-rate, you will battle through each one with little energy and strength to complete the tasks you have set yourself – you won't achieve much at all.

Over-training is really common, most people think that the more they do, the more they achieve. And this can be true for certain people on certain programs, but it needs to be done sensibly. Those doing vast amounts of exercise fall into only a few categories:

1. Professional, full-time or part-time athletes.

2. Amateur athletes.

3. People with health related issues, being closely supervised.

Coaches and relative experts will closely monitor all of those above, mostly so that they perform at their best and don't suffer burnout!

Believe it or not it is fairly easy to overdo it while following a training program. Listen to your body, if you experience any pain or discomfort while exercising – stop. If you experience difficulty with the same exercise during subsequent training sessions, get it checked. A physiotherapist or sports massage therapist is a good start.

Sports injuries can occur easily and if not seen to, can snowball. One small muscle injury can turn into something more serious when other muscles work overtime to compensate for that injury, thus causing further damage. So if you do experience a niggling pain, don't ignore it, see a sports therapist of some kind quickly. Injuries will slow down your training time and stop you achieving results as frequently as you would like.

Burnout is also quite common, if you find yourself feeling excessively tired or irritable, slow your training down by reducing session numbers per week, or take a break. We recommend you have one weeks break from your training every 12 weeks, so make sure you earn it! Set your goals to peak at the end of this period, take a break and enjoy it (without feeling guilty) and then start a new program with a new set of goals. This should prevent burnout and keep you fresh and interested in your training.

If you are simply exercising to burn off body fat, then training for an hour or two each day will probably be fine. But bear in mind that this type of training should be GENTLE, not too taxing on the body and easy to perform. It will probably involve mostly walking, with a small amount of resistance work thrown in to build muscle and therefore aid in speeding up the metabolism.

Concentrate on the quality of each workout, being fresh and energetic will allow you to get the most from everything you do, therefore assuring results for all that hard work.

Getting sick from being run-down because of over-training is avoidable. Be smart about your training, set realistic goals and know that these things take time. Have some fun along the way and enjoy the other benefits of exercise that are prevalent long before the physical changes are.

Regular long breaks from training are really important for everyone, for the same reasons as above, but also to give you a 'mental' break. We have designed your program and diary to run in 12-week blocks, when the 12 weeks are up, take a week off.

Your week off should be time to be away from your training and your healthy eating plan. OK, so that doesn't mean you just sit around and watch television all week while you eat chocolate and ice cream. It means you take a week off your regular routine to relax your mind and body. This should be a week to avoid your normal regime, if you feel like being active, do something different to normal, maybe a swim, bike ride or bushwalk. If you don't feel like being active, then take it easy, remember this is supposed to be time out so it's OK to be lazy for a while.

Avoid doing anything you would term 'training' during your week off. Take the break to renew your enthusiasm for your training. Review your last program along with your training diary and decide what to do next. You may resolve to advance to the next program level that has been suggested, or stay with the current program but make a few subtle changes to suit your needs.

Whatever your decision, remember that you should always be moving ahead and so be honest with yourself. If your current program is too easy, then an increase in intensity is required to keep your goals in view. Keep in mind that the biggest challenge involved in home training is the lack of encouragement from outside sources – there is no one else but you to do the assessing and re-writing of programs. So always stay focused on your goals and know that it takes hard work and determination to get there.

If your holiday falls right in the middle of your 12-week cycle, you have a decision to make. If there is a gym in or near where you will be staying, you could carry on as normal, although be warned, it will take a lot of will power to do so.

If you are going on a summer holiday, consider running or walking in the soft sand and/or a swim each morning. Do the best you can with your diet. If you are going on a winter holiday, it may involve skiing, if so your problem is solved. As long as you are injury free, skiing or snowboarding every day will keep you in shape.

Use your imagination to create challenging away-from-home training sessions to keep you going while you are away. Again, exercise every bit of will power you have to avoid over-indulgence in the food and alcohol department. Perhaps you could allow yourself a happy hour each day!

The key to healthy training is to keep track of energy levels and moods. If you notice undesirable mood swings or you are getting more head colds than normal, it may be time to reassess your training program or perhaps increase your rest times between sessions.

other benefits of exercise

OK so we all know that the main benefit from exercise (or perhaps the one we all place the most emphasis on) is that it makes us look better. But there are many other benefits to regular exercise, and most of them are apparent before you start to look better.

- Regular exercise will improve your circulation, making your blood flow throughout your body more efficiently.

- Toxins are also cleansed from the body more efficiently with increased blood flow and there will be plenty of life-giving oxygen in that blood. You will experience a high sense of well-being.

- Your energy levels will be increased as your body and it's systems cope better with the day-to-day stresses it has to deal with.

- You will experience better quality sleep.

- Stress should be reduced because of your training sessions, therefore resulting in lower levels throughout your day.

There are also other benefits to shedding a few kilos than those cosmetic. Decreased body fat around the mid-section (more predominant in men) can mean a decreased risk of heart attack. An overall reduction in body fat means less body weight, which in turn reduces the stress on joints, especially the knees. Not to mention the reduced risk of many other adverse medical conditions.

avoiding injury

Avoiding injury mostly means being sensible. Lengthy warm-ups and cool-downs at either end of your sessions and stretching each muscle group during your sessions are important safeguards.

During your sessions, listen to your body, if it is sending you a signal to slow down or ease up on the weight, then do it. Make sure it's not your brain kicking in instead though and telling you to slacken off!

Avoiding injury also means performing exercises – both cardio and strength – in a safe manner. Strength exercises should be performed smoothly with no 'jerky' movements and if you are not following one of the pre-set programs, make sure you give yourself a lengthy warm-up and cool-down and drink plenty of water. Cardio training should involve a smooth movement; your arms should glide back and forth beside your body, avoid crossing your arms in front of you.

Side and front railing on cardio machines are not there for you to constantly lean on either, contrary to what most people believe! Use the railings to steady yourself when taking a drink of water, but avoid resting heavily on them while you are exercising. This will impede your movement, making it jerky and uneven and put unnecessary amounts of stress on the muscles of the upper body. Using the railings for constant support will also decrease the intensity of the exercise, you will work away for the same length of time, but probably achieve less.

Of course before commencing any regular exercise program you should consult your medical practitioner to get the all clear. If at any time during your raining sessions you experience any pain, discomfort, dizziness or anything that you would deem unusual – stop. Get yourself a cool drink and sit quietly for a while. If the feeling recurs during subsequent training sessions, get it checked. It's not worth ignoring anything that may seem small and insignificant now, but if left unchecked could snowball.

ten ways to stay motivated

1. **Manage your time** – Find a few timeslots that will best suit you for training sessions and stick to them. Make an appointment with yourself; write it in your diary and DO IT! Train at the same designated times each week, that way it will become a habit.

2. **Play your favourite music** – There is no doubt that great music is highly motivating. Have a selection of your favourites on hand so that you can choose a CD to match your mood for the day.

3. **Train with a friend** – Having someone to train with may be your best source of motivation. Your training buddy will provide a bit of healthy competition and will also get you going on the days that you would probably give it a miss if you were on you own. It goes both ways too, so your training buddy will enjoy the same benefits.

4. **Set realistic goals** – Set yourself short-term goals that you know you can achieve. Short-term goals will keep you motivated because you will be achieving success on a regular basis and you will have something new to work towards. Be realistic; set yourself targets that are challenging but achievable.

5. **Brighten your surroundings** – Your physical training environment is also important for staying motivated. Vision is another sense, and just like your hearing, it needs stimulation to be excited. Make sure your training room is light and airy and hang pictures or posters on the walls that will be pleasing to your eyes.

6. Vary your training – Our programs are based on a 12-week cycle. Take a week off training once you finish a program and then start something new, the change will keep you interested.

7. Put a mirror in your studio – We know that this sounds a little tacky, but there are a few good reasons for it. Firstly, it will make checking your form a lot easier if you can see what you are doing in the mirror. Secondly, being able to see yourself in the mirror will motivate you to make changes, and when those changes come, you will be equally motivated to keep going.

8. Reward yourself - When you start to see results, go out and buy some new clothes that show off that flatter tummy, muscled arms or smaller bum. You will look and feel great in your new gear, and you will want to stay that way so that you can continue to wear your new flattering clothes – a little corny, but it works!

9. Accept compliments gracefully – Believe it when people tell you that you are looking great, smile and say thank you.

10. Think positive – Even if the results aren't coming as quickly as you would like, stay positive and keep going, everything you do is making a difference. Your mind and body have a very powerful link, so if you stay positive, motivation will be high and the results will keep rolling in.

SECTION TWO how to use this book

This book has been designed to cover most areas of training – from burning body fat to building muscle and from beginner through to the more advanced exerciser.

Even if you have done some training before, we suggest you still work through the beginner's section as well. The exercises in the beginners programs are all excellent choices for the more experienced trainer but have listed as starters because of their simplicity and ease of performance. Just increase the intensity to make the exercise more challenging.

There are lists of exercises throughout the book that will work the different muscle groups of your body, and some programs at the back to follow once you are familiar with the individual exercises.

There is a chapter on cardio training as well, which will give you advice on how much cardio work you should be doing and how often you should be doing it depending on your goals. Just about everyone needs to do some fitness and/or fat burning training, even those wanting to put on some muscle size – big muscles will look much better on a lean body. So read through the information and follow the heart rate chart.

Once you are familiar with the exercises and programs, select the exercise routine specific to your goals; one that suits you and that you will enjoy doing. Use the programs sheets and training diary to track your progress by photocopying the pages at the back of the book and then running off enough copies to do you for 12 weeks.

Fill these sheets in religiously. It really will make a difference to your level of motivation if you can see proof of your training goals being achieved. You will also be able to give yourself a big pat on the back at the end of the 12-week period when you can review the figures and see just what you have achieved; this is just how personal trainers do it with their clients.

We have also included some instructions for performing a basic fitness test to assess your strength, flexibility and fitness levels. Doing a fitness test before you begin your training program is a good idea. Once your 12 week training period is up, do another test to see how much you have improved.

It will not only be interesting to see what you have achieved, but it will be an excellent motivator as well. Hang on to all your records so that when you have worked through two or three 12-week programs you will be able to review and compare the whole lot.

Patterns should appear and you will then be able to see which areas require more work than others. Body fat levels may not be reducing as quickly as you would like for instance, perhaps it might be time to reassess your eating habits and the amount of cardio training you are doing to burn off that fat.

The fitness test also has another side – the lifestyle questionnaire. Take time answering these questions in order to get an accurate picture of your current health and approach to lifestyle and exercise. These questions, once answered will provide you with a clear-cut picture of where you are and where you want to be.

This book can also be used as an ongoing reference guide. Once you have some experience and extra knowledge on how to train your body to achieve your goals and what to eat to keep you on track, you may want a refresher. Perhaps a new take on a particular muscle group, a different training method or just some fresh ideas on modifying your current program.

You may want to advance to higher levels with your cardio training and so you could go back to the heart rate chart to monitor your progress or get some tips on how to boost your fitness levels.

Keep this book in your home training studio and use it as a handbook for ongoing information and motivation as you need it. We have designed and written it to become your training companion, not just something that is purchased on impulse, read and then forgotten.

using the forms at the back of this book

The forms contained in this book have been designed for you to be able to easily understand and relate to. They call for basic information on your current health and fitness. Some forms such as the medical questionnaire are one offs that only require you to fill them in once.

Others such as the food and training diary and 12 week planner are designed as an ongoing thing that should be filled in every day or with each training session. We have also included a blank program card to allow you to write your own training routines should you want to tackle it at a later date.

Taking the time to fill in these forms and follow the programs step by step will make the whole process a lot more interesting. It will also help you to understand how your body responds to exercise. Your training will seem easier and more enjoyable if you know what kind of an effect it is having on your body.

our favourite exercises

Look for our favourite exercises throughout the book. These exercises are listed for all levels and all forms of training. They are our favourites for a few reasons:

1. Ease of operation

2. Versatility

3. Enjoyment factor.

Some of these exercises have been chosen because they are easy to perform, for us, the basic will always win out. New exercises or new-takes on old exercises based on research are always great to try too, because technology is always advancing and we are always learning more about how our body's function and respond to movement. Looking for exercises that are safe and easy to perform but are also highly effective is a priority.

Versatility in an exercise is also important as it can provide the ability to work towards multiple goals with the one movement. Resistance training techniques can be especially versatile. Those that work more than one muscle group at once (compound exercises) can be great for when you don't have much time. These exercises can also be good in circuit or cardio training because they usually involve larger muscle groups that will maintain a higher heart rate.

Finally, the enjoyment factor. Yes that's right you are supposed to have fun while you are doing this stuff! Our favourites are enjoyable to do and will provide you with a sense of achievement. They are exercises that will be comfortable to perform and give you a strong sense of empowerment and success.

Of course the exercises that we have listed as our favourites may not necessarily be your favourites, so don't feel like you have to enjoy the exercises that we say you should. You will probably end up with a list of your own favourites.

setting goals long and short term

Goal setting can be difficult. Where do you start? How do you decide what you really want to achieve? And then how do you commit those desires to paper? More daunting still is the idea of tackling those goals, actually setting the wheels in motion to achieving something.

Goal setting is a major task that shouldn't be taken lightly. If you are willing to set goals then you need to be equally intent and focused on carrying them through and achieving what you set out to do.

You might now be wondering, why bother? Because goals keep us alive, continually helping us to strive for what we want from life. Goals themselves are a motivating force in our lives, it has been proven that people who regularly set and commit to goals in their lives are more motivated and energetic and achieve more out of life than those who do not.

The act of setting a goal, writing down what it is you want to achieve and when, will have you committing, trust us. Set yourself achievable goals and believe that you can do it, because you can.

As you record your goals remember, they don't have to be permanent. They can and should change as you make small achievements or alter your approach to your training. Review your goals regularly, and write down new ideas or fresh goals as they come to mind, this will give you something to continually work towards and keep you fresh and interested.

Most people will have an idea in mind, i.e. to lose five kilos before the start of summer, or gain some muscle size to look better in this seasons fashion. Maybe you are going on a trekking or snow skiing trip in a few months and you want to increase your fitness level so that you will experience a higher level of enjoyment.

Make sure that your goal is realistic and achievable to start with; dropping a dress size for a wedding in three months is one thing, but starving yourself to lose twenty kilos is out of the question. Set yourself something that you know you can achieve, but without being too easy on yourself.

Write down all the things that you are good at i.e. running, tennis or horse riding, anything that involves exercise or physical activity. This is a good way to find things that will motivate you and help you design goals that will not only improve your appearance and health, but also develop skills for your favourite pastime or leisure sport.

But what if you don't have any idea about what you want to gain or lose, you just know that you want to look and feel better. That's fine. Sit down with a pen and paper and write down everything you would like to change about yourself i.e. your bottom, your chest, your arms or legs etc. Also include other health related issues like giving up smoking or reducing stress levels. These can be tackled in succession and may even come naturally or more easily once you are exercising regularly.

Look for friends or relatives who have achieved something similar to what you want to achieve and ask their advice. Find out how they went about it and what sort of obstacles they came up against along the way. Don't be embarrassed to ask about these things, you will probably come away with some good ideas, and the person giving the advice will be pleased that they could share something positive with you.

Of course all bodies will react differently to exercise, so don't expect to adopt the very same routine and get the same results. What worked for them may do little for you, but you won't know that until you give it a go. One things for sure, will get something from making positive changes.

Be prepared for some form of failure, and don't be put off if it does happen. The only way to achieve what you want is to try your best, if you don't get the exact results you were after, re-assess and try again. Treat it as a learning process, each small failure will be a lesson, it can only make you wiser and more focused on success.

Finally, enjoy. Nobody is going to stick to an exercise routine that is downright hard work and no fun. Faced with that prospect, most people will give up.

It is possible to factor good times into your training though. Do it in ways that you like, choose your favourite exercises and adapt them to a routine that will satisfy your desires. Supplement your strength sessions with cardio exercises that you love i.e. dancing till dawn, walking or running a mini marathon or tennis competitions.

Try buying a healthy eating cook book, you'll be amazed at how many foods are not just low in fat and nutritious but really tasty too. Treat it as a challenge and enjoy the new and fresh flavours that healthy cooking has to offer.

Your game plan should be set out in 12-week blocks. Set yourself a goal that you will aim to achieve in those first 12 weeks, for example:

- If your aim is to reduce body fat, plan to lose between half to one kilogram a week. This is a realistic loss, any more than this will probably be attributed to the loss of lean muscle tissue and fluid (not good).

Weight yourself regularly during this period, but don't stress too much if you don't see 500 grams or more coming off. There are many factors that affect your weight reading, the time of day for instance. If you are the sort of person who is motivated be measuring something, replace your scales with a tape measure and watch the centimeters drop.

We personally do not place so much emphasis on weight loss, but would prefer to see you drop a dress size or bring the belt on your trousers in a notch. However, which ever works best for you is fine.

- Gaining muscle size and strength will depend on the individual, as each body will respond differently. Weigh yourself weekly and expect to see gains.

If you are also trying to lower your body fat levels at the same time, you may not see weekly weight gains. While your muscle mass is on the increase, your body fat is on the move, so your over-all weight gain may be slower. Again, replace your scales with a tape measure. Another option is to look in the mirror, physical appearance will be a better gauge and really motivating as well.

When setting a goal for gaining muscle size, think in terms of strength. Set a figure for what you would like to bench press, squat or whatever in 12 weeks. This of course should be based on what you can bench press etc now. An increase in strength will ultimately result in an increase in muscle mass, this will be a good gauge when the scales are not moving much.

Your 12-week goal will be your short-term objective. Your long-term goal should be something you want to achieve in the next 6 to 12 months. If your goal is simply to increase or decrease weight, multiply your 12-week goal by four to get a long-term objective. Add a couple of kilos either way just to keep you fired up.

Long term goals will be a little easier to set, simply because they are way off in the future sometime, an age away from where you are now. But think of it this way, your long-term goal should be the ultimate, what you really want to achieve, the one at the top of the staircase. Your short-term goals are just a series of stairs on the way up; at the top is your main goal.

Your short-term goals will be achievements in themselves, great things that you can say you have accomplished along the way. And without short-term goals your long-term goal would be un-achievable. How on earth could you make a statement like this...........

"In 12 months time I am going to be ten kilos lighter and much healthier and happier than I am now, but I have no idea how I am going to get there"

Understood this way you will see that your goals are also a map of the future, a guide for how you wish to get through the next six, twelve, twenty-four months. We see them as being the most important part of any training program.

tips on successfully setting and achieving goals

- Set realistic and achievable goals. If you can't see yourself achieving them, you won't.

- Write them down and review them regularly.

- Visualise yourself achieving them; see yourself doing whatever it is you set out to do.

- Have a time frame in mind, know when you want to achieve them by and be precise.

- Don't set too many goals at once, prioritise and decide which are the more important.

- Do something positive each day towards achieving your goals.

- Tell someone you respect and trust and ask for his or her support.

keeping a training diary

Every successful venture requires a solid plan of attack. Your commitment to improving your health and fitness and setting short and long term goals is no different.

Your training diary will tell its own story. It will be a map of your training progress. It will show ups and downs and provide you with the motivation to carry on when things are good and give you the answers to program modification when things aren't so good.

Without a firm plan and accurate records, you will wander around aimlessly, wasting time getting impatient and bored. Either that or you will go through each workout without any real idea of what you should do and how you should do it. And worst of all, doing nothing positive towards achieving the results you are really after.

The benefits of keeping a training diary are numerous. Knowing before beginning a training session which exercises will be performed, for how long and at what intensity level will make things just that little bit easier. If you walk into your training room with little or no idea of 'what to do today' you won't get far.

A training diary and program will take away the mystery. Your workouts will be planned, from which days you do cardio or strength, right down to the duration of each training session. Imagine how much easier it will be head off for a training session if you know exactly what you are in for, how long it will take and roughly how you will feel afterward. Before you know it, you'll be finished and in the shower thinking about what's next for the day.

Your training diary should not only exist for the purpose of recording what you have done so far, but also provide you with a strategy for what you will accomplish during future training sessions.

Through your records you will see a defined path. If you are not achieving results as quickly as you would like, you will have accurate records to review. These will hopefully provide you with the answers you need to correct any problems you are experiencing with your program.

You will see definite patterns to your training by recording your mood and energy levels at each session. You may decide that morning isn't the best time for you because your afternoon sessions all seemed to be productive and energetic, but in the morning you were lethargic and disinterested.

Perhaps increasing the intensity may be the answer, by looking back over previous training sessions you may honestly admit that you haven't been training hard enough, and so by reviewing your diary, you will be able to give yourself the kick in the butt you need!

Or maybe your training is going great, you are looking better, feeling fabulous and having a good time exercising. If so don't change a thing. You have found your winning formula, and it is all recorded for prosperity so you know exactly how to flick your switch in the future.

The forms provided have been designed for you to photocopy. We suggest you run off enough to keep you going for the duration of your 12-week program, being prepared makes the act of 'doing' a lot easier. You can also count down your sessions easily and map your progress as you go.

It will take little time at the end of each session to fill in your training diary and keep your records up to date, but will be well worth it. It will be without a doubt one of the most important steps along the way to a healthier mind and body and longevity of life.

rewarding yourself

On top of a regular holiday you should also enjoy the odd treat here and there. Rewarding yourself for all that dedication will make you feel like it is all worthwhile, and if your treat is of the forbidden food variety, then you will also feel less deprived.

When you start seeing results, go and buy yourself a new piece of clothing – what better reward than something new in a size smaller than normal. This will provide you with an incentive to work hard and achieve more – another excuse to buy something new! Your ongoing incentive to keep yourself in shape will be your new clothes, you want to continue to fit into them don't you?

OK, so that covers periodical rewards. What about something a bit more frequent? We suggest you have one relaxed day of eating and training each week. What better treat could you have than enjoying the high fat/sugar food that you love and know you can't eat any other day. We are only talking ONE day a week here though – no getting carried away!

Your 'treat day' should be on a weekend, or your equivalent day off during the week. This is also when you are most likely to be socialising, going out for meals and drinking more alcohol. Eat pizza, cake ice cream or whatever it is that you really love but know you shouldn't have. Enjoy it and don't feel guilty, a treat once a week will not jeopardize your chances of quick results too much. And as we said earlier, it will stop you from feeling totally bored and deprived.

SECTION THREE
equipment for your studio

how much room do you have

It doesn't matter whether you have put aside one corner of your bedroom or a whole garage, you will be able to fit out your home studio to effectively give you the workouts you want.

Space will be an issue if you have a certain multi-gym or equipment set-up in mind. Sticking a big gym in the middle of your living room is not a good idea. All it will do is annoy you every time you trip over it or sit down to watch the television in an awkward position because of it.

Likewise, if you decide to use your garage as a home studio instead of somewhere to house your car, think long and hard before taking action. Do you really want to leave your car on the street all the time in all weather conditions?

Find a space or room that is currently either not being used or could be re-arranged without troubling you or anyone else in the house.

What we are getting at here is that your studio should be set up somewhere that it is not going to inconvenience you, or cause you angst because you would rather be using the space for something else.

Once you have decided on an area, go ahead and design your home studio. If you have had a look around you will know what is on the market and how much space the stuff will take up. If you have been given some equipment, take into account how much space it will take up and then the space required for whatever you may want to buy to add on.

When calculating space for equipment, remember to allow room around the piece, not just the 'foot print'. Some machines will require more surrounding space than others – bars protruding from machines or room in front of the machine for sitting or standing for instance.

EQUIPMENT FOR YOUR HOME STUDIO

Your budget will also have a bearing on your provision for space. If you are restricted to spending minimal amounts, then look for a good quality bench and some free weights. This will be enough to provide you with a good all-round workout and you can do your cardio training outdoors while you save for a treadmill or bike! A set up like this will cost little and also take up only a small amount of room. You could also store a set-up like this in a corner somewhere and easily pull it out into the middle of the room when you are training.

Having said that, if your budget and/or space is unlimited, then go ahead and have some fun. There are some great machines and pieces of equipment available which will make your workouts adventurous, enjoyable and easy. If you have plenty of space, then use your artistic skills in setting up your studio. Perhaps you could design a small circuit of exercises that will keep you traveling effectively around the room in a clockwise direction.

Wherever you decide to set up your home studio, make sure you leave enough unobstructed room for floor work. You will need enough open floor space to place an exercise mat down flat for performing things like abdominal work and stretches.

a pleasant aspect

Setting the mood in your home studio is really important, because if you don't like the room or the surroundings, you are less likely to use it. Music is essential, either a small radio or the big fancy stereo, whatever. If you have your favourite music playing, you'll put yourself in the mood instantly and be ready to go. So make sure you take into account a power point for the tunes.

Try and make it a pleasant and motivating place to be as well. If it's the dungeon under your house that you are converting, a bright coat of paint and some wall hangings or pictures that you like to look at would be good. A good-sized freestanding fan or air-conditioner will also be important for ventilation.

If you have a large window in the room that provides direct sunlight, take care not to position cardio machines nearby. Two reasons why. Firstly, computer screens do not like direct sunlight. Over a period of time your display could fade and these things can be quite expensive to replace, especially if they are imported.

Secondly, training with the sun beating down on you for half an hour or so (even if you have air-conditioning) is not very pleasant, not to mention the risk to your health from de-hydration and heat stroke. If you have a pretty view out the window that you would like to take advantage of, try positioning your cardio machine on the other side of the room. This way you can enjoy the view and not get sizzled.

The sun will also quickly fade and damage upholstery on any machine that has to go under a window. So keep the binds/curtains closed when you are not training.

If you are setting up your equipment in your bedroom, make sure that corner of the room is set aside for training only. Don't hang clothes on your equipment and make sure that it is set up ready to use. Try and avoid partly dismantling equipment to make more room. It will be unattractive to look at, and will require extra effort to assemble before you can begin training which again will make the session seem like a less attractive option.

how much do you want to spend

The big question. Everything comes down to price doesn't it? Well, when it comes to money, it is like anything else, you get what you pay for. What you spend on equipment should be largely based on what your training requirements are (and anyone else who will regularly use the stuff too).

If your goal is mainly to lose body-fat, then you should look at a decent quality cardio machine e.g. bike, stepper or treadmill and a small selection of free weights. On the other hand, if you simply want to increase muscle size, then you should spend less on cardio equipment and more on weights and/or a multi-gym.

Deciding what you want to spend on equipment before you go shopping is a good idea. Set yourself a budget and stick to it. You will easily be able to get yourself some equipment that will do the job for you. And having set yourself a budget to stick to, you will be less likely to buy something that you don't really need.

what will you get for your money

Prices will obviously vary, but as with any other product, expect to find the lower end of the market to include a few less features and also be considerably cheaper. Top end stuff will be nice to look at, will be heavy-duty (sturdy looking) and finished well, including plenty of height and weight adjustments.

If you have plenty of money to spend and you like your equipment to look good, consider the chrome dumbells. although they look fantastic and wear well, they cost more. If you want to have a full range of weights, black cast iron weights cost a lot less and weigh exactly the same, they also offer the same ease of use as the former. Your budget will dictate which way you go here, either way you can't lose

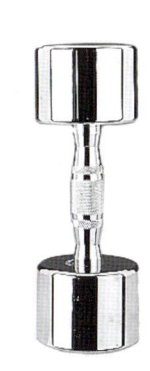

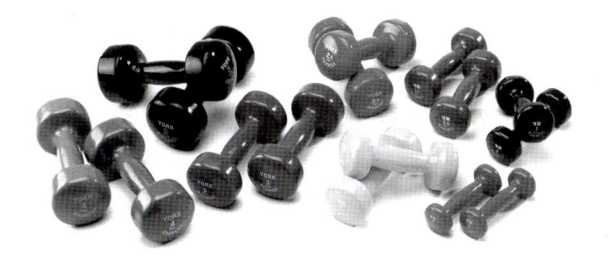

PVC dipped weights are a good alternative, they look great and are comfortable to use. And although they are still not cheap, they are a nice compromise between the standard black cast iron and the fancy chrome stuff. PVC and vinyl coated dumbells are also great to use. The fixed weight makes them quick and easy to handle and the coating is comfortable to grip.

Barbell and dumbell bars will not vary too much in quality or cost. There are several sizes, and which one you choose will depend on your size and what you want to use it for.

There are also plenty of accessories available which are cheap to buy and can make your workouts easier and more comfortable. Have fun shopping for things like sit-up bars, handgrips, exercise mats, push-up bars and skipping ropes.

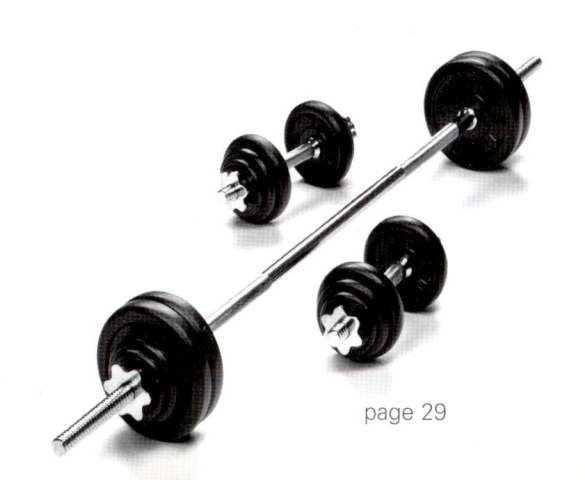

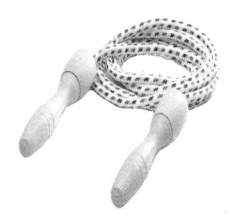

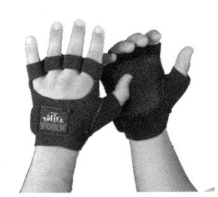

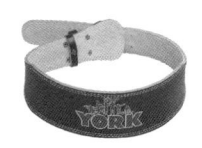

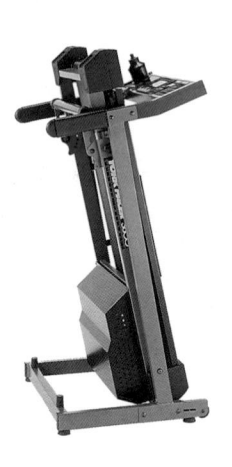

Weight lifting gloves are something that we highly recommend; they will give you a better grip and prevent slipping when you start to sweat. They also reduce the occurrence of calluses on the palms of your hands.

Weight belts are also a good idea and should be used mostly for doing any exercise that requires you to lift a heavy weight above your head, although they can be used for support during any strength exercise. These belts provide excellent support for anyone with a lower back weakness or injury, but again, check with a professional before starting any form of training if you do have a back injury.

When buying cardio equipment, our advice is to spend as much as your budget will allow. As we have already said, you get what you pay for and in the case of cardio gear, quality is pretty important if you want it to last. The quality of internal parts and computerised functions will increase with the price tag.

Although if you intend on only spending short periods on the machine, warming up and cooling down for instance, then a cheapie will be fine. As with any form of equipment, get on and try it out first, especially with bikes – uncomfortable seats aren't much fun for anyone! You want it to be comfortable to use. Treadmill mats should be wide enough for you to safely run or walk on. Elliptical trainers and step machines should feel easy enough for you to sustain the movement for an extended period of time.

Multi-gyms are pretty straightforward, the more exercises you can perform on it, the more expensive it will be. If you are looking for something that just does a few exercises, perhaps to combine with some free-weights (a scenario we highly recommend) then again, the low-range machines will be fine. Get on and have a play. Look for smooth movements, height adjustments and an easy transition from one exercise to the next.

EQUIPMENT FOR YOUR HOME STUDIO

Maximum weight stacks are also an issue. You can't add weight to the original stack; the machine has been designed to carry only what it was assembled with. Adding extra weight is dangerous and over and above anything else, will void your warranty. So make sure there is more than enough weight for you to handle, even after you have grown big and strong from all that training!

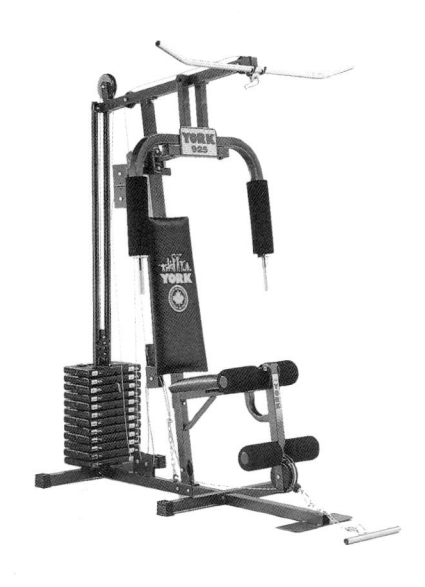

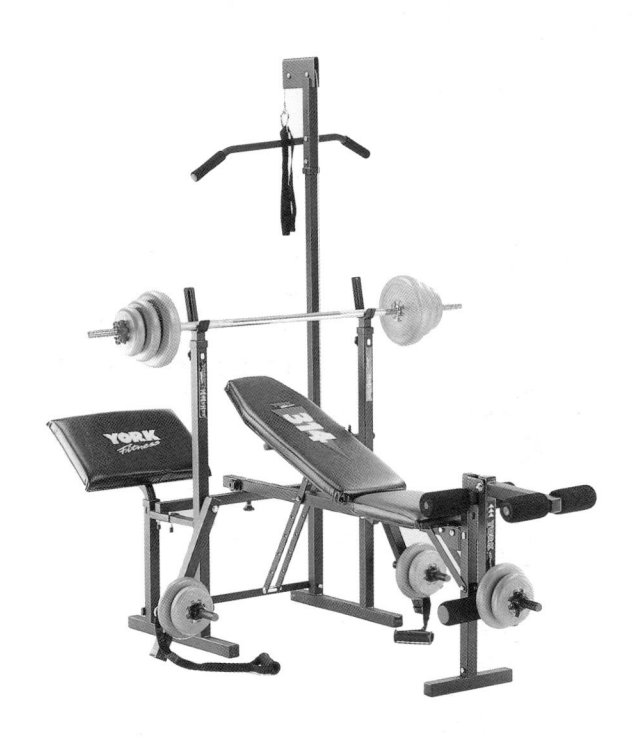

As we mentioned earlier, it doesn't really matter whether you have allowed yourself only a small amount to spend or you have an endless supply of cash to buy the latest and greatest. You will be able to set yourself up with the right equipment to achieve the kind of results you are after, and we will show you how.

the basics

Regardless of your budget, if you just want some basic equipment to perform the essentials, you can't go past a decent quality bench, a selection of free weights and a couple of bars.

There are plenty of benches to choose from including some that can fold up to be stored easily and others that include items such as a squat rack added on. Most will include a basic leg curl/leg extension attachment. And if you intend on working with only a bench, then we recommend you get one with this particular attachment. A leg curl/extension allows you to work the two major muscle groups of the legs - quadriceps and hamstring – effectively and simply.

Your bench should also include uprights to support a barbell bar for doing exercises such as flat and incline bench press and an adjustable backrest, again for variety of exercises. These are the basic needs when purchasing a bench. There are plenty of extras that can be purchased separately and added on, or that may come with the bench that you decide to buy, these include squat racks and butterfly and arm curl attachments.

A simple cable system is available which will give you the ability to perform exercises that aren't possible with free weights, lat pull down for example. This machine doesn't have a weight stack and so you can also utilise your free weights with it. Combined with a bench and weights it is an excellent alternative to the full multi-gym.

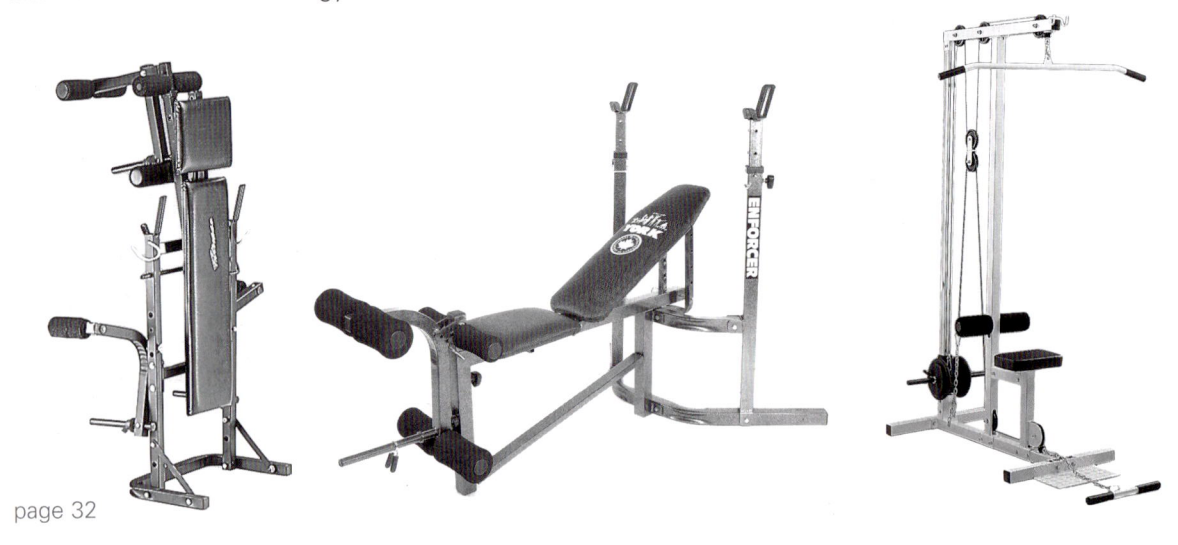

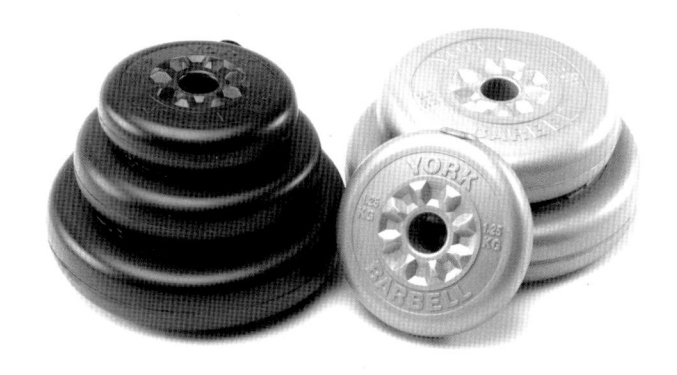

Added extras will make your workout more extensive and probably more efficient but they are definitely not essential to an effective workout. The choice is yours.

Free weights are free weights. As we discussed earlier, there are different shapes, sizes and colours but they all do exactly the same thing and they weigh in exactly the same as well. Again, the choice is yours, let your budget and preference dictate here. One word of advice though, the standard cast iron weights will last a little longer than the PVC coated or sand filled ones. And if they start to look shabby, rub them back and give them a paint job!

When deciding on weight ranges, you will need to take into account your current and future strength levels. If you are a female starting on a weight training program for the first time, obviously you wont need to buy half a dozen 20kg plates. Stick with the small stuff, you probably won't need to go any bigger than 10kg.

A male will undoubtedly require larger weights and so a couple of 20kg plates wouldn't go astray. Don't buy anything smaller than 2.5kg because again, they probably wont get used, unless of course a smaller person in the household intends on joining in as well. Barbells and dumbells don't vary too much.

There are four basic types:

1. Solid bars

2. Hollow bars

3. Bars with 'T' or 'L' collars

4. Bars with spinlock collars

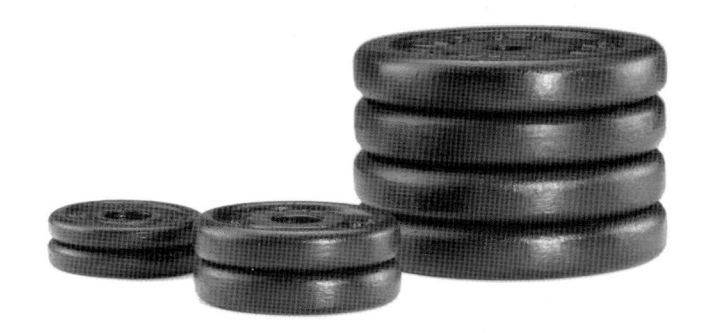

Hollow bars will be cheaper than the solid ones but are not as strong. Choose hollow bars only if you are not intending on loading heaps of weight on to them. Choosing plain or spinlock bars should be left up to personal preference. Both are as good as each other. Although the spinlock system is a little safer because of the way the collars screw down.

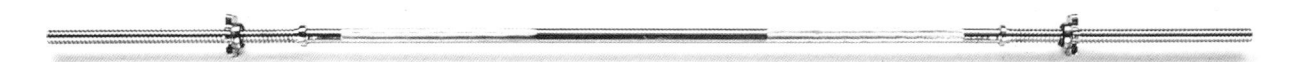

Fixed or welded dumbells are easy to use because there are no adjustments to make, you just pick them up and away you go. They are quick and efficient and particularly easy to use. They're only downfall is the fixed weight, once you outgrow that particular weight value, there is no challenge. This means advancing to the next level, and if you don't have heavier dumbells, you will have to go and buy them.

There are also other gadgets available like quick-release spring collars, rubber grips for dumbell bars and vinyl coated spinlock collars. Go and have a look at all these things, have a play and ask lots of questions of sales staff. And then decide what is going to best suit your needs.

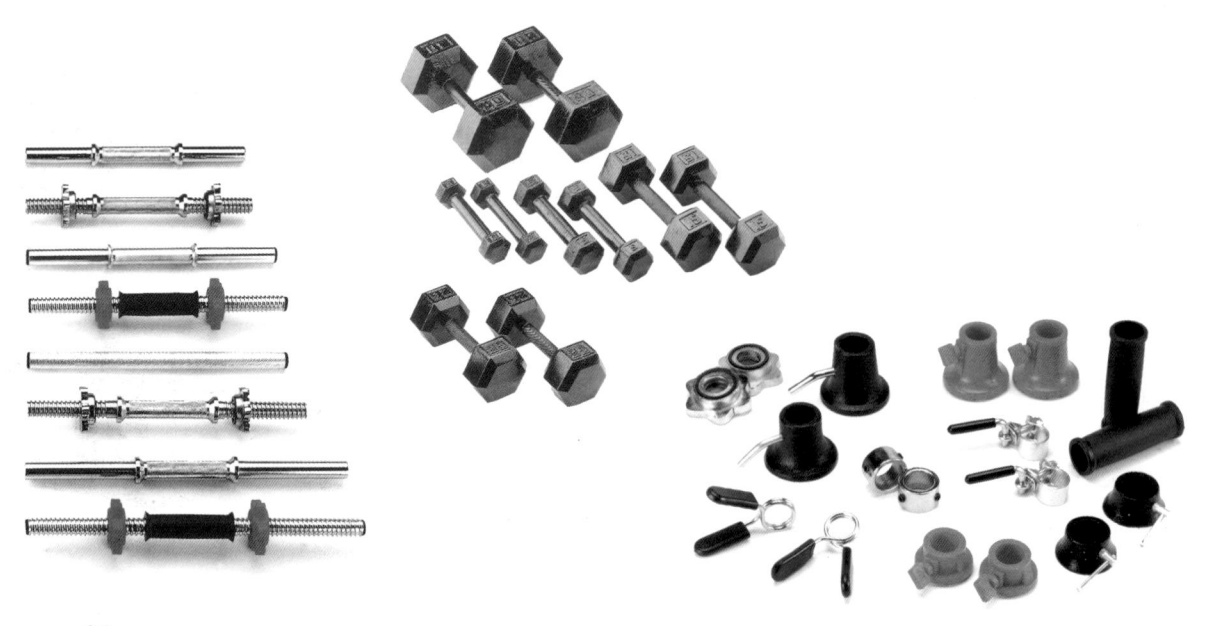

EQUIPMENT FOR YOUR HOME STUDIO

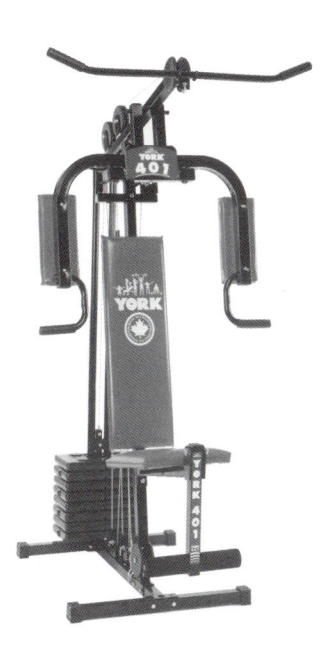

a multi gym

If you have a bit more money to spend and more room to spare, the next option is to buy a multi-gym. There are plenty to choose from. Starting with those that have few attachments but will still have a common weight stack and a cable system allowing for upper and lower body exercises, and ranging through to the top of the range machines that allow you to perform a couple of dozen exercises.

Multi-gyms are a great choice, they can be easy to use, especially if you are training on your own – you wont require someone to spot you as you would with free weights. This also means that they are a good deal safer than handling free-weights especially for beginners.

There is also no playing around with loading weights on and off barbell and dumbell bars and screwing and unscrewing collars. This can make for a quicker and more efficient training session.

Buying multi-gyms can be a little tricky though. There are more considerations to take into account than with a bench and weights. You will need a machine that does all or most of the things that your training will require. If you are overly tall or short, height adjustments will be a must for you to perform exercises correctly and safely. Space will also be an issue, some of these machines will require a good deal of space for full performance.

You don't necessarily need to buy the machine that offers the most amount of exercises either, chances are you will only perform about half of them on a regular basis. Again your decision should be based upon who is going to use the machine and what their training requirements/goals are.

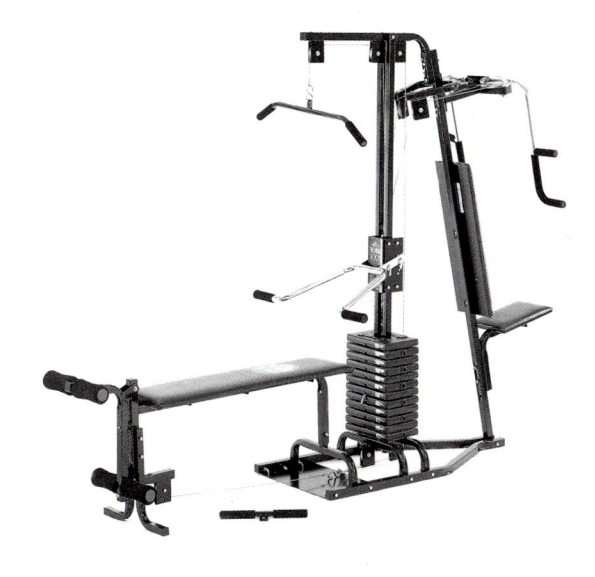

page 35

If you are purchasing a gym for fitness and toning, look for a machine that offers some or all of the following:

- Little or no cable changes. This will allow for a quick and easy transition between one exercise and the next.

- A good range of exercises for large muscle groups (legs, back and chest). Training large muscle groups will keep your heart rate high using the low weight–high repetition principal.

- A machine that is easy and comfortable to work around.

If you are looking at a strength-training program, a machine that offers a good range of exercises - both compound and isolation - will be important. Height adjustments will also be important, as full-range of movement with all exercises is always encouraged. And finally a good-sized weight stack, which may seem unimportant now, but down the track when your strength has increased, it will be disappointing if you outgrow your machine.

As a rule, the more features or exercise stations the gym has, the more expensive it will be. Some machines have extra attachments that can be purchased at a later date, but most will come as they are.

Top of the range multi-gyms will give you the enjoyment and variety of many different exercises performed with ease on a better quality set-up including larger foam rollers and smooth cable systems. Heavier weight stacks are another bonus with top range machines. Most attachments will come inclusive with the machine, with little else to be purchased on top, except possibly some fixed dumbells for use with free weight exercises.

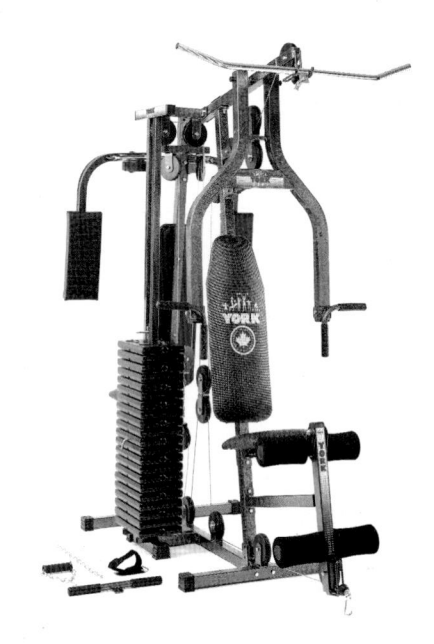

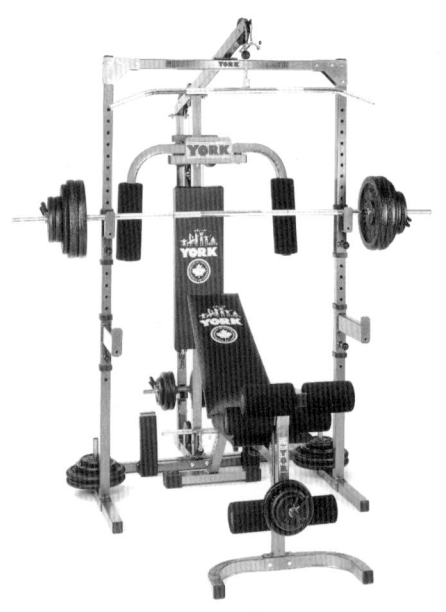

EQUIPMENT FOR YOUR HOME STUDIO

If you would like to mix both free-weights and cable exercises, consider getting yourself a small gym that allows you to perform the basics. This kind of machine will offer you a cable pull-down, chest-press/pec dec and leg extension, which can also be used for standing leg curls.

Add to this a flat bench and some free weights and you will have an effective set up which will give you a good mix of exercises – smooth cable exercises that can't be performed any other way, and good quality free weight movements which, in our belief, are essential to any program.

advanced machines for advanced exercises

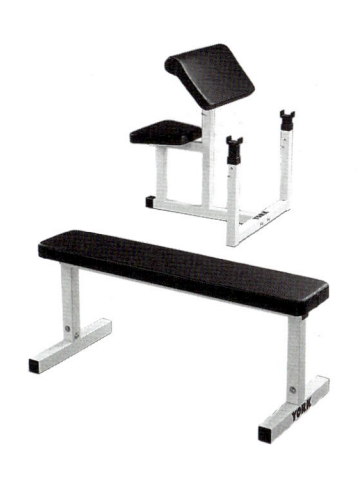

OK, so these are machines that are used for advanced techniques or exercises. The stuff you only tackle once you know a bit about what you are doing and why you are doing it. You will also need a good feel for the weight in your hands and what it will feel like when you move through a full range.

Advanced exercises are more difficult to perform, mainly because of the level of control required to move the weight from point A to point B and back again.

Advanced machines fall into a couple of categories,

1. attachments for benches or multi-gyms and;

2. freestanding machines designed to be used singularly.

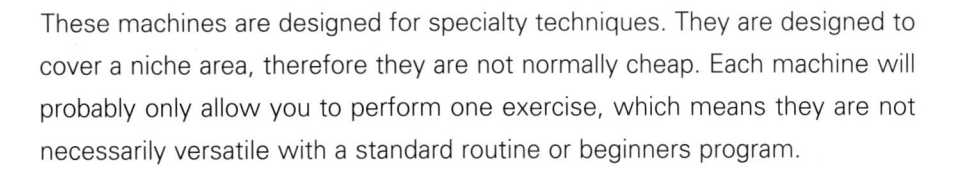

These machines are designed for specialty techniques. They are designed to cover a niche area, therefore they are not normally cheap. Each machine will probably only allow you to perform one exercise, which means they are not necessarily versatile with a standard routine or beginners program.

If you have some training knowledge and experience, then these machines will give you the opportunity to perform exercises that would otherwise be impossible or awkward to do on an irrelevant machine.

cardio equipment

Choosing which type of cardio machine to purchase will probably be fairly easy – it's a matter of preference. What you most enjoy using. There are of course other considerations to take into account. For instance, if you have an injury or disability, there may be some machines that require a certain movement through your legs or hips that will be difficult, painful or damaging, especially when using the machine for an extended period of time.

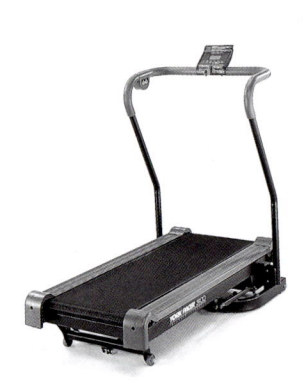

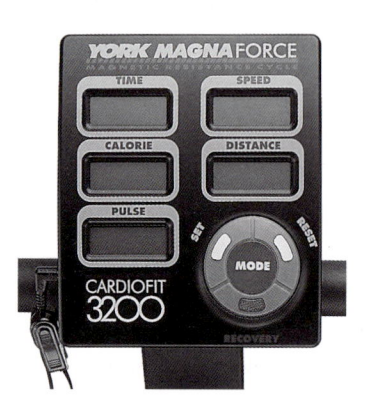

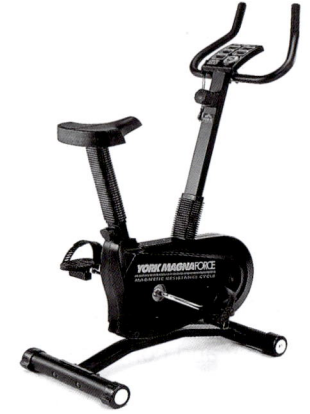

If you do fall into a special category, seek professional advice before making any decisions. See your usual sports doctor, physiotherapist or other specialist and discuss with them what you intend on doing. They may have a helpful suggestion on what type of machine or movement would be best suited to your needs. Do a bit of homework first and collect some brochures from retailers on the machines you are interested in. Take these along to your specialist for an appraisal.

Knee troubles, which are extremely common, could pose a problem with machines such as steppers and elliptical trainers. These machines can cause stress to the knee joint because of the constant movement going back and forth and the strength required for operation. If you have some form of weakness, diagnosed or not, using these types of machines could be detrimental. Again, seek advice from a physiotherapist or other sports therapist before making your purchase.

If you do not have any special requirements, then go ahead and try them all! All cardio machines will do one thing – keep your heart rate up – so that's one criteria you don't have to worry about when making a decision.

One of the best things about using cardio machines for your fitness and fat burning work is that you are at little risk of injury from impact. Unlike walking, running or stair-climbing outdoors these machines virtually eliminate the impact factor if used correctly.

Some of the machines will have an in-built heart rate pick up to allow them to automatically read from a chest band, others will have an earlobe-attachment that plugs into the computer console. We highly recommend you get yourself a heart rate monitor of some sort if your program will involve a lot of fitness/fat burning training (see heart rate monitors in chapter three).

exercise bikes

Bikes are probably the most favoured of the cardio equipment. They are easy and comfortable to use, they don't take up a great deal of space and they don't require a high level of skill or co-ordination.

Yet they supply the user with an excellent cardio workout through elevated heart rate while relying on all the muscles in the lower body to keep those pedals moving. If used correctly you should also get stabilization work through the mid-section (mid and lower back and abdominal). Exercise bikes can also be used for warming up and cooling down and make an effective component in a circuit program.

When choosing a bike, keep in mind what you will mainly use it for. If you intend on using it for fitness and fat burning, then a good variety of programs will be important. If your bike will be used for warm ups and cool downs and some supplementary work in between, you won't need the fancy programs. This also means that you won't need something super comfy either, so look at the smaller models which may still include a heart rate monitor. These smaller bikes will be fine to use for shorter periods of time and should still provide a smooth, quiet movement.

Some of the York bikes can also be converted to a rowing machine, this will provide you with a bit of variety if you will be using your machine quite often. They also have the feature of folding away, so that minimal room is required when the machine is not in use.

treadmills

The second most favourite piece of equipment! A treadmill will take up more space when in use, but all York models will fold away for easy storage when not in use.

The biggest consideration when buying a treadmill is deciding whether or not you need a machine to run on. The smaller, lower end treadmills are walkers only, most will go as fast as 6.5kph which is OK if walking is all you want to do. But if you do wish to do some running, you will need a treadmill which goes at least 10kph, a little faster even, so that the motor isn't working overtime.

If you are tall, make sure that the mat is long enough for a full stride. Getting on the machines and trying them out is the easiest way to find out.

Don't be afraid to wind the machine up to see how it performs.

Larger treadmills also come with larger motors, which means less stress on the mechanical components, and most importantly, less noise. The smaller treadmills can be a little noisy.

Last of all, the elevation factor. Most will have an elevation system of some kind, manual or automatic. The lower range machines have a manual system that needs to be adjusted while the treadmill is not in use. The larger machines have an automatic system that can be controlled from the computer, both systems work well.

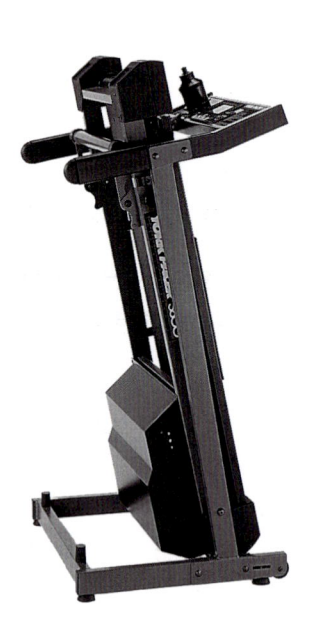

stepping machines

Steppers will require a bit more balance and co-ordination than the bike or treadmill. Your legs have to work independently of each other and the pedals should not touch the top of the machine or the floor during the movement, thus avoiding any impact and providing a smooth exercise. The big challenge is doing all this and maintaining a high heart rate at the same time - imagine walking upstairs non-stop for half an hour or so. It's certainly not just for the ultra-fit and not that hard to get the hang of either. It may just take a little practice.

Most domestic step machines will work on hydraulic cylinders for resistance. This system works fine, but does have to be maintained regularly, so make sure you follow any care instructions provided. They will have tension adjustments on the cylinders to make the exercise easier or harder, and computer console to monitor such things as time and steps per minute.

As with other machines, get on and try the stepper out. Don't buy anything without first being sure that you are confident and stable on the machine and comfortable with using it for extended periods of time.

If you are looking for a machine to spend lengthy periods of time on, fat burning training for instance, we would advise against buying a stepper. It is our belief that a stepping machine used over extended bouts of exercise could be damaging to the knees. If you are strong and fit you may have no problems however those with a tendency to weak knees could find themselves literally wearing the joint out.

Step machines will elevate the heart rate very quickly and so in our opinion are more appropriately used for interval or fitness training where you will spend 20 to 30 minutes maximum on the machine.

elliptical trainers

This machine will require a similar level of skill to the stepper. You will need the co-ordination involved in moving upper body and lower body at the same time.

The upper body muscles are used to move the arms of the machine backward and forward, providing an efficient pushing and pulling movement. At the same time, the lower body muscles are used to move the pedals of the machine around.

These machines can be used in either a forward or backward movement, giving the muscles variation in the way they are required to work to keep the machine moving. The one big selling point for this type of machine is that it is virtually impact-free when used correctly. There should be no risk to knees or any other major joint with correct form, although caution should be taken with shoulders if using the machine for long periods of time.

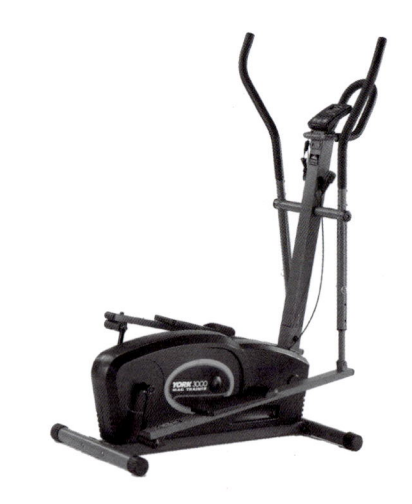

Heart rate monitors are included with some and are available as an added extra with others. All will come with pedal and arm adjustments, and should have a tension adjustment as well.

boxing equipment

Boxing gear in a home situation is primarily used for elevating the heart rate and increasing fitness. Upper body strength will improve and it is also a good way to develop better co-ordination.

The basics required are a good pair of gloves and a bag. If you just want to have some fun and let off some steam, a punching bag will serve you well, remember you can kick it as well as punching it.

If you want something a bit more advanced, try a speedball, or a floor to ceiling ball. These balls require a fair bit of co-ordination and concentration as the ball itself is quite small and will swing unpredictably, but once mastered can be a lot of fun. Have a chat with someone who knows they're stuff and again, don't be embarrassed about trying it all out. This will ensure you get something that will work well for you. Keep in mind that these punching bags and balls are all ceiling mounted, so find yourself somewhere to hang it first. Make sure that you are attaching the bag to a beam or something of similar strength that will support its weight and the impact of your punches and kicks. Speedballs are not as heavy but will still require a sturdy position, floor to ceiling balls, as the name suggests, will require a solid anchor position at both ends.

Freestanding punching bags are available, and are a great alternative if you can't find a hanging position. The range will be a little limited though and the bag itself will feel different to hit but will provide you with just as good a workout as a hanging bag.

accessories

Accessories have been designed to make exercising easier and more comfortable. They also tend to make it more expensive because you will want to go off and buy all sorts of gadgets. Beware the gadget that promises miracles in the training stakes. Anything that suggests you will get bigger, leaner or fitter in half the time it would normally take simply by using this 'amazing product' should be treated with some trepidation.

Some of these accessories really are useful though and these will make your training sessions more effective, safer and in some cases, more fun. You will also find that having an accessory like a heart rate monitor will mean that you are better informed as to how your workouts are progressing. Below we have listed some of the accessories that we recommend.

There are so many different accessories on the market that it would take up half of this book to review them all. Instead we have chosen some of the most popular ones and those that we think are well worth investing in.

weight training belts

Training belts give effective support through the mid to lower back and are used mostly with resistance training. Anyone pushing large amounts of weight, especially during exercises where the weight is being lifted above the head should consider wearing a training belt.

Training belts can be used for support with any resistance exercise as long as you feel comfortable wearing it. The belt should be pulled in as tight as possible when performing an exercise and then loosened between sets. Remember that the belt should feel comfortable at all times, don't pull it in so tight that you can't breathe or feel sick.

Most belts are available in four sizes – small, medium, large and extra large – and are available in leather or synthetic materials.

The choice is yours when it comes to deciding on a style of belt. The leather belts will obviously last a lot longer than the synthetic version, but they do take a while to 'break in'. The leather will remain a little stiff for while, this makes it a bit uncomfortable, but it should definitely not be a major consideration when deciding which one to purchase.

Synthetic belts tend to be lighter and cooler to wear in warmer temperatures. Although they are made from an artificial fabric and will probably promote sweating, they will feel a little lighter and more comfortable to wear once your body core temperature starts to rise and the blood is pumping. Good quality synthetic and leather belts will probably cost around the same, so the choice will be based entirely on your preference.

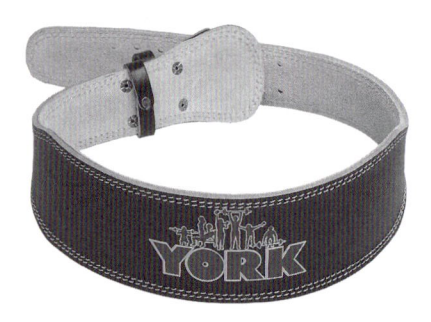

weight training gloves

Training gloves are one of those accessories that we recommend for anyone doing resistance work, regardless of their goals. A good pair of gloves will provide you with a solid grip, reduce the chances of slipping and decrease the incidence of calloused hands.

They will also protect jewellery from being damaged by bars, although we strongly recommend you remove any rings, watches etc before beginning your training session.

As with training belts, gloves are available in small, medium, large and extra large. Fabric options are leather and neoprene (similar to wetsuit material). Again both will cost about the same. Durability wise, the gloves probably do not differ much regardless of whether they will get an absolute pounding or are only worn once a week.

exercise mats

If you have a carpeted training area, then you will probably have no need for an exercise mat. However if you will have your training gear set up on concrete or floor boards, you will need somewhere soft and comfortable to stretch. And yes, everyone needs to stretch, even those on advanced resistance programs.

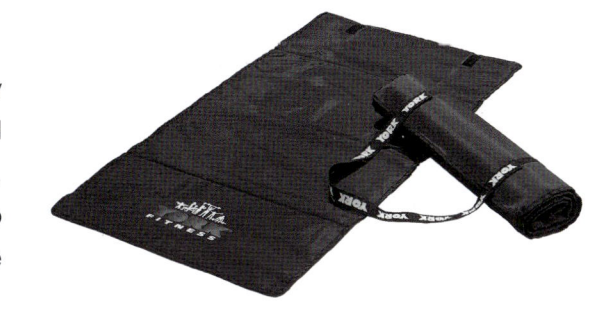

Your training mat can also be used for doing any form of floor work that calls for you to lie or sit on the floor. They make a great yoga mat too.

We don't recommend you use an exercise mat for performing exercises where your weight will shift from one leg to the other. In this situation the mat will serve as an unsteady surface and could see you flat on your back with a pair of dumbells on top of you.

Exercise mats are made from vinyl and contain foam padding to make them soft and comfortable to lie on. They also roll up for easy storage.

ankle and wrist weights

Ankle weights come in various shapes and sizes and are useful for several forms of training. We don't recommend you strap them on to go walking or running as the impact and excessive joint wear and tear is just not worth the minimal advantage gained. Your heart rate will be further elevated because of the extra weight you are carrying but form can be easily compromised, especially once you become fatigued.

Use ankle weights for gentle strength training exercises, lighter weights are also quite good for rehabilitation work. We have listed some exercises for you to perform with ankle weights under the lower body strength section.

Ankle weights are by no means essential to a strength or resistance training program. They will make a great supplement to standard exercises that can be performed on a bench or multi-gym and will also target smaller muscles groups in the legs efficiently.

They come in several different fabrics, the most common being vinyl and neoprene. Weight ranges start at 0.5kg and go up to 2kg, that's for each leg. Adjustable ankle weights are available; these have a maximum weight of 5kg.

skipping ropes

Jump ropes are a great supplement to a cardio program, they also work really well with boxing training. You will need a good deal of co-ordination to keep the momentum going for a period of time though, and that comes with practice.

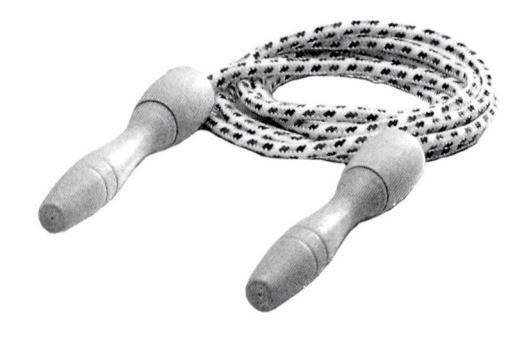

We know it's hard to picture adults skipping for exercise when all you can see is kids having a great time in the playground. But remember how much energy and enthusiasm you had when you were a kid? Not to mention staying power when it comes to exercise. Instead picture those super-fit boxers, who rely on skipping for fitness, co-ordination and endurance.

Monitoring your heart rate during skipping will give you an idea of how effective this exercise is for increasing fitness levels. It will also give you a change of pace and focus when the standard cardio stuff becomes a little glum.

Jump ropes come in leather and cotton. Leather will be a little more expensive but will obviously last longer, because the rope hits the floor with each rotation. If you are new to skipping a cotton rope might be a good idea, because it isn't quite as heavy and will be easy to spin around.

heart rate monitors

OK this is where it gets a little more specialised. First of all, if your goal is simply to gain muscle and strength, you have no need to monitor your heart rate and so you won't need one of these. If you are using resistance and/or cardio machines in a circuit or other fashion with the goal of increasing your fitness we highly recommend you invest in one.

When you buy a heart rate monitor, you will get a chest band and a watch. These things work on a telemetry signal that is sent from the chest band and picked up by the watch. The chest band has two or more electrodes on the inside that will pick up a direct signal from your heart, so positioning and a snug fit is important for getting a clear signal and accurate reading.

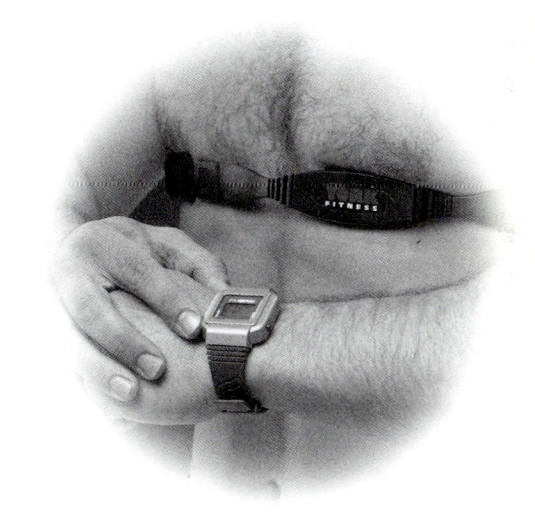

From experience we have found that a little lubrication initially will have your monitor producing a clearer and more accurate signal faster. Once your heart rate and body core temperature are increased you will begin sweating and lubrication won't be a problem.

There are a few models to choose from, so knowing what you are going to use it for is important, also take into account the needs of anyone else who will be using the monitor on a regular basis.

A base model heart rate monitor will read your heart rate and that's about it. If you simply want to keep track of your heart rate during training sessions to see how it reacts to different loads, then this one is for you.

Anything above the standard model will include upper and lower zone limits. This function enables you to set your minimum and maximum heart rate for your training session (you can get this information from the charts supplied with your monitor or chapter eleven in this book). While you are inside your 'training zone' your heart rate monitor won't make any noise, but if you go above or below those limits, an alarm will sound to let you know. This means you can speed it up or slow it down accordingly.

Mid range models will include features such as the following:

- Watch settings for time of day
- Calendar (day and month)
- Alarm
- Stopwatch

Top of the range models will have the same features as the mid and lower range, but have the added advantage of being PC compatible. This means that the monitor is capable of downloading training information straight onto your computer for storage and/or analysis. These monitors aren't cheap and really won't be necessary unless you get super serious about your training.

All the heart rate monitors include standard features such as LCD light, bike mount for watch and instruction manual. They are all also water resistant to 20 meters, so you can take your monitor swimming if you like.

Don't be dazzled by all the features when purchasing one of these things. Be honest with yourself about what you really need it for and buy something that suits both your needs and that of your wallets.

SECTION FOUR
designing your home studio

Laying out your studio should be done with some thought and imagination. Of course you could throw it all into a room and go for it, no problem. You'll soon discover though that constantly moving heavy gym equipment around isn't much fun! If your training area is well organised and efficiently designed and laid out, it will be a much more enjoyable place to train.

Making a few designs in advance will pay off. Although you are the only person who can ultimately decide on the final layout (based on your training requirements), it will help to have a bit of professional advice and some tried and tested ideas.

If you are planning on a mix of cardio, resistance machines and free weights, it will be best to group like machines together. Don't forget that you will need plenty of room around multi gyms and free weight benches, so locate cardio machines well away. Free weights are dangerous to handle and should be positioned against a wall on a rack if you have one, if not in a corner of the room away from where you will be moving around.

Power points will be a consideration if you intend on purchasing an electricity-driven cardio machine. Rewiring is expensive unless you are an electrician, and trailing cables across the floor is extremely dangerous. So place anything that requires power at the wall nearest the outlet.

Finally, the structure of your training area or room should be taken into account. If you intend on setting up your studio in an upstairs location, it would be a good idea to have an engineer assess the stability of the floor. This will probably only be an issue if you intend on purchasing a large multi-gym, plenty of free weights and a motorised treadmill. But you never know, its better to be safe than sorry – you wouldn't want your home studio ending up downstairs in the living room.

layout

We have put together three scenarios for you; hopefully your space will fit into one of these following categories.

1. Section of an existing room e.g. the corner of a bedroom or living room
2. Spare room
3. Garage

These are the three most common places for people to set up their equipment. A spare room could be a bedroom, office or sunroom. A basement or cellar would both come under the heading of a garage, and part of an existing room could be any small space in the house.

1. section of an existing room

This set up will suit anyone who only has a small amount of space to spare for their home training studio. It could be part of a living room, kitchen, study or bedroom as we have used in our scenario.

We do advise against setting up your equipment on a verandah or balcony unless it is completely protected from the weather. Any steel components e.g. bars, weights and bench parts will rust over an extended period of time.

You will require basic equipment that provides you with enough options for a full workout routine including cardio training. Lets look at your options:

- Combination cycle/rower
- Foldaway bench
- Exercise mat
- Fit ball
- Free weights and bars

DESIGNING YOUR HOME STUDIO

[Floor plan diagram showing a bedroom layout with: CYCLE/ROWER, FOLDAWAY BENCH, FIT BALL STORED ON BENCH, WEIGHTS & BARS in one corner; EXERCISE MAT, BED, WINDOW, CHEST OF DRAWERS, and BUILT-IN WARDROBE occupying the rest of the room.]

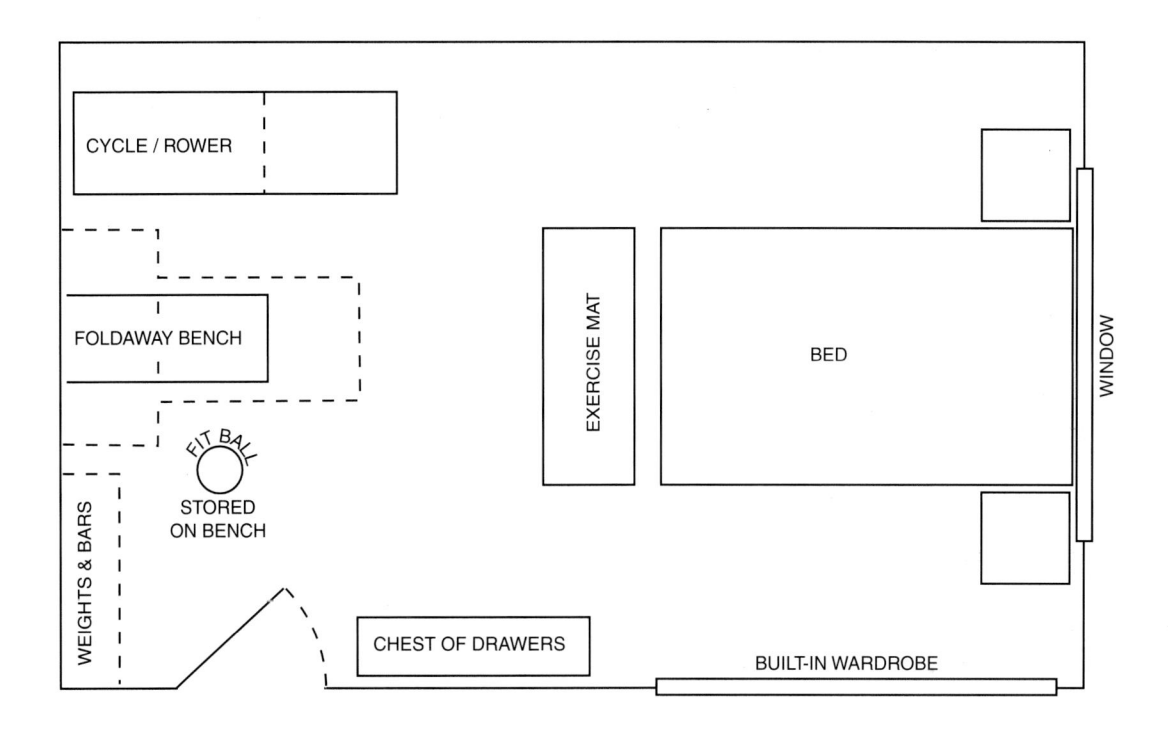

The trick to this set up is to put the equipment in a corner that is out of the way. If you are constantly tripping over the stuff, or climbing over it to get to whatever is behind, you will quickly tire of the whole thing. Try not to obstruct doorways either, for the same reasons.

We have dedicated one end of this bedroom to training; the other half remains the same. The wardrobe and chest of drawers can still be accessed without any hassle and the area at the end of the bed has been kept clear for floor work when you are training and ease of movement when you are not.

Obviously this setup is designed for one user at a time because of the lack of room to move. Although if you have a training partner who is following the same routine and you can train 'set for set', it would probably be fine.

The cardio machine performs two exercises, rowing and cycling, which provides a bit more versatility in a small space. It has been placed in the corner away from the weights for safety and also to allow more room around the bench. When not in use it can be stored in the cycle position, which takes up less space.

The bench folds away, which also allows for more space when not in use and the weights and bars can be stored on the floor behind the door. The exercise mat can be rolled up and stored in any small space, and the fit ball can be stored in front of the folded bench.

Ventilation may be an issue in a small space and so you may want to consider including a fan to keep you cool if your room isn't air-conditioned.

We used:
York Cycle Rower 2 in 1
York Foldaway 230 Bench Space Saver
York fit ball-65cm
1 x York 6ft Barbell Bar with collars
2 x York 14 inch Dumbell Bars with collars
York Cast Iron Weight Plates - 2 x 10 kg, 4 x 5kg, 4 x 2.5kg, 4 x 1.25kg

2. the spare room

Devoting a whole spare room to your training studio means that you will probably have enough space for the following;

- One piece of cardio equipment e.g. bike or elliptical trainer
- Small multi gym
- Small selection of free weights and bars
- Fit ball
- Exercise mat for floor work

Obviously what you purchase for your spare room will depend largely on the size of the room and the size of your budget. What we have laid out below is based on a room that is 3 meters x 5 meters. The cost involved in this kind of set up isn't huge, although it is a larger investment than that of a bench and weights only.

DESIGNING YOUR HOME STUDIO

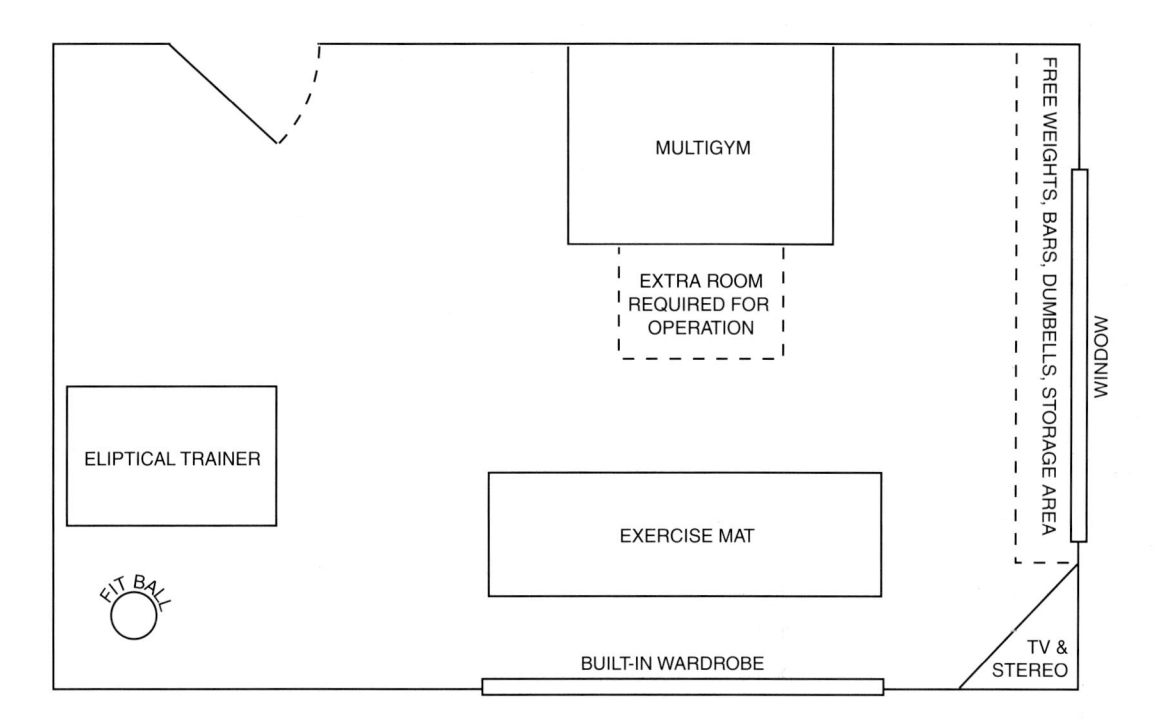

```
┌─────────────────────────────────────────────────┐
│                                                 │
│         ┌──────────────┐                        │
│         │   MULTIGYM   │    FREE WEIGHTS,       │
│         │              │    BARS, DUMBELLS,     │
│         └──────────────┘    STORAGE AREA        │
│           EXTRA ROOM                            │
│           REQUIRED FOR           WINDOW         │
│           OPERATION                             │
│                                                 │
│  ┌──────────────┐                               │
│  │  ELIPTICAL   │                               │
│  │   TRAINER    │                               │
│  └──────────────┘                               │
│                   ┌────────────────┐            │
│     ⊙ FIT BALL    │  EXERCISE MAT  │            │
│                   └────────────────┘   TV &     │
│                                       STEREO    │
│              BUILT-IN WARDROBE                  │
└─────────────────────────────────────────────────┘
```

Adapt where necessary to make this design appropriate for your situation. Take special note of where each machine is situated. This will make a big difference when you are actually moving around the room during a training session. For example, the free weights and bars have been placed under the window where they won't get in the way. We have also placed them close to the multi-gym and allowed some free space right next to them for performing free weight exercises.

The cardio machine is at the other end of the room with plenty of space surrounding it for ease of getting on and off. Your cardio machine is also best located away from the gym and free weight area.

The television and stereo have their own corner away from the action but are still easily accessed. Make sure you have a clear line of sight from your cardio machine to the television.

The fit ball has been placed in the corner next to the cardio machine and can be taken out into the middle of the room when in use.

Last of all, the designated stretching area has been placed in front of the wardrobe doors. This area will need to be kept clear for you to access your wardrobe, so this is a great place for the exercise mat. Roll the mat up when you are not using it and store it in the corner next to the cardio machine.

We used:
York Compact-901 multi gym
York Mag Elliptical Trainer
York Exercise Mat
York fitball-65cm
York Hexagonal Dumbells - 2 x 2kg, 2 x 5kg, 2 x 10kg

3. the garage

OK now we're getting down to the serious stuff! If you have set aside a garage for your training room, you have either decided to tackle the whole thing with a full-on approach or you will be sharing your equipment with a friend or two.

Maybe you are setting up a gym that you and your family can use. Either way, a larger space means more freedom when purchasing equipment (provided the budget will allow such freedom).

Again, lets look at your options:
- Treadmill
- Small exercise bike
- Large multi gym
- Free weights and bars
- Punching bag
- Skipping rope
- Fit ball
- Exercise mat for floor work

DESIGNING YOUR HOME STUDIO

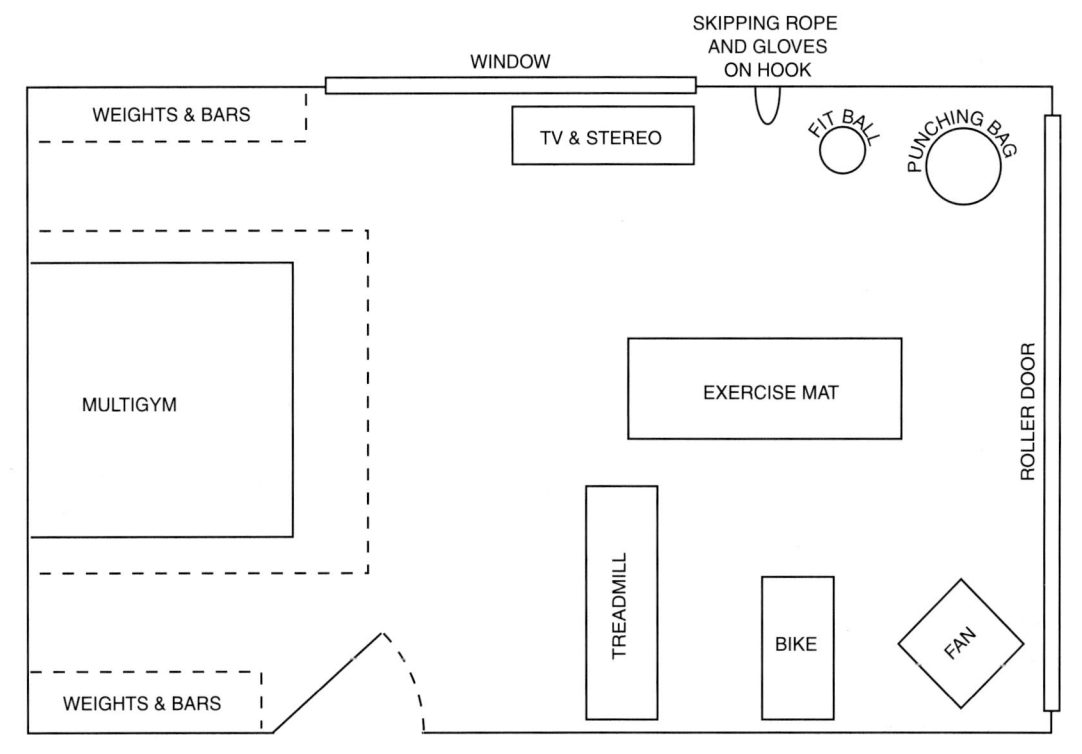

We have designed this training room around a space that is pretty much a standard single car garage size.

This set up will cost more because of the amount of equipment that will be in your training room. The things that we have included are also a step above the standard stuff and so will set you back a little more.

We have included in this setup, a freestanding fan to keep you cool. If you have a roller door and aren't too shy, perhaps you could have it open in summer when you are training, this will provide plenty of flow through air to keep the temperature down; or if you wish you could install an air conditioner.

The television and stereo are located in an easily accessible position and the television can be clearly seen from the cardio gear. Weights and bars are stored on either side of the multi gym for ease of use and safety. The multi gym is backed up against the wall at one end so that two or three people could easily exercise together – while one party is on the cardio gear, the other is using the gym without getting in anyone's way.

The punching bag has been located closest to the roller door, which is the furthest point from all other equipment. This will allow for plenty of swinging room when hitting or kicking the bag. The skipping rope and mitts are stored on hooks attached to the wall nearest the bag. Skip rope can be done in the floor space provided for the exercise mat, this is also close to the punching bag as these two can be used in conjunction with each other.

The fit ball is stored on the floor under the mitts and skipping rope. The ball can be used in the middle of the room where open floor space has been provided.

We used:

York Power Station 3000 multi gym
York Pacer 3600 treadmill
York Cardiofit 3200 cycle
22kg Boxing Bag
York Exercise Mat
York fit ball-75cm
York leather skipping rope
Neoprene bag mitts
1 x York 7ft Barbell Bar with collars
2 x York 14 inch Dumbell bars with collars
York Cast Iron Weight Plates - 2 x 20kg, 4 x 10kg, 4 x 5kg, 4 x 2.5kg, 4 x 1.25kg

SECTION FIVE strength training

why lift weights?

A few years ago, if someone mentioned the words weight training, most people would conjure up an image in their heads of a muscle-bound guy or girl who couldn't stand with their legs together or hold their arms directly by their sides!

Things have changed a little since then.

Research has done some great things for resistance training over the years. It has been discovered that resistance training can benefit most people, regardless of their age or ability, in some way.

The fitness industry has changed over the years too, and although there is still room for improvement, gyms are now a much friendlier place to visit. Gone are the days when the gym was the domain of the young and super-fit, when you felt like you needed to get into shape before you signed up for a membership.

For these reasons, more and more people are discovering the many benefits of resistance training for themselves. There are many more reasons for training with weights than just to grow big muscles, take the following for instance.

Regular resistance training will

a. Improve or maintain the health of your bones

b. Improve strength and stability

c. Burn more calories through increased muscle mass

d. Increase prevention of injuries through increased muscle mass

e. Provide a leaner more athletic appearance

Through our years of experience as personal trainers, we have certainly seen both younger and older adults achieve brilliant results from a specifically designed resistance program. Younger guys fill out their clothes better, especially suits, younger females tend to be more confident about wearing shorts and sleeveless tops or dresses. All feel and look a good deal better because of the exercise.

The older client will experience increased flexibility and control over muscle movement and prolonged staying power during leisure activities. Existing injuries can be worked out through gentle resistance training, and the incidence of new injuries is reduced. Resistance training is also an excellent stress buster. There are great physical results to be had too, imagine showing off your hard earned biceps and triceps and age 50!!

Remember though, that it is extremely important to seek approval from a Medical Practitioner or physiotherapist before starting on a resistance program.

how long will it take ?

This is the question that everyone asks. How long do I have to keep doing this before I start to see some rewards?

The answer is a little complex. There are a couple of variables to take into account, the first is your level of body fat. Everyone has muscles, one of the big differences between us is the level of body fat that is covering those muscles. If your body fat level is low, any muscle you gain through resistance training will be apparent pretty much straight away.

If your body fat level is high, your muscle growth may be the same but will be less apparent because of the layer of fat covering those muscles. Overall size may actually increase slightly, but this is due to an increase in muscle size not in body fat. Cardio training is a good way to speed up the process and therefore ensure physical results sooner. Don't be discouraged by the weight gain, be encouraged by the fact that everything is on the move and you are well and truly on the way to a new you.

The other variable, which probably plays the biggest role in muscle growth is your genetic make up. Regardless of how quickly you want to build your physique, if your body isn't capable of fast growth it won't happen. Take runners as an example.

- The short distance sprinter requires maximum power in minimum time to get him from point A to point B. Big explosive movements from plenty of muscle is essential and so his build will be bulky.

- The long distance runner requires staying power and energy to make her go the distance. Bulky muscles will impede and slow her down. The energy required for carrying large amounts of muscle that far is huge and so her build will be slim and lean.

A large bulky runner will probably never make a great long distance racer because of his or her genetic make up. The same can be said of a small lean framed person aspiring to be a short distance sprinter.

The point we are trying to make here is that each body will respond differently to resistance training. The level of results and the time required to achieve those results will differ between one person and the next.

There is one thing that you can be sure of though, regardless of your current physique and your ability to build muscle and burn body fat, you will change your appearance for the better. You can improve your build through regular resistance work, you may not be capable of looking like Mr. Universe, but everyone can build some muscle and look stronger, fitter and healthier.

advantages and disadvantages of machines

the good

- Machines are a great start for beginners. Cables will guide the user through the movement. Although it is still possible to perform the exercise with bad form, training on machines will take away some of the extra challenges early on.

- Machines are also great if you are training on your own without a partner to spot you and correct your form. Muscle failure through heavy sets can still be achieved without the risk of getting stuck with a weight on your chest that you can't move.

- No wasted time changing free weights. Selecting your chosen weight on the stack is a lot quicker than moving weight plates on and off bars, especially during circuit training or when backing up sets on different machines.

- Everybody has days when that training session never seems to end, when it feels like you will never get through it. On down days, cable machines can be great to get you through your workout safely and quickly without the focus required for free weight training. Great for when the alternative may have been not training at all.

- Machines can be great space savers. A multi gym with a small footprint will provide a good selection of exercises but still only take up a limited amount of space.

the not so good

- Machines in our opinion can change the 'feel' of the exercise by not allowing the muscle group you are working to move through a completely natural sequence.

- Machines can make it more difficult for the left and right side of a muscle to work independently.

- Machines will restrict you to one plane or arc of movement.

advantages and disadvantages of free weights

the good

- Training with free weights allows for a freedom of movement that is as natural as possible, therefore providing the user with a good feel for how the muscle naturally shifts a weight.

- A free weight set up will always cost less than a machine, making it an excellent starting point for anyone.

- Free weights on the whole occupy minimal space compared to even the most compact of machines.

- Free weight training develops a high level of skill related movements that machines can't.

the not so good

- Free weights are dangerous. Care has to be taken when handling weights and especially with children around.

- Free weights require a slightly higher level of skill, and so can be challenging for beginners.

- Heavy training with free weights is best done with a partner who can get you out of trouble should the need arise.

- Free weights are hard to store. Unless you take the time to unload bars and store weights when you finish your training session, you will find the room soon becomes cluttered and untidy. There is then the potential danger for tripping over or slipping.

- It is time consuming changing weights on bars a few times during your training session, especially if you have a training buddy who has a different level of strength to yourself.

Having pointed out the pros and cons of both, it is fair to say that neither set up has any major drawbacks. If asked frankly which set up we prefer, we would both honestly say that a mix of some free weights and a cable assisted multi gym is best. This will provide you with the ability to perform a huge range of exercises and do away with the restriction of not having one or the other.

The other major variable to keep in mind here is self-preference. You will probably in your travels meet people who swear by the old system of a bench and free weights. Then there will be others who believe that a modern multi gym is the only way to go, it comes down to what you believe will be best for your goals and enjoyment.

reps and sets

These are the two most common terms in resistance training. Repetition is the number of times you perform a particular exercise, and sets are groups of repetitions (reps for short). For example, if you were asked to do three sets of ten reps you would perform the exercise ten times then take a break, then perform another ten and take another break, then the third set of ten.

Most weight training programs will be broken down into reps and sets. The numbers of reps and sets performed will vary greatly depending upon the individual's goals and abilities.

how many reps should I do?

The number of repetitions you perform with each set will depend mostly on your goals, but also on your strength and stamina. As a rule, when using resistance training to increase fitness and aid body fat loss your program should be based on high repetitions and low weights.

For example: 3 sets of 20 reps with no more than 30 seconds rest between and using a weight which allows you to work comfortably through those reps while still providing a challenge.

If your primary goal is to build muscle, your repetitions will be lower and you should be working to full capacity, that is, close to muscle exhaustion by the end of each set. A heavy program may allow up to one minutes rest between sets and anywhere from 2 to 4 sets may be performed.

There are also many different techniques to explore with resistance training, no matter what your goals, these include:

Pyramiding: Increase the weight and decrease the reps with each set

Super setting: Combine two exercises for the same muscle group and perform one set of each without a rest in between.

Giant setting: Combine two or more exercises for different muscle groups and perform one set of each without a rest in between.

Drop sets: Perform two or more sets of an exercise without a rest between sets and reduce the weight slightly each time. A drop set should be performed after training that same muscle group. It is designed for total fatigue.

how many sets should I do?

The same rules apply here, as with the above it will depend upon your goals. Multiple sets are necessary to fatigue the muscle during a resistance program that is designed to build size and strength. Multiple sets are also necessary during circuit or fitness training because they are used to keep the heart rate high while also stimulating muscle growth.

One bit of advice is not to do a dozen sets for each exercise. If you want to concentrate on one particular muscle group, vary your training by using several different exercises for the same group. That way you will have variety in your training and the muscle group will be hit from different positions and levels of intensity.

how much rest do I take between sets?

Most fitness professionals will have their own opinion on how much rest we should take between sets, latest research also plays a big part in what we should be doing. However, as a guideline for a heavy program designed to build maximum muscle, take between 45 and 60 seconds rest between sets. If you are training for fitness and fat burning, somewhere between 15 and 30 seconds rest will be fine. Refer to your chosen program card for guidelines.

how do I know when I am ready for more weight?

If you are thinking the obvious, then you are right – when the exercise feels too easy. When you can comfortably push out all of your sets and reps without too much trouble, you are ready for more. If you have to cheat for those last couple of reps with bad form, it may be a good idea to stay with the same weight. Try perfecting the exercise, getting every rep in safely and with good form, when you can do that, then increase the weight.

Increasing the weight may mean that you can't push out the same amount of reps that you could with the lower weight. That's fine, just decrease the amount of reps you perform each set. It won't be long before your strength will improve and you will be getting the original number of reps in, at which time you can increase the weight again.

fast reps and slow reps

Some trainers will swear by the benefits of slow reps – three seconds up, three seconds down. Other trainers believe that heavy is the go, push lots of weight and get the reps in with good form but as quick as possible.

Both concepts are OK and as with everything else, it will depend upon your goals. Slow reps are really only of benefit in a muscle building routine, and if you can handle the intensity and discomfort during the set, it is an excellent way to train. The down side, if you look at it that way, is that this type of training will require a lot of focus and more time as the sets will take longer to get through. The theory is that the muscle is held under load for a longer period of time, therefore more effectively achieving the point of fatigue.

If you are using resistance training for fitness and fat burning, fast reps are the go. The aim of the game here is to keep the heart rate high, that isn't going to happen if it is taking you six seconds to complete one repetition!

Fast reps should be performed with good form and in a safe manner, don't go recklessly charging through your session, just to keep your heart rate in your target zone. If you find that your heart rate is not elevated to the level it should be, increase the weight slightly, but only to a point where you can still push out a decent amount of reps per set. This will maintain your heart rate training zone whilst keeping you on the move for the duration of your session.

order of exercises

What order do you perform all this stuff in? Again there are many different theories about how it should be done. There is one tried and tested theory though, and that is largest to smallest muscle group. Here is the basic layout of this theory:

* Perform the exercises in the order below, first working the largest muscle group that requires maximum power and blood volume. Work through to the smaller muscle groups in the body which require less blood volume and power (energy)

1. **Legs** – quadriceps and hamstrings
2. **Back** – latissimus dorsi, trapezius, and rhomboids
3. **Chest** – pectorals
4. **Shoulders** – front, mid and rear deltoids
5. **Arms** – biceps and triceps
6. **Torso** – abdominal, lower back

There are many different variations to this standard routine; muscles can be split into pushing and pulling groups or upper and lower body or broken down into opposing sets (working opposites).

We suggest that you start with a standard routine and get a feel for the way your muscles work during your training sessions. Time will provide you with more experience and knowledge and you will be able to move on to some of the more advanced techniques.

The amount of times you intend on training per week will play a large role in how your program should be laid out. For instance, if you will only train once or twice a week, then full body workouts each session will be the go. If you intend on training three or more times per week, you will need to break your muscle groups down and only work certain groups on certain days. This will prevent muscle tiredness and avoid you becoming run down, it will also allow you extra time for each muscle group, therefore increasing your chances of better results earlier.

how many times per week should I train?

The answer to this question should be left up to yourself. How many hours a week can you spare for your training without it seeming a chore?

Each training session should last about one hour, any longer and you are taking too much rest between sets, or you are simply trying to do too much at once. If you are really keen on achieving results in a hurry, concentrate on the quality of your workouts and not the quantity. Honestly, if you try to do too much, you will probably achieve less. You will not be giving your body the chance to recover, you will probably become run down and suffer from constant muscle soreness – you need a healthy body to achieve results.

In most cases you will need to commit to at least two training sessions per week to continually achieve results. However there is no doubt that with some hard work, you can achieve results with just one one-hour session per week. So if that is all you can spare, then go for it, it's a much better option than doing nothing.

For maximum results, we recommend three to four sessions per week, again depending upon your goals and your desired time frame. Keep in mind that once you see some results and you are achieving what you initially set out to, things will slow a little and your goal setting may not be as frantic. Two full body weight sessions combined with two or three 30-minute cardio sessions per week is a nice combination and attainable by most people.

how often should I change my routine?

We have designed all the programs in this book around a 12-week working period, followed by a one-week break, then the start of a new 12-week program.

Variation is very important to any training program, your mind will need new stimulation to keep you interested, and your body will also require new stimulation to keep it growing.

Some people find that following the same program over and over again is the best way to keep them going because it is predictable and requires no brain power during training. If this is you, persevere, 12 weeks is plenty of time for you to settle into a routine and you should find that it will only take a couple of weeks to get used to a new routine. It really is important to vary the exercises you perform so that your muscles are hit from different directions each program, this will stimulate growth and also aid full range of movement when training.

If you are the type of person that needs constant change and you find yourself wanting to vary each session, that's OK too. Try sticking to the same program for the 12 weeks, but vary the exercises you do for each muscle group, rather than the order or technique.

For example: do a machine chest press instead of free weight bench press, but in the same order as your program suggests e.g. super-setting or drop sets.

dealing with muscle soreness

Muscle soreness is unavoidable in the early stages we're afraid to say. However as your training sessions advance and your muscles become accustomed to being placed under load, the amount of post training muscle soreness you experience should decrease.

After the initial bouts of soreness, you will probably experience discomfort after performing an exercise you haven't done for a while, for the first couple sessions into a new program, and after increasing the weights in a current program. Muscle soreness should be worst the day after your training session and should last no more than three or four days at the most.

It is not unusual to experience enough pain the day after your training to make it difficult to walk down stairs or perform normal duties with your upper body, however this kind of pain should last no more than a couple of days.

Although every body is different, that is, some may experience little or no muscle soreness even after the most intense training session, ongoing severe discomfort or pain is not normal. If you are experiencing excessive amounts of muscle soreness on an ongoing basis, your training program and form during each session should be assessed by a qualified fitness professional.

Adequate warm ups and cool downs can aid in the reduction of muscle soreness following a training session. Gentle cardio exercise will help once you are actually experiencing soreness in the muscles. Try a gentle 20 minute walk outdoors, or the equivalent indoors on a your cardio equipment. Follow this up with a full body stretch, being careful not to force sore muscles into too deep a stretch.

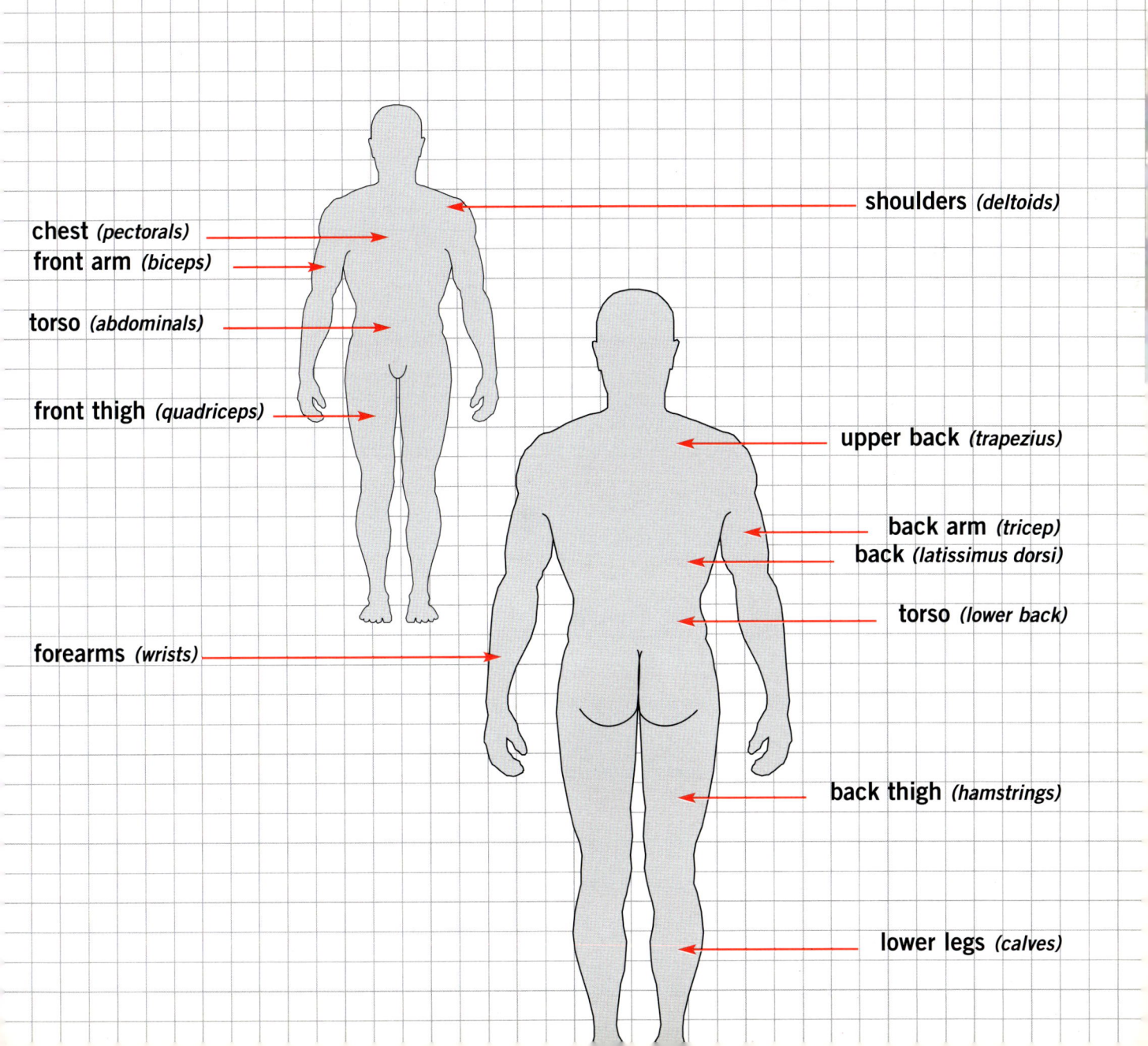

SECTION SIX exercise guide

- chest *(pectorals)*
- front arm *(biceps)*
- torso *(abdominals)*
- front thigh *(quadriceps)*
- forearms *(wrists)*
- shoulders *(deltoids)*
- upper back *(trapezius)*
- back arm *(tricep)*
- back *(latissimus dorsi)*
- torso *(lower back)*
- back thigh *(hamstrings)*
- lower legs *(calves)*

major muscles of the lower body

FRONT THIGH (quadriceps)

Compound
- Squats (barbell)
- Squats (dumbell)
- Lunges (forward)
- Lunges (reverse)
- Lunges (pulsing)
- Lunges (walking)
- Horizontal press bar squats

Isolation
- Leg extension

Advanced
- Squats (single leg)

BACK THIGH (hamstrings)

- Leg curls (standing)
- Leg curls (lying)
- Leg curls (standing ankle weights)

Advanced
- Straight leg deadlift

LOWER LEG (calves)

- Calf raise dumbell double leg (standing)
- Calf raise dumbell single leg (seated)
- Calf raise single leg (standing)
- Horizontal press bar calf raise

EXERCISE GUIDE

major muscles of the upper body

BACK (latissimus dorsi)

Compound
- Single arm dumbell row
- Pulldown (under-hand close grip)
- Pulldown (over-hand wide grip)
- Low cable seated row

Isolation
- Dumbell pullovers
- Pulldown (straight arm)

Advanced
- Chin up (under-hand close grip)
- Chin up (over-hand wide grip)
- Low cable bent over row
- Bent over barbell row
- Low cable long bar seated row

Upper back (trapezius)

- Barbell upright row
- Dumbell upright row
- Low cable upright row
- Dumbell shrugs
- Low cable shrugs
- Barbell shrugs
- Horizontal press bar shrugs

CHEST (pectorals)

Compound
- Bench press (barbell)
- Bench press (dumbell)
- Vertical machine bench press
- Incline press (barbell)
- Incline press (dumbell)
- Lying machine bench press

Isolation
- Straight-arm pec deck
- Dumbell flyes (flat bench)
- Dumbell flyes (incline bench)
- Pec deck

Advanced
- Decline press (barbell)
- Decline press (dumbell)
- Decline flyes

SHOULDERS (deltoids)

Compound
- Overhead press seated (barbell)
- Overhead press seated (dumbell)
- Overhead press standing (barbell)
- Overhead press standing (dumbell)
- Overhead machine press

Isolation
- Deltoid dumbell raises (front)
- Deltoid dumbell raises (side)
- Deltoid dumbell raises (rear)
- Deltoid cable raises (front)
- Deltoid cable raises (side)
- Deltoid cable raises (rear)

Advanced
- Rear pec deck

major muscles of the arms

FRONT ARMS (biceps)

    Barbell curls (standing)
    Low cable curl (standing)
    Dumbell curl (seated)
    Dumbell curl (seated incline)
    Dumbell hammer curl (seated)

Advanced
    Reverse curls ez bar
    Cable reverse curls
    Concentration curls (dumbell)
    Preacher curls (barbell)
    Twisting curls dumbell seated

BACK ARMS (triceps)

    Lying ez bar extensions
    Lying dumbell extensions
    Single dumbell seated over-head extension.
    Single dumbell kickbacks
    High cable pushdowns
    Flat bench dips

Advanced
    Rope pushdowns
    Under-hand pushdowns
    Single handle pushdowns
    Parallel bar dips
    Single hand dumbell extension (seated)

EXERCISE GUIDE

FOREARMS (wrists)

Dumbell double wrist flexion

Dumbell double wrist extension

midsection exercise listing

TORSO (abdominals)

Crunches (feet flat on floor)

Crunches (feet on bench)

Crunches (feet elevated, no bench)

Crunches (knee raise)

Floor knee raise

Crunches (knees over)

Vertical knee raise (machine)

Decline sit-ups

Horizontal abdominal hold (knees)

Horizontal abdominal hold (toes)

Hanging knee raise

TORSO (lower back)

Lower back hyperextension

Single arm/leg raise

SECTION SEVEN lower body

front thigh - quadriceps

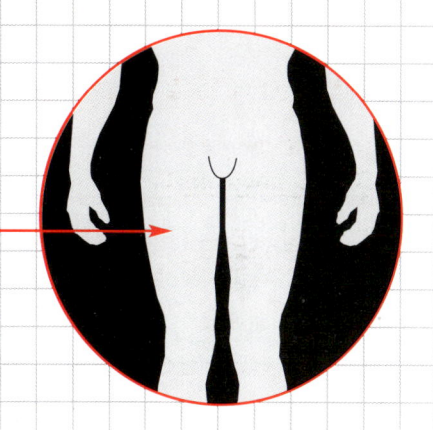

s-t-r-e-t-c-h Don't forget to stretch. Every muscle you strengthen, you should also stretch. Hold this stretch for at least 10 seconds between each set. See page 263

REMEMBER Keep your abdominal and lower back muscles tight through out the movement and remember to exhale during the lifting phase.

Tips The weight should always be under your control and if you need to cheat, you are probably trying to lift too much weight.

A lifting belt may also be of assistance to you in some squatting and lunging exercises when the weights you are lifting become more challenging (see accessories).

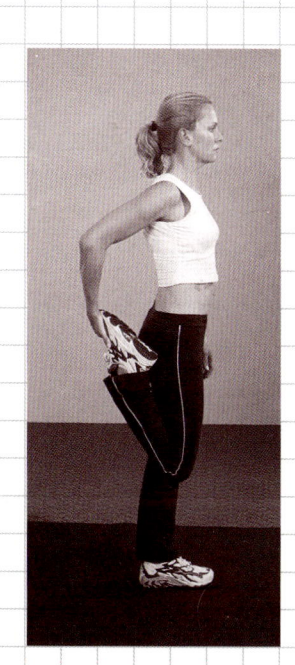

barbell squats

muscles working: Quadriceps (front thigh)

Glutes (buttocks)

Hamstrings (back thigh)

Erector spinae (lower back)

The start/finish position: Approach the squat rack and position the barbell on the solid section of your upper back, not your neck. Grasp the bar with an over hand grip (palms facing away from you) about double your shoulder width and place your feet about shoulder width apart with your toes angled slightly outward. Keep your head up and your eyes focused ahead while keeping your body weight directly below the bar. Lift the barbell from the rack and take 2 steps backward. Reposition your feet as above and keep your back straight with your eyes still focused ahead.

The movement: With your head up, start to bend from the knees and slowly lower your hips toward the floor until your thighs are parallel with the floor. Hold the midpoint position for a count of one, then push your heels hard against the floor and slowly control the barbell back to the start/finish position. Hold again for a count of one and repeat. If you find your heels are lifting from the floor as you squat, try using 2 weight plates below your heels to give you firm support.

Tip As the weight you are lifting increases, try to have someone assist you as a 'spotter' just in case you get into trouble.

NOT RECOMMENDED FOR THOSE WITH LOWER BACK PROBLEMS

Try to avoid leaning forward during the squat as this will place too much stress on your lower back.

LOWER BODY

dumbell squats

muscles working:
- Quadriceps (front thigh)
- Glutes (buttocks)
- Hamstrings (back thigh)
- Erector spinae (lower back)

The start/finish position: Approach the dumbells on the floor and position your feet between the two dumbells. Grasp the dumbells with your palms facing toward your ankles and place your feet about shoulder width apart with your toes angled slightly outward. Keep your head up and your eyes focused ahead. With your back straight and shoulders back, stand to an upright position.

The movement: From the upright position, start to bend from the knees and slowly lower your hips toward the floor until your thighs are parallel with the floor. Hold the midpoint position for a count of one, then push your heels hard against the floor and slowly lift yourself back to the start/finish position. Hold again for a count of one and repeat.

Tip As the weight you are lifting increases, try to have someone assist you as a 'spotter' just in case you get into trouble.

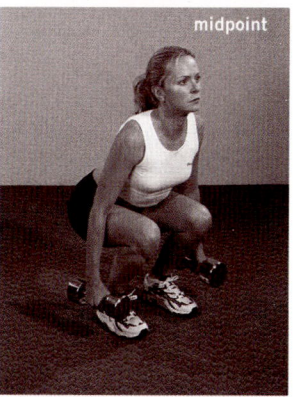

> **Try to avoid leaning forward during the squat as this will place too much stress on your lower back.**

NOT RECOMMENDED FOR THOSE WITH LOWER BACK PROBLEMS.

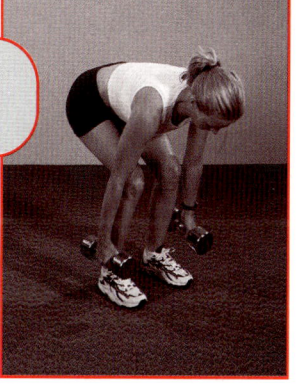

page 77

forward lunges

muscles working: Quadriceps (front thigh)

Glutes (buttocks)

Hamstrings (back thigh)

The start/finish position: Grasp a dumbell in each hand with your palms facing in toward your thighs. Stand with your feet together and keep your head up with your eyes focused ahead.

The movement: From the standing position, step forward with your right foot. Bend your right knee and begin to lower your left knee towards the floor stopping a few inches from the floor. Be sure your foot placement is such that your left knee is positioned diagonally behind your right heel ensuring a 90-degree angle in both your right and left knees. Hold the midpoint position for a count of one, then push your right heel hard against the floor and slowly push yourself back to the start/finish position. Hold again for a count of one and repeat until you complete the required repetitions for the right side and then do the same for the left side.

Tip Try to make sure your foot placement is correct with every footfall with your toes pointing straight ahead.

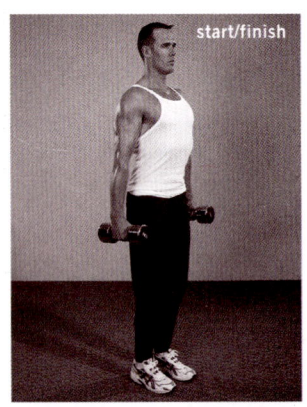

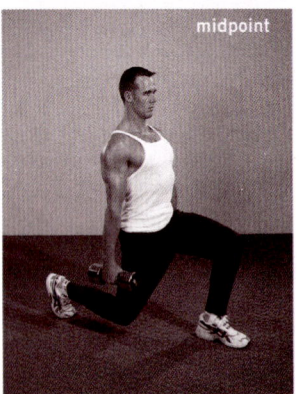

Try to avoid leaning forward during the lunge, keep your back straight and eyes forward and make sure that your knee doesn't extend over and past your front foot as this will place too much stress on the knee.

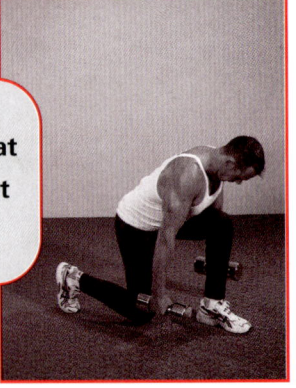

LOWER BODY

reverse lunges

muscles working:	**Quadriceps (front thigh)**

Glutes (buttocks)

Hamstrings (back thigh)

The start/finish position: Grasp a dumbell in each hand with your palms facing in toward your thighs. Stand with your feet together and keep your head up with your eyes focused straight ahead.

The movement: From the standing position, step backwards with your right foot. Bend your left knee and lower your right knee towards the floor stopping a few inches from the floor. Be sure your foot placement is such that your right knee is positioned diagonally behind your left heel ensuring a 90-degree angle in both your right and left knees. Hold the midpoint position for a count of one, then push your left heel hard against the floor and slowly push yourself back to the start/finish position. Hold again for a count of one and repeat until you complete the required repetitions for the right side and then do the same for the left side.

Tip Be careful with your foot placement as you learn to judge the correct distance behind and keep your toes pointing straight ahead.

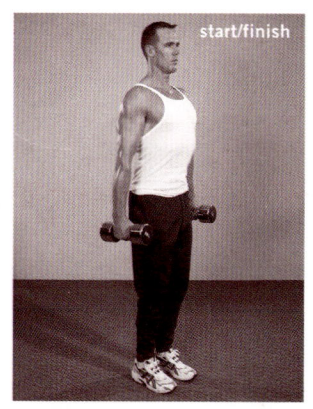

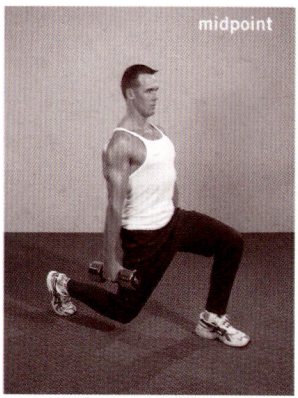

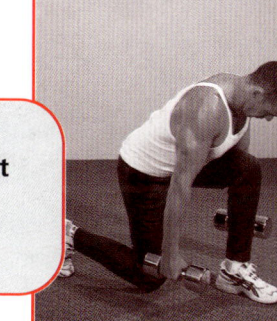

> **Try to avoid leaning forward during the lunge, keep your back straight and eyes forward and make sure that your knee doesn't extend over and past your front foot as this will place too much stress on the knee.**

page 79

pulsing lunges

muscles working: Quadriceps (front thigh)

Glutes (buttocks)

Hamstrings (back thigh)

The start/finish position: Grasp a dumbell in each hand with your palms facing in toward your thighs. Stand with your feet together and keep your head up with your eyes focused ahead. From the standing position, step forward with your right foot.

The movement: Bend your right knee and begin to lower your left knee towards the floor stopping a few inches from the floor. Be sure your foot placement is such that your left knee is positioned diagonally behind your right heel ensuring a 90-degree angle in both your right and left knees. Hold the midpoint position for a count of one, then push your right heel hard against the floor and slowly push yourself up until your right leg is straight with your right foot still positioned out in front. Continue to 'pulse' lunge on your right foot until you complete the required number of repetitions then return back to the start/finish position. Repeat for the left side.

Tip Try to make sure your foot placement is correct and your toes are pointing straight ahead.

> Try to avoid leaning forward during the lunge, keep your back straight and eyes forward and make sure that your knee doesn't extend over and past your front foot as this will place too much stress on the knee.

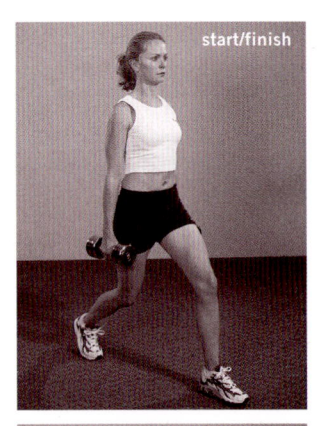

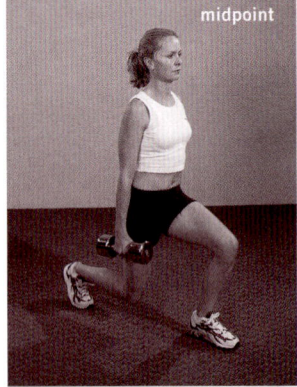

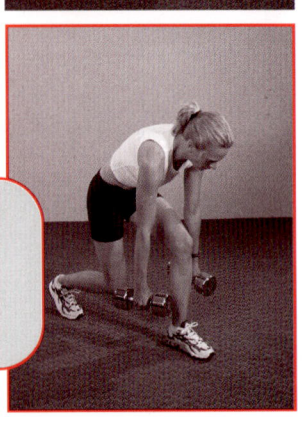

walking lunges

muscles working: **Quadriceps (front thigh)**

                                       Glutes (buttocks)

                                       Hamstrings (back thigh)

The start/finish position: Grasp a dumbell in each hand with your palms facing in toward your thighs. Stand with your feet together and keep your head up with your eyes focused straight ahead.

The movement: From the standing position, step forward with your left foot. Bend your left knee and begin to lower your right knee towards the floor stopping a few inches from the floor. Be sure your foot placement is such that your right knee is positioned diagonally behind your left heel ensuring a 90-degree angle in both your right and left knees. Hold the midpoint position for a count of one, then push your left heel hard against the floor and slowly walk yourself forwards until your feet are side by side. Alternate legs in a walking action until the completion of the desired number of repetitions and finish at the start/finish position.

Tip Try to make sure your foot placement is correct and your toes are pointing straight ahead.

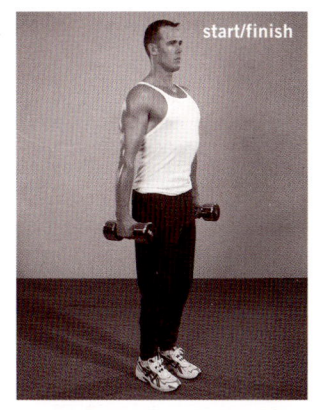

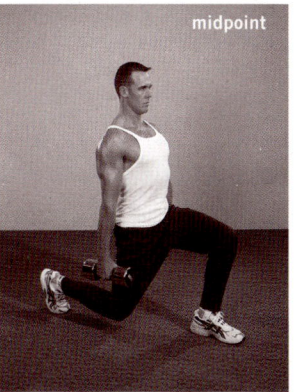

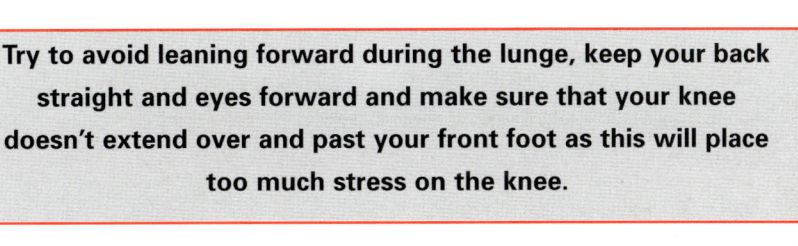

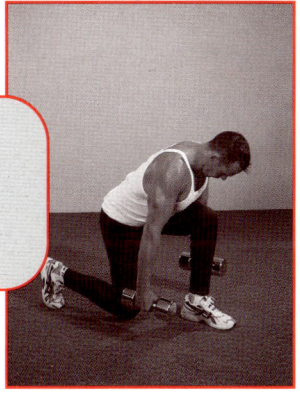

> **Try to avoid leaning forward during the lunge, keep your back straight and eyes forward and make sure that your knee doesn't extend over and past your front foot as this will place too much stress on the knee.**

horizontal press bar squats

muscles working: Quadriceps (front thigh)

Glutes (buttocks)

Hamstrings (back thigh)

The start/finish position: Approach the horizontal press bar with the bench removed. Position yourself with the press bar resting on the upper portion of your back - not your neck - and grasp the handles. Position your toes angled slightly out and feet about shoulder width apart. Keep your head up and your eyes focused straight ahead while keeping your body directly below the bar.

The movement: With your head up, start to bend from the knees and slowly lower your hips toward the floor until your thighs are parallel with the floor. Hold the midpoint position for a count of one, then push your heels hard against the floor and slowly control the press bar back to the start/finish position. Hold again for a count of one and repeat.

Tip As the weight you are lifting increases, try to have someone assist you as a 'spotter' just in case you get into trouble.

NOT RECOMMENDED FOR THOSE WITH LOWER BACK PROBLEMS

> **Try to avoid leaning forward during the squat as this will place too much stress on your lower back.**

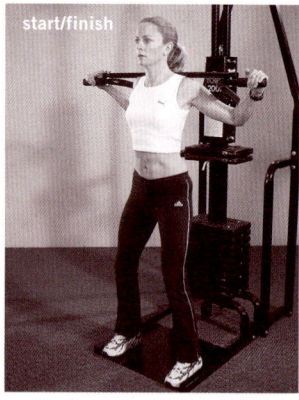

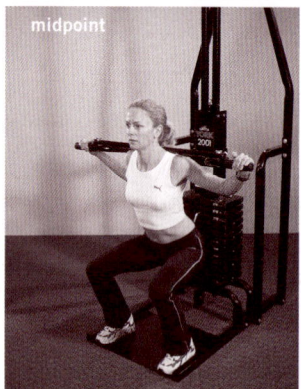

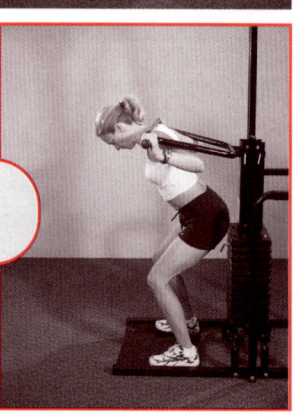

leg extension

muscles working: Quadriceps (front thigh)

The start/finish position: Sit down in the leg extension chair and position your feet behind the extension pads at the front of your ankles and make sure that the back of your knees are against the edge of the seat. Grasp the edge of the bench, point your toes forward and keep your head up and your back straight.

The movement: From the start/finish position, begin to straighten your legs with a smooth controlled lift until your legs are straight but without locking your knees out. Hold the midpoint position for a count of one, then slowly control the weight back to the start/finish position being careful not to allow the weight stack to touch or rest down. Hold this position again for a count of one before commencing the next repetition. At the completion of the desired number of repetitions, slowly lower the weight back down to the start/finish position.

Tip Try to keep both feet pointing straight ahead and your toes lifted towards to your shins. Make sure you lower the weight all the way down.

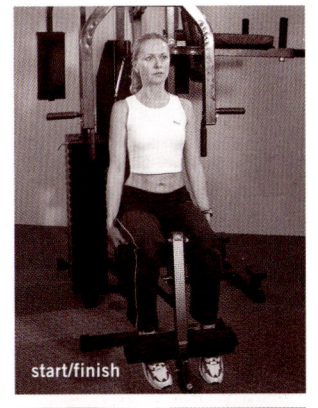

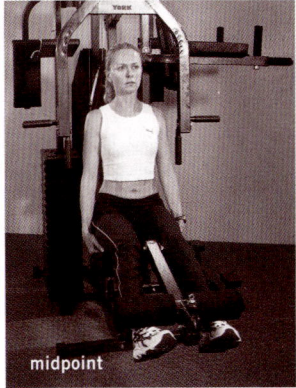

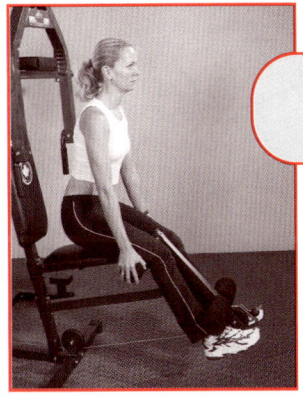

Try to avoid "kicking" the weight up and make sure your backside stays firmly against the bench.

LOWER BODY

start/finish

midpoint

page 83

single leg squats

muscles working:
- Quadriceps (front thigh)
- Glutes (buttocks)
- Hamstrings (back thigh)
- Erector spinae (lower back)

The start/finish position: Grasp a dumbell in each hand with your palms facing in toward your thighs. Place the top of your left foot on the surface of a flat bench. The top lace of your shoe should just clear the edge of the bench. Your right foot should be flat against the floor far enough away from the bench to allow your knees to be side by side. Keep your head up with your eyes focused ahead.

The movement: From the upright position, start to bend the right knee and slowly lower your hips toward the floor until your right thigh is parallel with the floor. Hold the midpoint position for a count of one, then push your heel hard against the floor and slowly lift yourself back to the start/finish position. Hold again for a count of one and repeat. Complete the desired number of repetitions for the right side and repeat for the left.

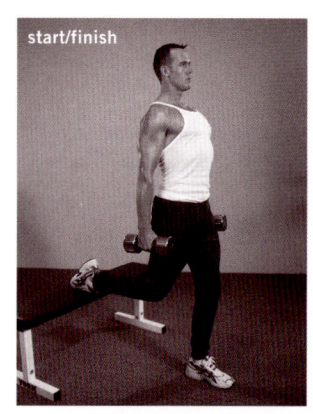

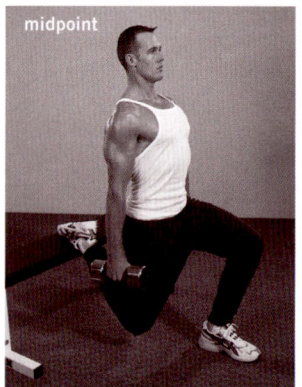

FOR ADVANCED LIFTERS ONLY

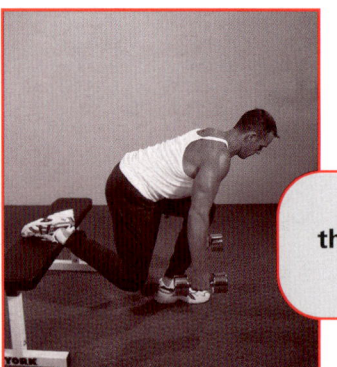

Tip Try to focus on aiming your back knee toward the floor and keeping your back straight.

> Try to avoid leaning forward during the squat and make sure that your knee doesn't extend over and past your foot as this will place too much stress on your knee.

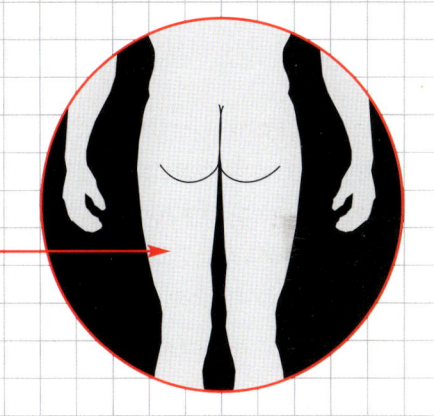

back thigh - hamstring

s-t-r-e-t-c-h Don't forget to stretch. Every muscle you strengthen, you should also stretch. Hold this stretch for at least 10 seconds between each set. See page 265

REMEMBER Keep your abdominal and lower back muscles tight through out the move and remember to exhale during the lifting phase.

Tips The weight should always be under your control and if you need to cheat, you are probably trying to lift too much weight.

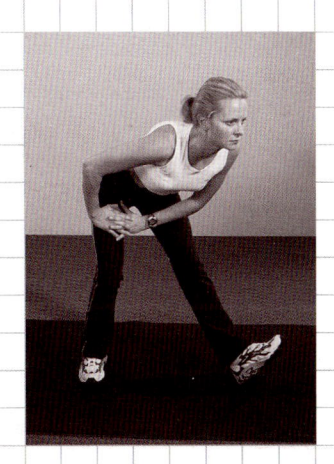

leg curls standing

muscles working: Hamstrings (back thigh)

The start/finish position: Approach the leg section of the machine and slide your right ankle behind the low ankle pads and ensure the top pads support your right thigh. Lean slightly forward, keep your eyes focused straight ahead and grab hold of the machine for balance and support.

The movement: With your head up, start to slowly curl your right ankle in towards your glutes, squeezing your hamstrings as hard as you can at the top and hold for a count of one. Slowly return the ankle pad to the start/finish position, being careful not to allow the weights to touch the stack, and hold for another count of one. At the completion of the desired number of repetitions for your right leg, swap sides and repeat for the left leg.

Tip Try to keep your toes pointing straight ahead and on your working leg, lifted up towards your shins. This will give a greater contraction on the hamstring muscle.

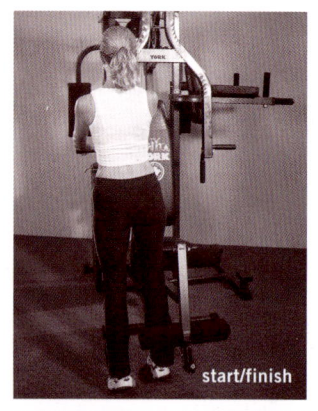

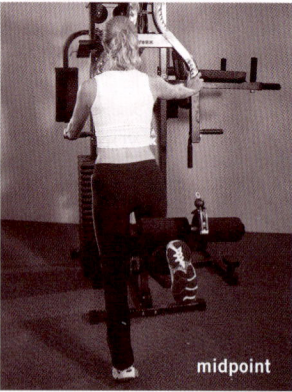

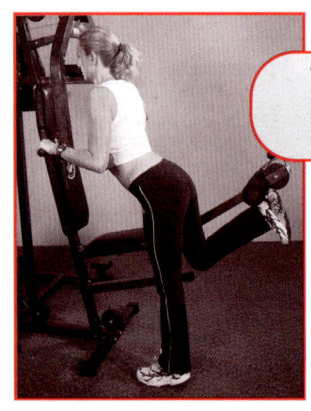

Try to avoid leaning forward and arching your back as this will place excess stress on your lower back.

leg curls lying

muscles working: Hamstrings (back thigh)

The start/finish position: Lie face down on the leg curl section of the bench with your knees just free of the edge of the bench and your ankles positioned under the ankle pads. Reach forward to grasp a section of the bench to keep your body hard against the bench.

The movement: Start to slowly curl the ankle pads in towards your glutes, squeezing your hamstrings as hard as you can at the top and hold for a count of one. The ankle pads should touch the top of your hamstrings. Slowly return the ankle pads to the start/finish position, being sure to get full range of motion but careful not to allow the weights to bottom out. Hold again for a count of one and repeat.

Tip Try to pull your body and hips down hard against the bench and keep your toes pointing straight ahead and lifted up towards your shins. This will give a greater contraction on the hamstring muscle.

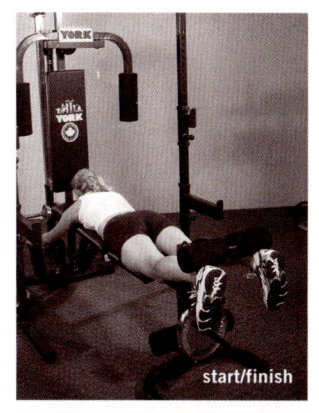

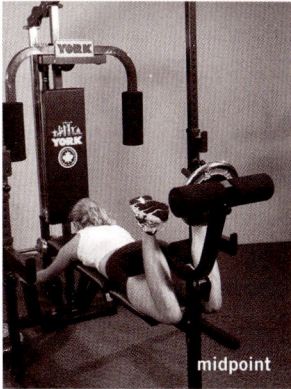

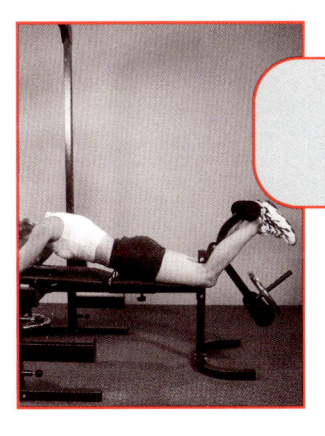

Try to avoid arching your lower back and lifting your hips and body off the bench as you curl the weight in as this will place excess stress on your lower back.

leg curls standing ankle weights

muscles working: Hamstrings (back thigh)

The start/finish position: Attach the appropriate ankle weight (if required) to your right leg and stand upright with hands supported at waist height. Stand with feet together, eyes focused straight ahead and your right toe lifted towards your right knee.

The movement: With your head up, start to slowly curl your right ankle in towards your glutes, keeping your knees side by side. Squeeze your hamstrings as hard as you can at the top and hold for a count of one. Slowly return to the start/finish position, being careful not to allow your foot to swing through and hold for another count of one. At the completion of the desired number of repetitions for your right leg, swap sides and repeat for the left leg.

Tip Try to keep your toes pointing straight ahead and on your working leg, lifted towards your shins. This will give a greater contraction on the hamstring muscle. Standing on a weight plate with your support leg will give your working leg a bit of ground clearance.

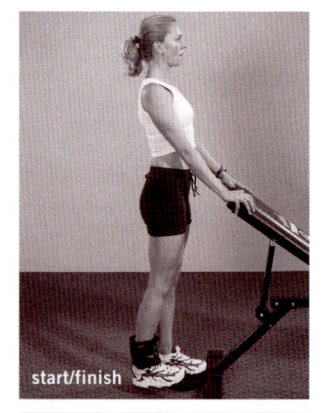

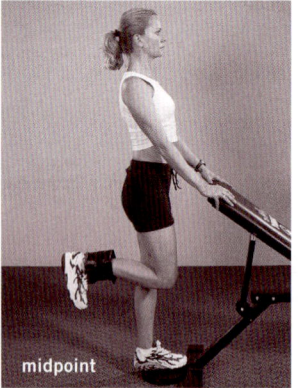

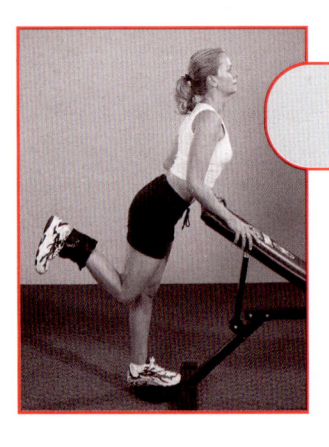

Try to avoid leaning forward and arching your back as this will place excess stress on your lower back.

LOWER BODY

straight leg dead lift

muscles working: Hamstrings (back thigh)
Lower back

The start/finish position: Approach a barbell on the floor and grasp with an over hand, shoulder width grip. With your knees bent and your head up, stand to an upright position with your feet at shoulder width. Keep your eyes focused straight ahead and the barbell resting against your thighs.

The movement: With your eyes focused straight ahead, bend forward at your hips and slowly lower the barbell towards the top lace of your shoes. Keep your back straight with your eyes focused ahead and hold for a count of one. While focusing on the muscles in the back of your legs, begin to stand upright to the start/finish position. Hold again for a count of one and repeat.

FOR ADVANCED LIFTERS ONLY

Tip Try to forget the weight in your hands and place all your mental focus on the lengthening of the hamstrings as you drop and the shortening of the hamstrings as you stand. Standing on a slightly elevated surface will allow ground clearance for the barbell plates. This exercise can also be done with a dumbell in each hand.

NOT RECOMMENDED FOR THOSE WITH LOWER BACK PROBLEMS

> **Try to avoid letting your head drop and your back round as this will place excess stress on your lower back.**

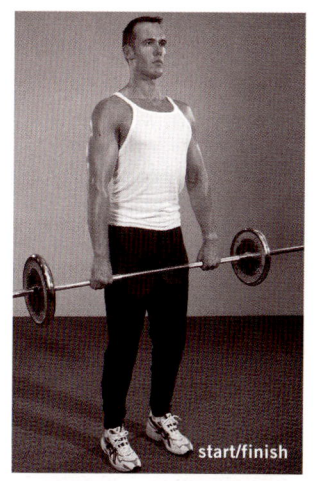

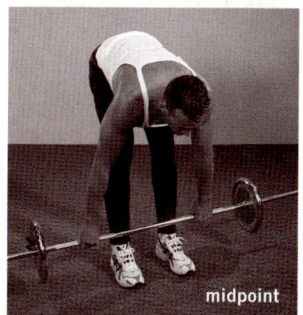

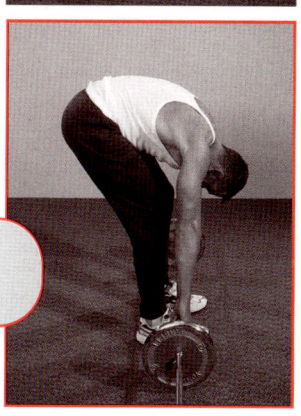

page 89

www.yorkfitness.co.uk

lower leg - gastrocnemius

s-t-r-e-t-c-h Don't forget to stretch. Every muscle you strengthen, you should also stretch. Hold this stretch for at least 10 seconds between each set. See page 264

REMEMBER keep your abdominal and lower back muscles tight through out the move and remember to exhale during the lifting phase.

Tips The weight should always be under your control and if you need to cheat, you are probably trying to lift too much weight.

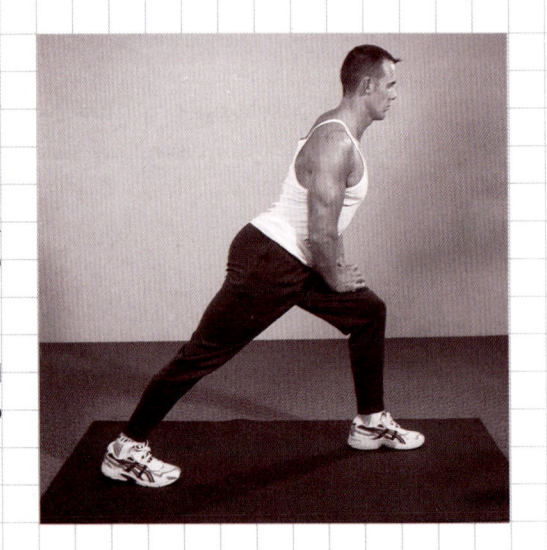

calf raise standing double leg

muscles working: Calves (lower leg)

The start/finish position: Grasp a dumbell in each hand and stand upright making sure you lift from your legs while keeping your back straight. Position your feet approximately shoulder width apart with your toes pointing straight ahead. The dumbells should be held with your palms facing your thighs in an arms fully extended position. Keep your back straight and your eyes focused straight ahead.

The movement: With your head up, start to rise up onto the balls of your feet, squeezing your calves at the top and hold for a count of one. Slowly return your heels to the start/finish position, ensuring a full stretch but being careful not to allow your heels to touch the floor. Hold again for a count of one and repeat.

Tip Try to keep your toes pointing straight ahead and avoid rolling towards your little toe.

> **Try to avoid any movement in the knee joint and avoid arching your back.**

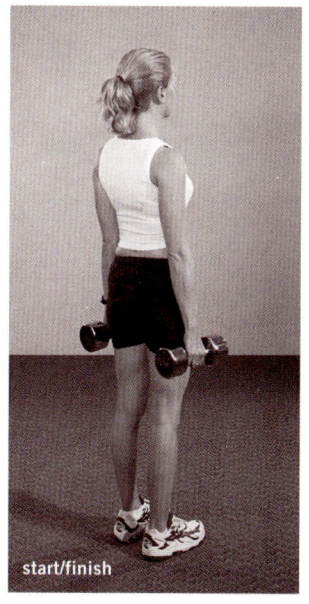

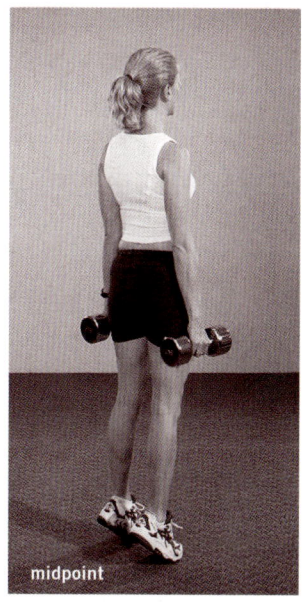

calf raise seated single leg

muscles working: Calves (lower leg)

The start/finish position: Take a seat on the end of a flat bench with a dumbell resting on end on your right knee. Position your right foot on a weight plate approximately one inch thick with your toes pointing straight ahead. The dumbell should be held with both hands while you keep your back straight and your eyes focused straight ahead.

The movement: With your head up, start to rise up onto the ball of your right foot, squeezing your calf muscle at the top and hold for a count of one. Slowly return your right heel to the start/finish position, ensuring a full stretch but being careful not to allow your heel to touch the floor. Hold again for a count of one and repeat.

Tip Make sure you place the dumbell right over your knee and not too far down your thigh. This exercise can also be done both calves at once.

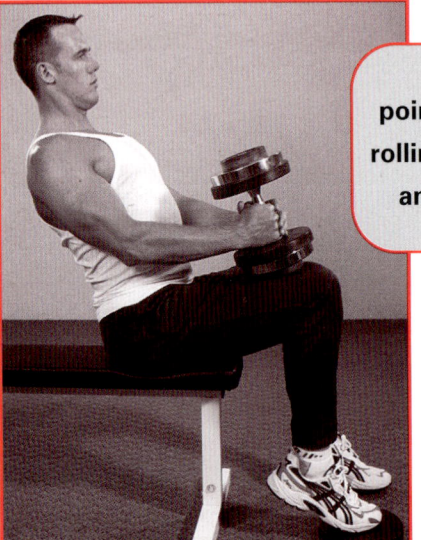

Try to keep your toes pointing straight ahead without rolling out towards your little toe and avoid arching your back.

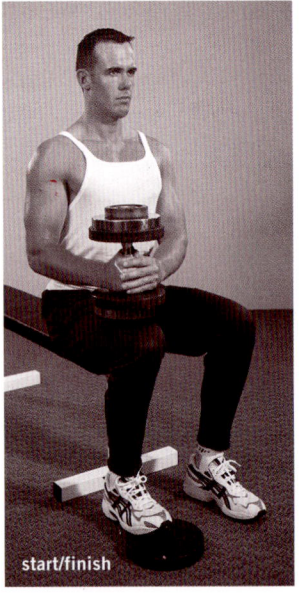

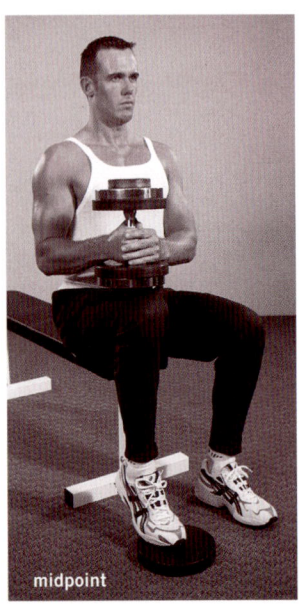

start/finish

midpoint

calf raise standing single leg

muscles working: Calves (lower leg)

The start/finish position: Grasp a dumbell in your right hand and stand upright on your right leg whilst supporting yourself against something vertical with your left hand. Tuck your left toe in behind your right calf. Position your right foot on a weight plate approximately one inch thick with your toes pointing straight ahead. The dumbell should be held with your palm facing your thigh in an arms fully extended position. Keep your back straight and your eyes focused straight ahead.

The movement: With your head up, start to rise up onto the ball of your right foot, squeezing your calf muscle at the top and hold for a count of one. Slowly return your right heel to the start/finish position, ensuring a full stretch but being careful not to allow your heel to touch the floor. Hold again for a count of one and repeat.

Tip Try to avoid any movement in the knee joint and avoid arching your back.

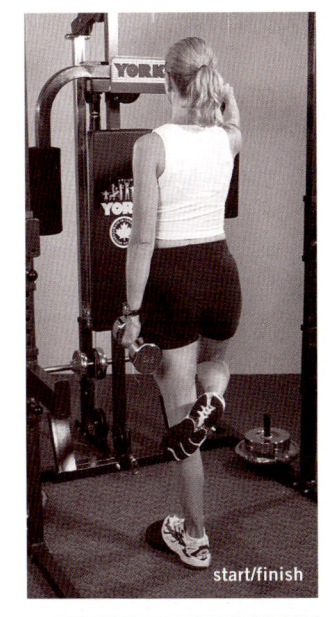

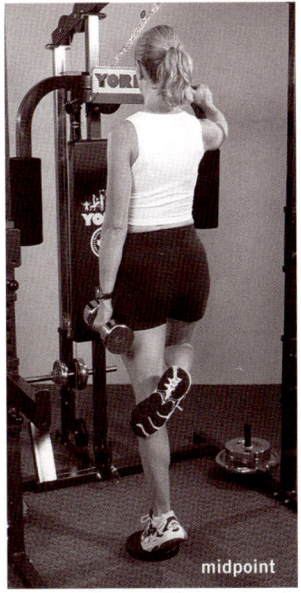

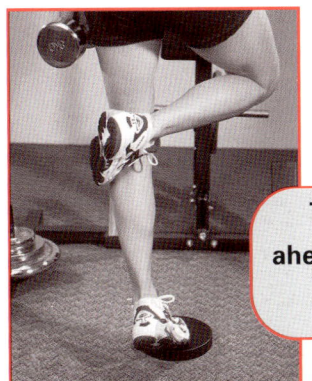

Try to keep your toes pointing straight ahead without rolling out towards your little toe and avoid arching your back.

horizontal press bar calf raise

muscles working: Calves (lower leg)

The start/finish position: Position yourself beneath the press bar in squat stance position with the weight resting across your shoulders. With your back straight and your head up, bring yourself to an upright standing position. Place your feet approximately shoulder width apart with the balls of your feet on a weight plate approximately 1 inch thick and your toes pointing straight ahead and your heels directly below the press bar. Grasp the machine anywhere that is comfortable and keep your back straight and your eyes focused straight ahead.

The movement: With your head up, start to rise up onto the balls of your feet without bending at your hips or your knees and squeeze your calves at the top and hold for a count of one. Slowly return your heels to the start/finish position, ensuring a full stretch but being careful not to allow your heels to touch the floor. Hold again for a count of one and repeat.

Tip Try to keep your toes pointing straight ahead and avoid rolling towards your little toe. Try to avoid any movement in the knee joint.

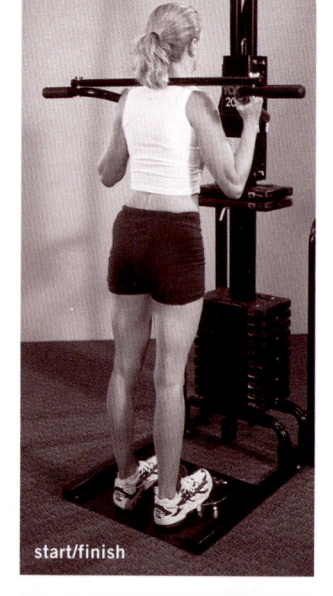

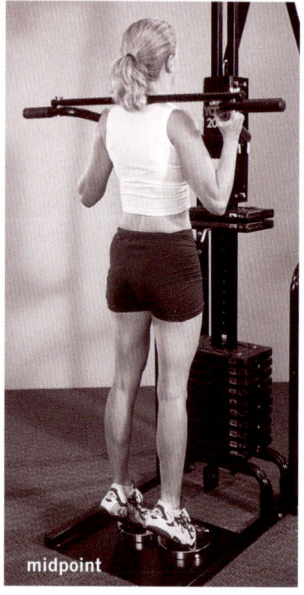

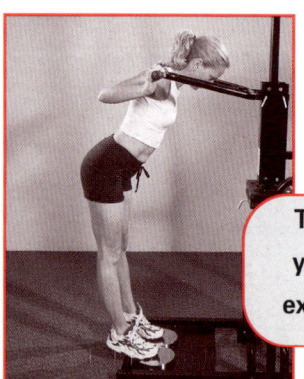

Try not to let your head drop or your back arch as this will place excess stress on your lower back.

CHAPTER EIGHT upper body

upper back - trapezius

back - latissimus dorsi

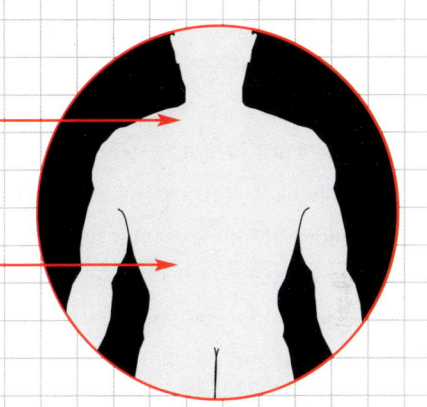

s-t-r-e-t-c-h Don't forget to stretch. Every muscle you strengthen, you should also stretch. Hold these stretches for at least 10 seconds between each set. See pages 256, 265

REMEMBER Keep your abdominal and lower back muscles tight through out the movement and remember to exhale during the lifting phase.

Tips A thumbs over grip (thumbs the same side as your fingers) will decrease the tendency to pull with the biceps and forearms and instead place more emphasis on the larger back muscles. Try to visualise your hands being 'welded' to the bar and instead of pulling with your arms, focus more on pushing down or back with your elbows to place more emphasis on the larger back muscles. The weight should always be under your control and if you need to cheat, you are probably trying to lift too much weight.

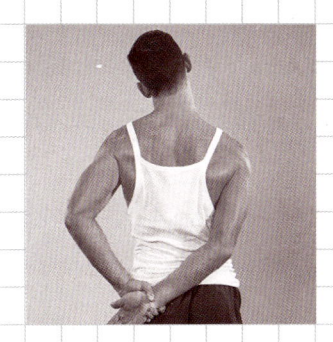

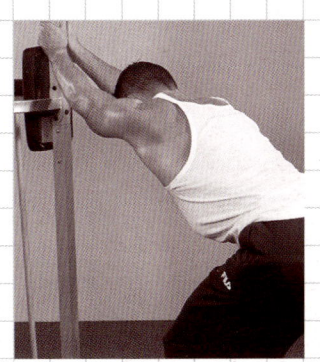

single arm dumbell row

muscles working: Latissimus dorsi (sides of upper back)
Bicep (front arm)

The start/finish position: Approach a flat free weight bench and place your left knee on the bench and your right foot flat on the floor. Lean forward to place your left hand on the bench to create a good triangle shaped base e.g. left knee, right foot and left hand. This combination should ensure your back is almost parallel to the floor. Reach down to pick up your dumbell in your right hand and hold it with a straight arm a few inches off the floor to keep your shoulders square and parallel. Keep your eyes up and look straight ahead, not down on the floor. Start and finish in an arms fully extended position, not allowing the dumbell to touch the floor.

The movement: Pull the dumbell towards your body squeezing your elbow back as far as it can go without twisting your upper body. The dumbell should finish almost in line with your navel. Remember to keep your elbows tight by your side and hold the midpoint position for a count of one, then slowly control the dumbell back to the start/finish position. Hold again for a count of one and repeat. At the completion of your desired number of repetitions, place the dumbell on the floor, swap sides and repeat for the left arm.

Tip: Be sure to pull your shoulders back and push your chest out at the midpoint of the movement

Try not to bend or round the lower back as you pull the dumbell in.

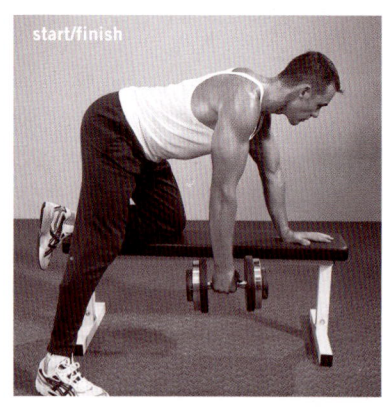

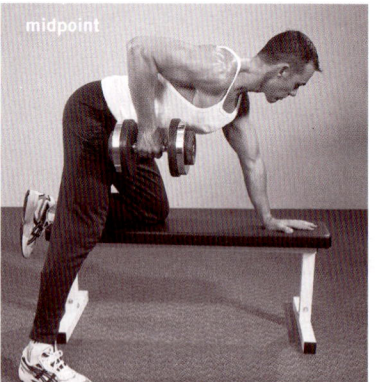

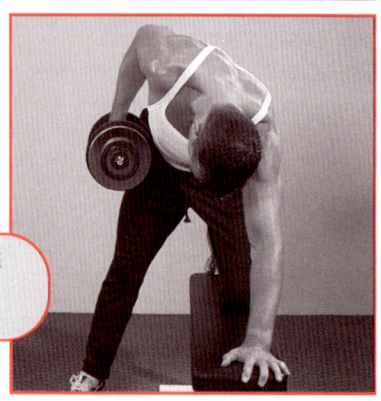

pull down underhand close grip

muscles working: Latissimus dorsi (sides of upper back)

Bicep (front arm)

The start/finish position: Approach the pulldown station facing the machine and grasp the pulldown bar with a shoulder width, underhand grip (palms facing toward you). Drop down onto the seat and slide your thighs under the kneepads (if applicable) ensuring a snug fit. Start and finish in an arms fully extended position.

The movement: Keeping your head up and your eyes focused straight ahead, pull the bar down to your upper chest, keeping your elbows close by your side and your chest high. Hold the midpoint position for a count of one, and then slowly control the bar back to the start/finish position. Hold again for a count of one and repeat.

Tip Remember to pull the bar down all the way to your upper chest to maximize the benefit of the exercise.

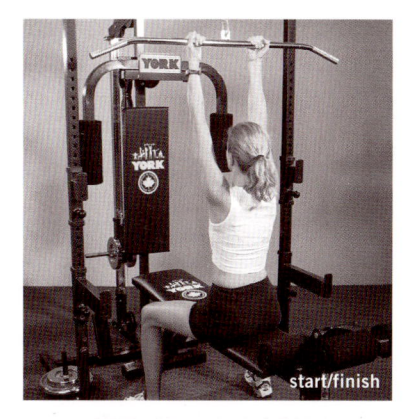

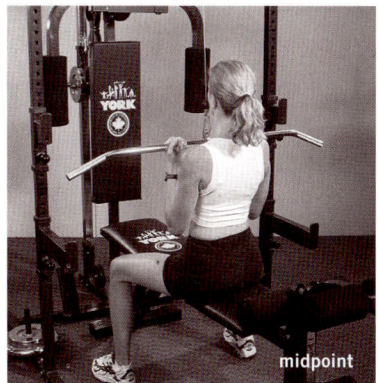

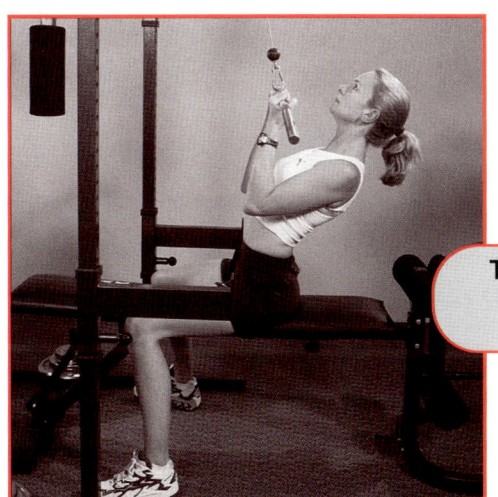

Try to avoid leaning back excessively or swinging with momentum.

pull down overhand wide grip

muscles working: Latissimus dorsi (sides of upper back)

Bicep (front arm)

The start/finish position: Approach the pull down station facing the machine and grasp the pull down bar with a slightly wider than shoulder width grip, palms facing away. Drop down onto the seat and slide your thighs under the kneepads (where applicable) ensuring a snug fit. Start and finish in an arms-fully extended position.

The movement: Keeping your head up and your eyes focused on the top pulley, pull the bar down to your collarbone, keeping your elbows below the bar at all times. Hold the midpoint position for a count of one, and then slowly control the bar back to the start/finish position. Hold again for a count of one and repeat.

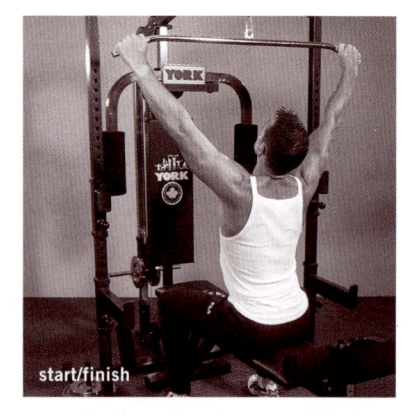

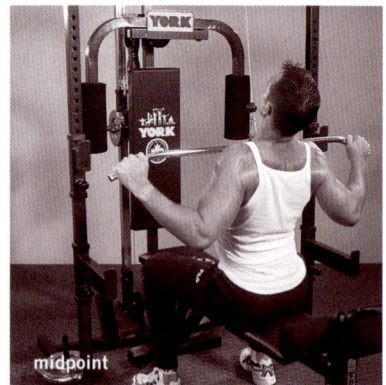

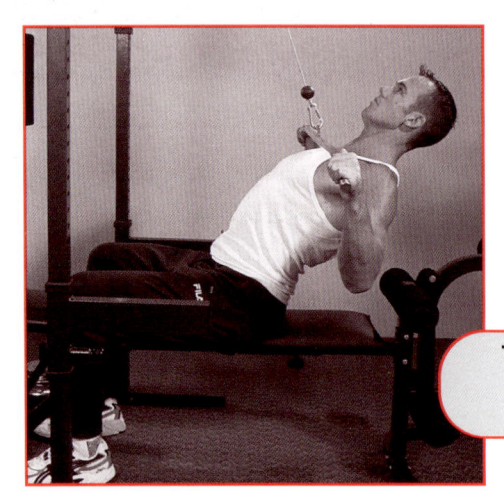

Tip Try not to pull the bar down too far past your collarbone to your sternum. The bar only needs to travel to your collarbone.

Try to avoid any excessive lean back or swinging with momentum

low cable seated row

muscles working: Latissimus dorsi (sides of upper back)
Bicep (front arm)

The start/finish position: Sit on the floor facing the low pulley station with your feet braced firmly against the machine. Grasp the low row bar (palms facing down) and slide yourself back until your legs are only slightly bent. Ensure your back is straight and your head is up. Start and finish in an arms fully extended position.

The movement: Keeping Your head up and your eyes focused straight ahead, pull the row bar into your midsection keeping your elbows tight by your side. Hold the midpoint position for a count of one, and then slowly control the bar back to the start/finish position. Hold again for a count of one and repeat.

Tip Remember to pull your shoulders back and push your chest out at the midpoint of the movement.

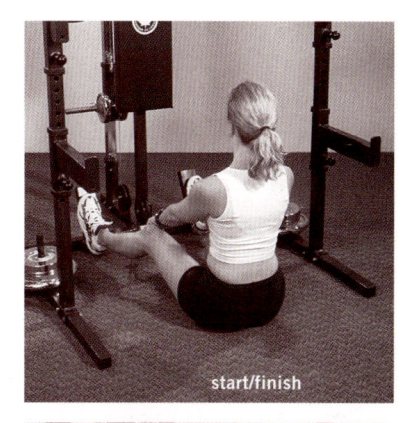

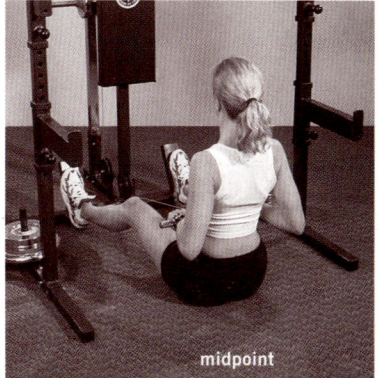

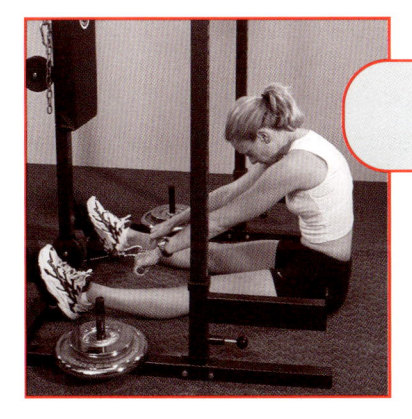

Try not to bend or round the lower back as you reach forward and be sure to keep your legs slightly bent.

dumbell pullovers

muscles working: Latissimus dorsi (sides of upper back)

The start/finish position: Use a flat free weights bench to lie your body across ensuring only your upper back makes contact with the bench and your head hangs just off the bench. Position your feet flat against the floor about shoulder width apart with your hips lower than your knees. Hold the weight with a palms flat grip at the top end of the dumbell and lift the weight overhead at arms length and hold in the start/finish position.

The movement: Keeping your hips lower than your knees, lower the dumbell in a controlled arc while keeping your elbows slightly bent. At the midpoint of the exercise (full-stretch), hold for a count of one, then follow the same arc back to the starting position. Hold again for a count of one and repeat.

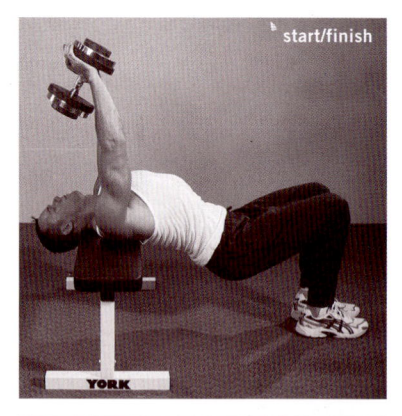

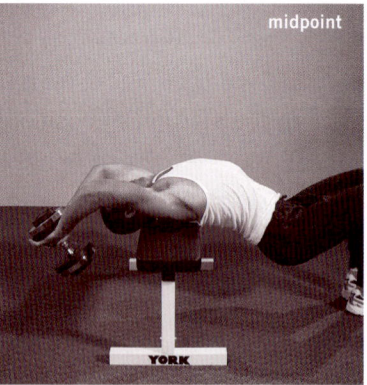

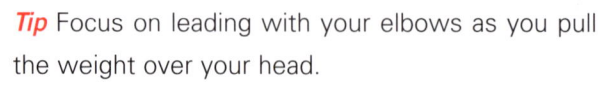

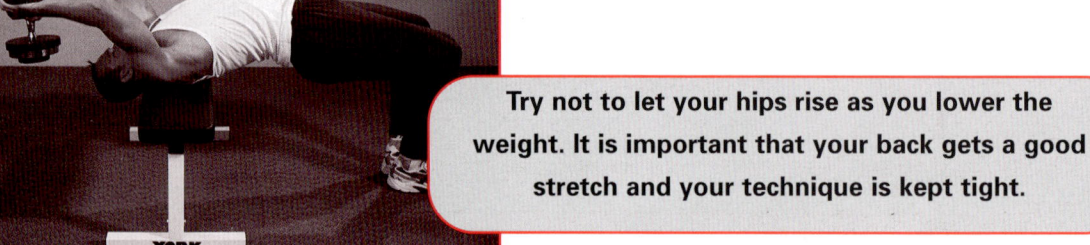

Tip Focus on leading with your elbows as you pull the weight over your head.

Try not to let your hips rise as you lower the weight. It is important that your back gets a good stretch and your technique is kept tight.

UPPER BODY

pull down straight-arm

muscles working: Latissimus dorsi (sides of upper back)

The start/finish position: Approach the pull down station and grasp the pull down bar with a slightly wider than shoulder width grip, palms facing away and arms straight. Make sure the pull down bar is just above chest level and your feet are shoulder width apart. Start and finish just above chest level with arms straight.

The movement: Keeping your lower back and abdominal muscles tight, begin to push the bar down towards the floor keeping your back straight and your eyes focused straight ahead. The bar should travel as close to your thighs as the machine will allow. Hold the midpoint position for a count of one, then slowly control the bar back to the start/finish position. Hold again for a count of one and repeat.

Tip Try to ignore what your hands are doing and place all your focus on the larger back muscles running from underneath your arms down towards your waist while forcing your arms down towards your sides.

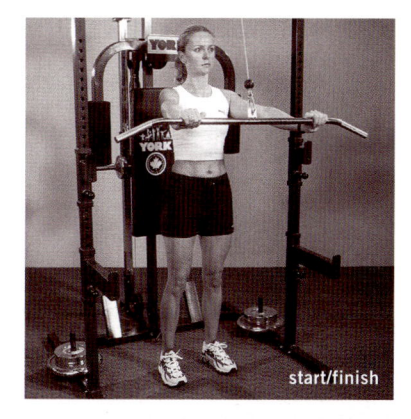

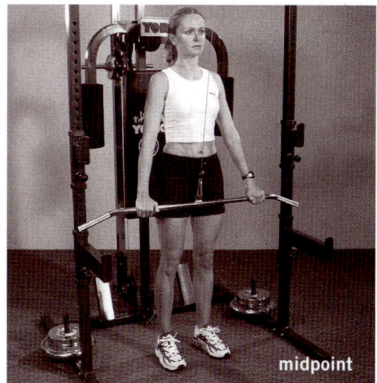

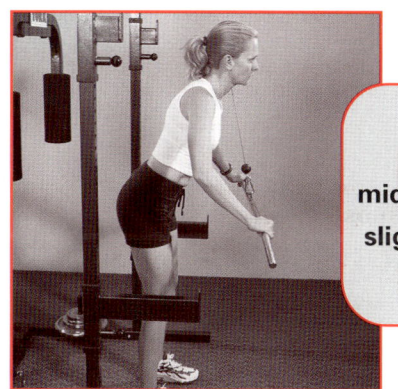

Try not to bend at the waist as you push the bar down. It is most important to keep your midsection tight at all times and to keep your knees slightly bent. This will ensure that the muscles you are trying to isolate will get the work.

page 101

chin up underhand close grip

muscles working: Latissimus dorsi (sides of upper back)

Biceps (front arm)

The start/finish position: Approach and grasp the chinning bar with a shoulder-width, underhand grip (palms facing toward you). Allow your arms to take your body weight as you lift your feet off the floor and cross your ankles. Start and finish in an arms fully extended position.

The movement: With your head up and your eyes focused on where you are going, slowly pull your body towards the chinning bar. To complete one full repetition your chin should reach above the height of the bar, hold for a count of one then slowly control your body back to the start/finish position. Hold again for a count of one and repeat.

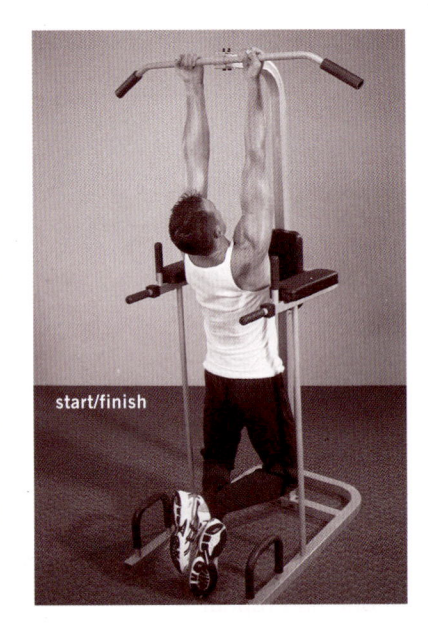

FOR ADVANCED LIFTERS ONLY

Tip Try to pull your body weight up with a slow controlled movement to avoid any body swing that will come with untidy technique.

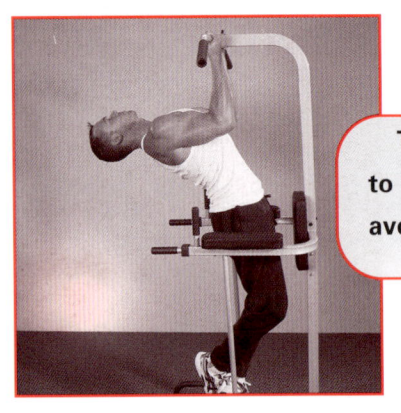

Try not to allow your legs to 'kick out' during the lift and avoid any excessive lean back.

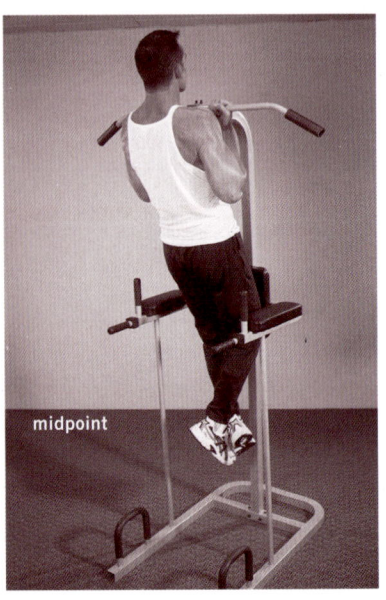

chin up overhand wide grip

muscles working: Latissimus dorsi (sides of upper back)
Biceps (front arm)

The start/finish position: Approach the chinning bar and grasp the bar with a slightly wider than shoulder width, overhand grip (palms facing away from you). Allow your arms to take your body weight as you lift your feet off the floor and cross your ankles. Start and finish in an arms fully extended position.

The movement: With your head up and your eyes focused on where you are going, slowly pull your body towards the chinning bar. To complete one full repetition your chin should reach above the height of the bar, hold for a count of one then slowly control your body back to the start/ finish position. Hold again for a count of one and repeat.

FOR ADVANCED LIFTERS ONLY

Tip Try to pull your body weight up with a slow controlled movement to avoid any body swing that will come with untidy technique..

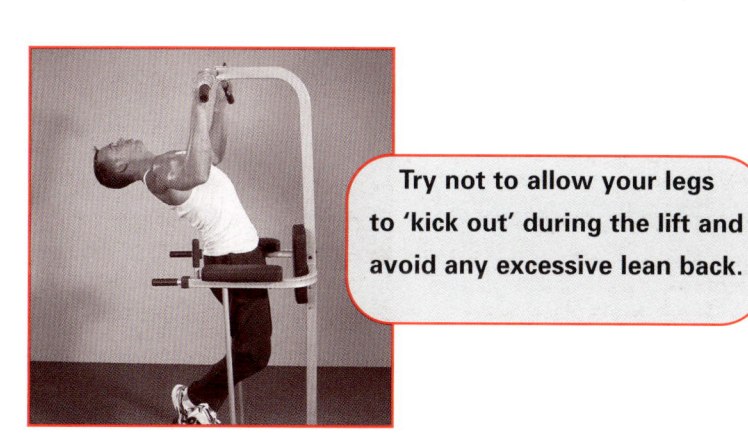

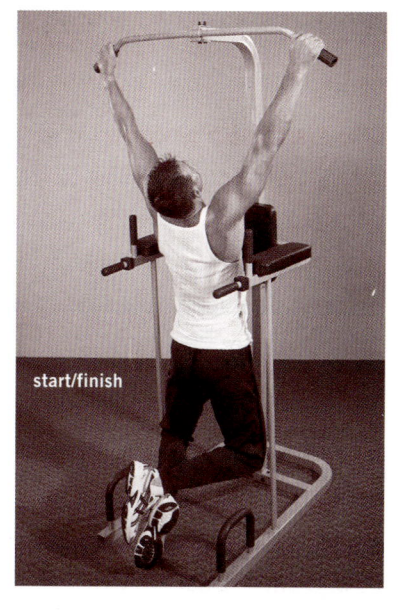

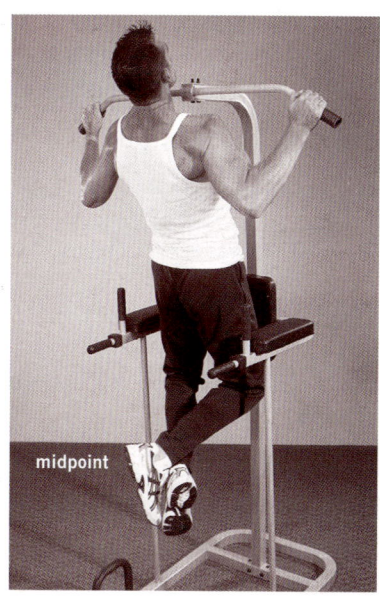

Try not to allow your legs to 'kick out' during the lift and avoid any excessive lean back.

low cable bent over row

muscles working: Latissimus dorsi (sides of upper back)
Bicep (front arm)

The start/finish position: Approach the low cable with the pull down bar already attached. Grasp the pull down bar at arms length with a wider than shoulder width, overhand grip (palms facing you) and your feet positioned at shoulder width. Stand up to a bent over position bending at the waist until your upper body is almost parallel with the floor and slightly bend your knees. Keep your eyes up and look straight ahead, not down on the floor. Start and finish in an arms fully extended position, keeping the cable tension tight and not allowing the weight stack to rest.

The movement: Pull the bar towards your body, keeping your back straight and without swinging your torso. The bar should touch your belly button as you squeeze your elbows back as far as they can go. Hold the midpoint position for a count of one, then slowly control the bar back to the start/ finish position. Hold again for a count of one and repeat.

FOR ADVANCED LIFTERS ONLY

Tip Be sure to pull your shoulders back and push your chest out at the midpoint of the movement.

NOT RECOMMENDED FOR THOSE WITH LOWER BACK PROBLEMS

> **Try not to bend or round the lower back as you pull the bar in.**

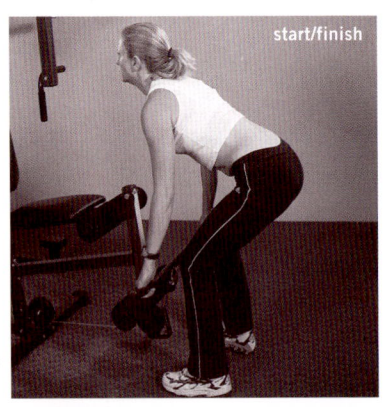

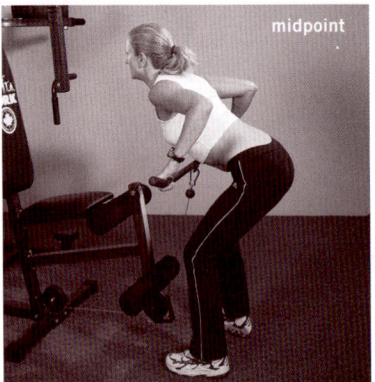

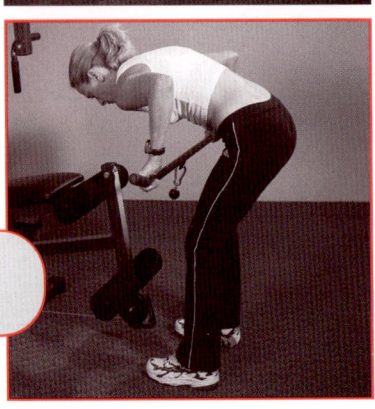

bent over barbell row

muscles working: Latissimus dorsi (sides of upper back)

Bicep (front arm)

The start/finish position: Stand with feet positioned at shoulder width apart holding a barbell at arms length with a wider than shoulder width, overhand grip (palms facing you). Bend over at the waist until your upper body is almost parallel with the floor and slightly bend your knees. Keep your eyes up and look straight ahead. Start and finish in an arms fully extended position, not allowing the barbell to touch the floor.

The movement: Pull the barbell towards your body, keeping your back straight and without swinging your torso. The barbell should touch your navel as you squeeze your elbows back as far as they can go. Hold the midpoint position for a count of one then slowly control the barbell back to the start/finish position. Hold again for a count of one and repeat.

FOR ADVANCED LIFTERS ONLY

Tip Be sure to pull your shoulders back and push your chest out at the midpoint of the movement.

NOT RECOMMENDED FOR THOSE WITH LOWER BACK PROBLEMS

Try not to bend or round the lower back as you pull the barbell in.

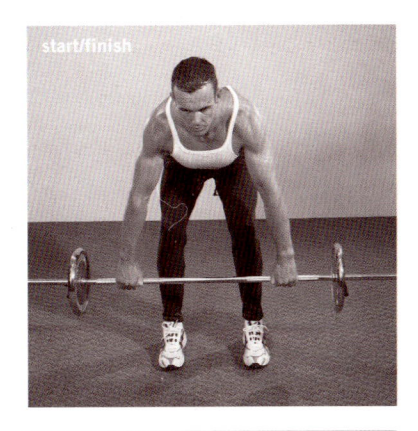

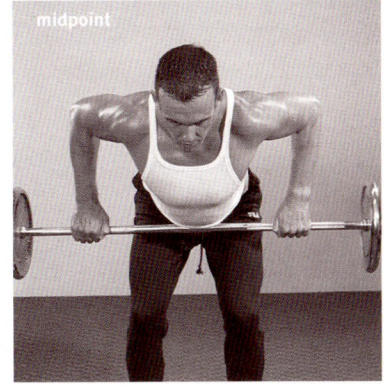

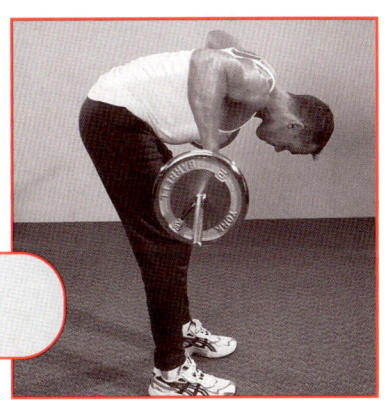

low cable long bar seated row

muscles working: Latissimus dorsi (sides of upper back)
Bicep (front arm)

The start/finish position: Take a seat on the floor facing the low pulley station with the long pull down bar already attached and your feet braced firmly against the machine. Grasp the long bar (palms facing down) at a wider than shoulder width grip and slide yourself back until your legs are only slightly bent. Ensure your back is straight and your head is up. Start and finish in an arms fully extended position.

The movement: Keeping your head up and your eyes focused straight ahead, pull the long bar into your midsection keeping your elbows directly behind your hands. Hold the midpoint position for a count of one, then slowly control the bar back to the start/finish position. Hold again for a count of one and repeat.

FOR ADVANCED LIFTERS ONLY

Tip Remember to pull your shoulders back and push your chest out at the midpoint of the movement.

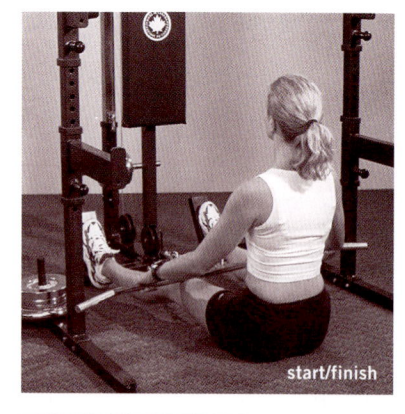

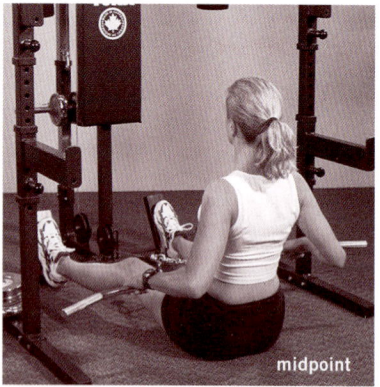

> **Try not to lean back too far at the midpoint.**

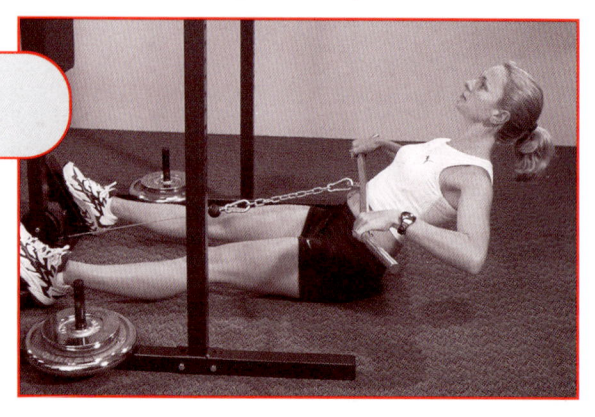

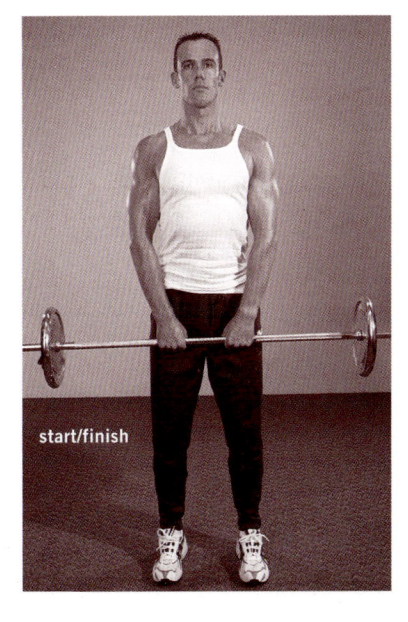

barbell upright row

muscles working: Trapezius (upper back)

Deltoids (shoulders)

Bicep (front arm)

The start/finish position: Grasp the barbell with an overhand grip (palms facing you) and about a 1 to 2 hand space gap between your hands. Stand upright with your feet shoulder width apart and your knees slightly bent. Your arms should be straight with the bar resting at the top of your thighs. Keep your eyes up and look straight ahead. Start and finish in an arms fully extended position.

The movement: Pull the bar up to the midpoint position just below your chin by bending your elbows and using the larger muscles of the upper back and neck area. The bar should almost touch your chin as you squeeze your elbows and shoulders up as high as they can go. Hold the midpoint position for a count of one, then slowly control the bar back to the start/finish position. Hold again for a count of one and repeat.

Tip Your elbows should always be the highest point in the movement.

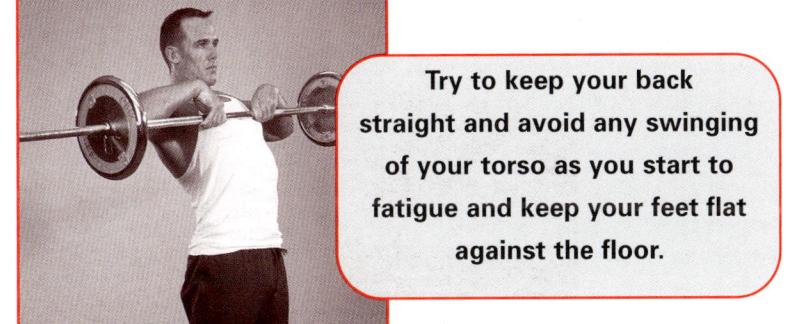

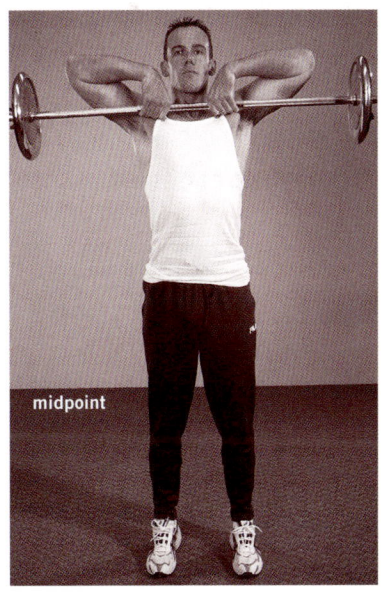

Try to keep your back straight and avoid any swinging of your torso as you start to fatigue and keep your feet flat against the floor.

dumbell upright row

muscles working: Trapezius (upper back)

                                    Deltoids (shoulders)

                                    Bicep (front arm)

The start/finish position: Grasp one dumbell in each hand and allow them to touch end to end with an overhand grip (palms facing you). Stand upright with your feet about shoulder width apart and your knees slightly bent. Your arms should be straight with the dumbells resting on the top of your thighs. Keep your head up and look straight ahead. Start and finish in an arms fully extended position.

The movement: Pull the dumbells up to the midpoint position, just below your chin, by bending at the elbows and using the larger muscles of the upper back and neck area. The dumbells should just separate as you reach the midpoint while you squeeze your elbows and shoulders up as high as they can go. Hold the midpoint position for a count of one, then slowly control the dumbells back to the start/finish position. Hold again for a count of one and repeat.

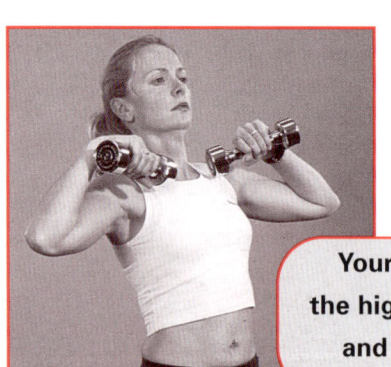

Tip Try to keep your back straight and avoid any swinging of your torso as you start to fatigue and keep your feet flat against the floor.

Your elbows should always be the highest point in the movement and try to avoid leaning back.

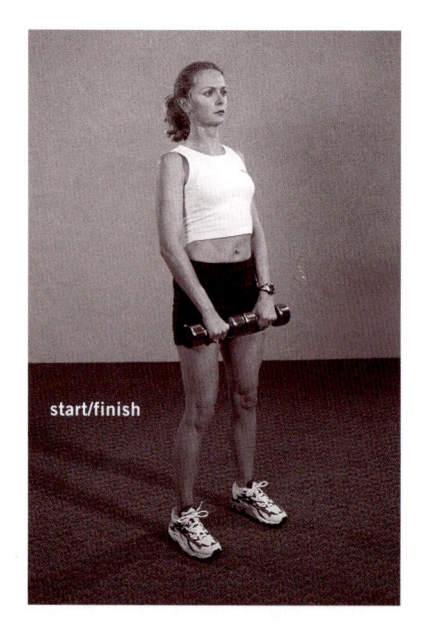

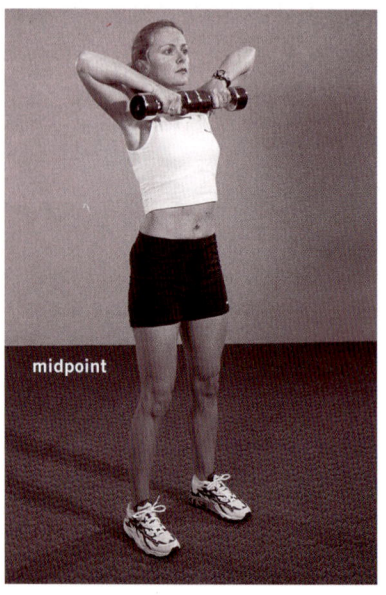

page 108

low cable upright row

muscles working: **Trapezius (upper back)**
                               Deltoids (shoulders)
                               Bicep (front arm)

The start/finish position: Grasp the bar with an overhand grip (palms facing you) with about a 1 to 2 hand space gap between your hands. Stand upright with your feet shoulder width apart and your knees slightly bent. Your arms should be straight with the bar resting on the top of your thighs. Keep your eyes up and look straight ahead. Start and finish in an arms fully extended position.

The movement: Pull the bar up to the midpoint position just below your chin by bending at the elbows and using the larger muscles of the upper back and neck area. The bar should almost touch your chin as you squeeze your elbows and shoulders up as high as they can go. Hold the midpoint position for a count of one, then slowly control the bar back to the start/finish position.Hold again for a count of one and repeat.

Tip Try to keep your back straight and avoid any swinging of your torso as you start to fatigue and keep your feet flat against the floor.

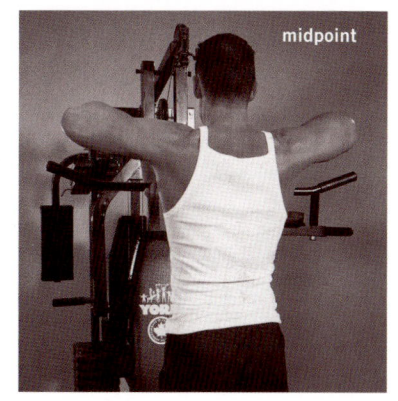

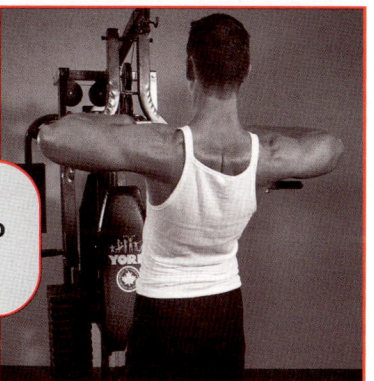

> **Your elbows should always be the highest point in the movement and try to avoid leaning back.**

dumbell shrugs

muscles working: Trapezius (upper back)

The start/finish position: Hold one dumbell in each hand as you stand upright with your feet about shoulder width apart and your knees slightly bent. Your arms should be straight with your palms facing in towards your thighs. Keep your eyes up and look straight ahead. Start and finish in an arms fully extended position.

The movement: Raise the dumbells up by keeping your arms straight and lifting with a 'shrugging' action of the upper back and neck area. Hold the midpoint position for a count of one, then slowly control the dumbells back to the start/finish position. Hold again for a count of one and repeat.

Tip As you elevate the dumbells toward the midpoint, imagine you are trying to touch your ears with your shoulders as your hands stay welded to the bars and your arms remain straight.

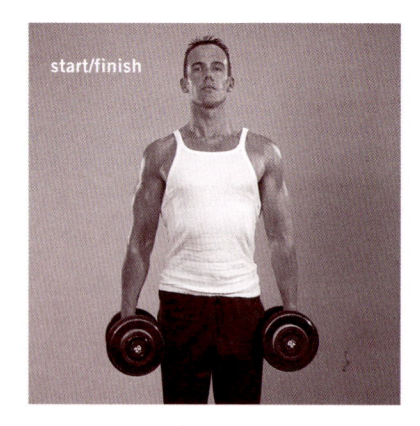

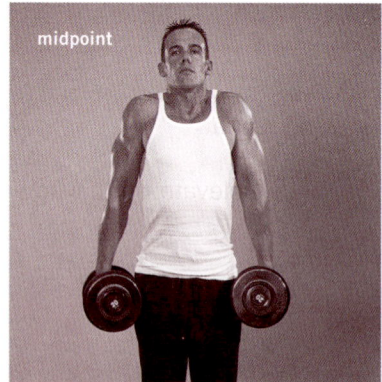

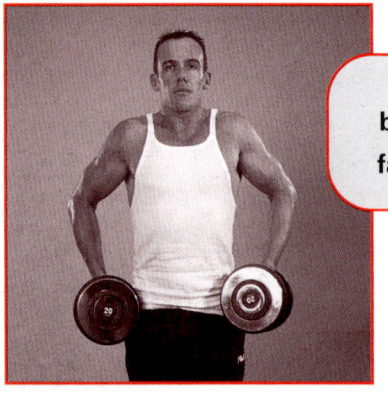

Try to keep your back straight and avoid bending your arms at the elbow as you start to fatigue and keep your feet flat against the floor.

low cable shrugs

muscles working: Trapezius (upper back)

The start/finish position: Grasp the pulldown bar attached to the low cable with a slightly wider than shoulder width, overhand grip (palms facing you). Stand upright with your feet shoulder width apart and your knees slightly bent. Your arms should be straight with the bar resting on your thighs. Keep your eyes up and look straight ahead. Start and finish in an arms fully extended position.

The movement: Raise the bar up by keeping your arms straight and lifting with a 'shrugging' action of the upper back and neck area. Hold the midpoint position for a count of one, then slowly control the bar back to the start/finish position. Hold again for a count of one and repeat.

Tip As you elevate the bar toward the midpoint, imagine you are trying to touch your ears with your shoulders as your hands stay welded to the bar and your arms remain straight.

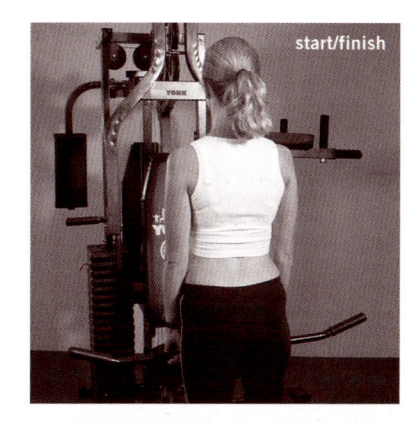

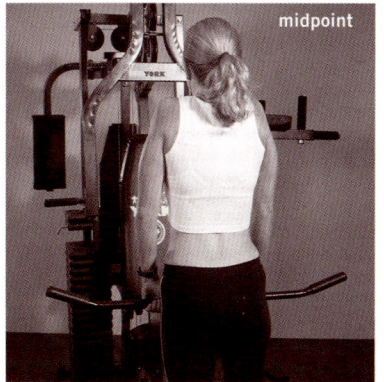

Try to keep your back straight and avoid bending your arms at the elbow as you start to fatigue and keep your feet flat against the floor.

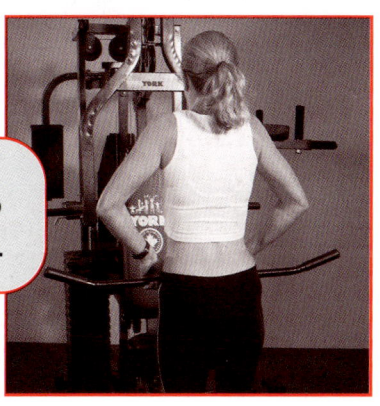

barbell shrugs

muscles working: Trapezius (upper back)

The start/finish position: Grasp the barbell with a slightly wider than shoulder width, overhand grip (palms facing you). Stand upright with your feet shoulder width apart and your knees slightly bent. Your arms should be straight with the bar resting on your thighs. Keep your eyes up and look straight ahead. Start and finish in an arms fully extended position.

The movement: Raise the bar up by keeping your arms straight and lifting with a 'shrugging' action of the upper back and neck area. Hold the midpoint position for a count of one, then slowly control the bar back to the start/finish position. Hold again for a count of one and repeat.

Tip As you elevate the bar toward the midpoint, imagine you are trying to touch your ears with your shoulders as your hands stay welded to the bar and your arms remain straight.

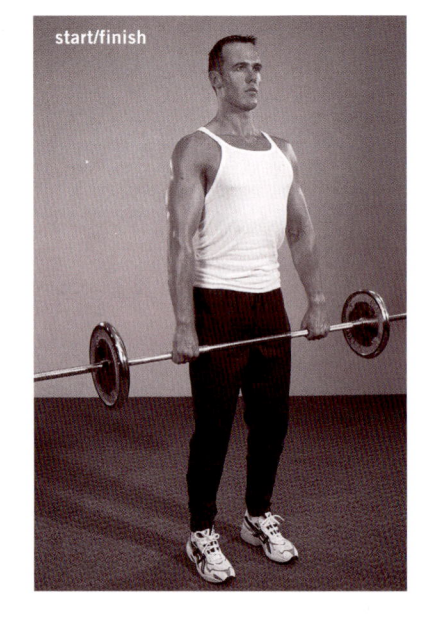

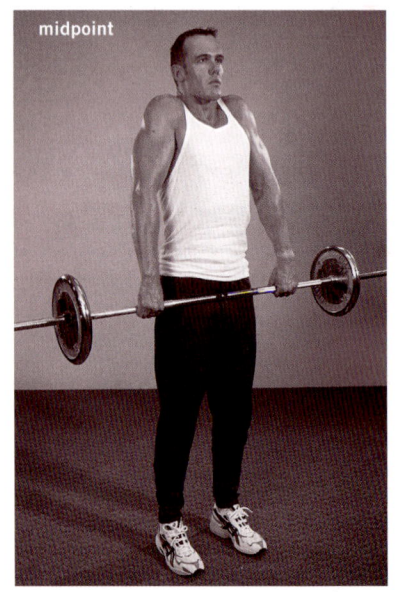

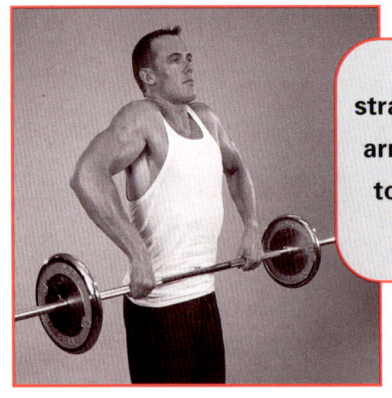

Try to keep your back straight and avoid bending your arms at the elbow as you start to fatigue and keep your feet flat against the floor.

horizontal press bar shrugs

muscles working: Trapezius (upper back)

The start/finish position: Approach the horizontal press bar of the machine weight stack. Grasp the handles with an overhand grip (palms facing you). Stand upright with your feet shoulder width apart and your knees slightly bent. Your arms should be straight with the handles as close to your thighs as possible. Keep your eyes up and look straight ahead. Start and finish in an arms fully extended position.

The movement: Raise the press bar up by keeping your arms straight and lifting with a 'shrugging' action of the upper back and neck area. Hold the midpoint position for a count of one, then slowly control the press bar back to the start/finish position. Hold again for a count of one and repeat.

Tip As you elevate the press bar toward the midpoint, imagine you are trying to touch your ears with your shoulders as your hands stay welded to the handles and your arms remain straight.

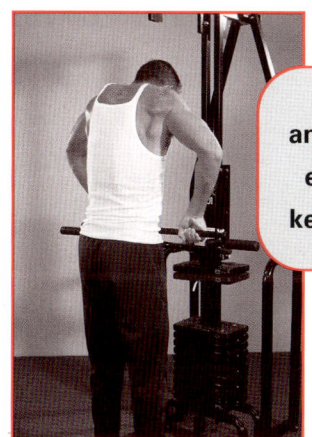

Try to keep your back straight and avoid bending your arms at the elbow as you start to fatigue and keep your feet flat against the floor.

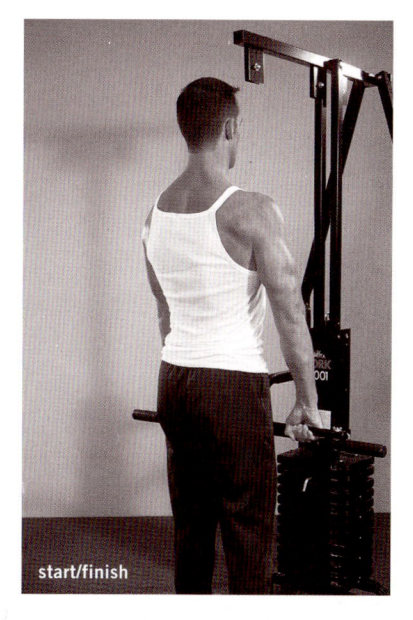

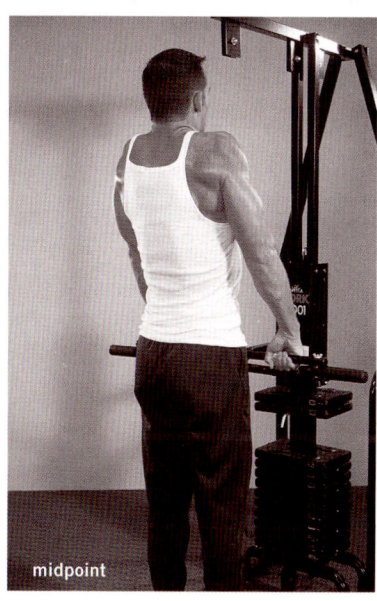

www.yorkfitness.co.uk

chest pectorals

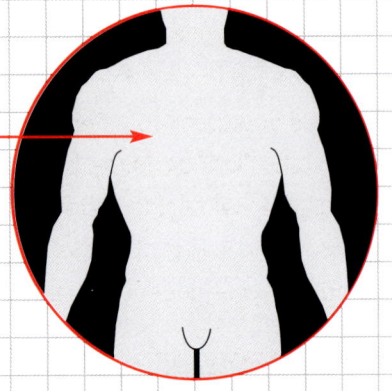

s-t-r-e-t-c-h Don't forget to stretch. Every muscle you strengthen, you should also stretch. Hold this stretch for at least 10 seconds between each set. See page 259

REMEMBER Keep your abdominal and lower back muscles tight through out the movement and remember to exhale during the lifting phase.

Tips The weight should always be under your control and if you need to cheat, you are probably lifting too much weight.

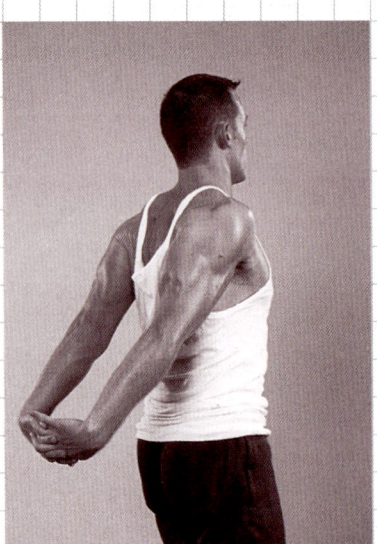

UPPER BODY

barbell bench press

muscles working: Pectorals (front of chest)

Deltoids (front shoulder)

Triceps (back arm)

The start/finish position: Lie on the flat bench with the barbell positioned in line with your eyes. Position your feet anywhere that enables your back to have full-time contact with the bench, either flat on the floor or on the bench at a comfortable angle. Grasp the bar slightly wider than shoulder width with an overhand grip and press the bar out of the racks to a held position right over the middle of your chest with your arms straight.

The movement: With your eyes fixed on a spot directly above you on the ceiling, slowly lower the bar to just touch your chest at about the nipple line. Hold for a count of one then press the weight back to the start/finish position. Hold again for a count of one and repeat.

Tip As the weight you are lifting increases, try to have someone assist you as a 'spotter' just in case you get into trouble.

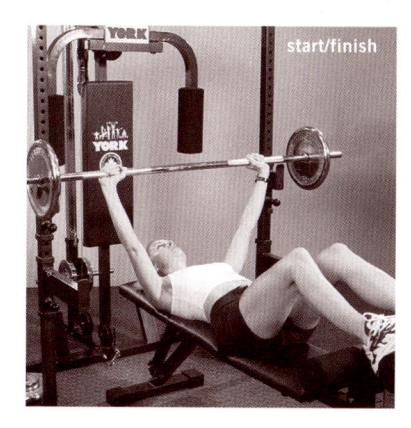

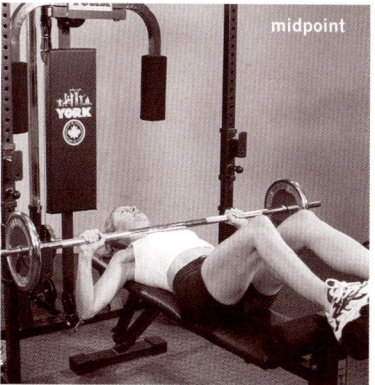

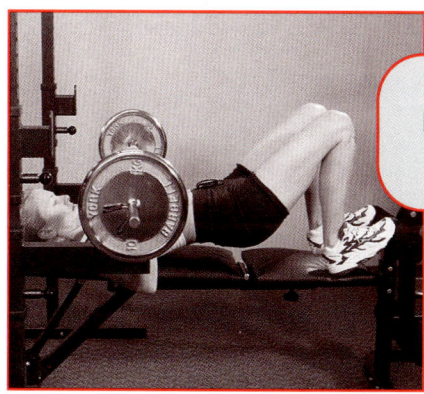

> Try to avoid lifting your buttocks and lower back off the bench as you press and don't allow the barbell to bounce off your chest.

page 115

dumbell bench press

muscles working: Pectorals (front of chest)

Deltoids (front shoulder)

Triceps (back arm)

The start/finish position: Lie on the flat bench with a dumbbell in each hand. Bring the dumbells end to end directly above your shoulders with straight arms and your elbows pointing out to the sides. Position your feet anywhere that enables your back to have permanent contact with the bench, either flat on the floor or flat on the bench.

The movement: With your eyes fixed on a spot on the ceiling, slowly lower the dumbells to just above your shoulders. Pause for a count of one then press the dumbells back to the start/finish position. Hold again for a count of one and repeat.

Tip Your elbows should at all times stay directly beneath your wrists.

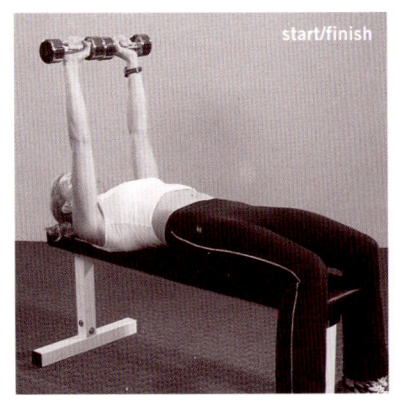

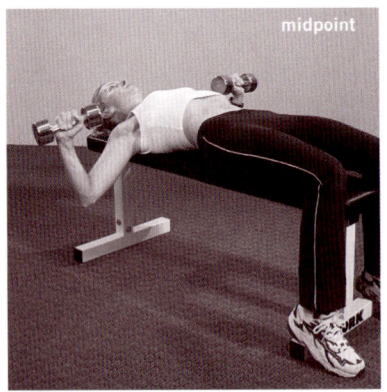

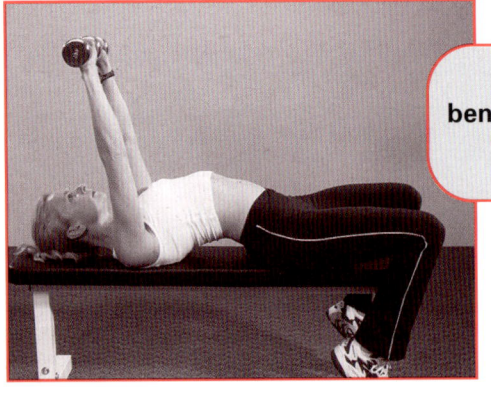

Try to avoid lifting your hips off the bench as you press and try to keep control of the dumbells as they travel.

vertical machine bench press

muscles working: **Pectorals (front of chest)**

                                            Deltoids (front shoulder)

                                            Triceps (back arm)

The start/finish position: Sit on the vertical bench press machine with the handles positioned across the middle of your chest and your head supported against the bench. Position your feet flat against the floor with your lower back hard against the machine. Grasp the handles with an overhand grip and find a focal point across the room.

The movement: Keeping your lower back straight and your hips and shoulders against the seat, press the handles forward away from you until your arms are fully extended and hold for a count of one. Slowly lower the weight back to the start/finish position being careful not to let the weight stack touch down, this will decrease the intensity and increase the chance of injury. Hold again for a count of one and repeat.

Tip If you use the vertical handgrip on the press bars, you will bring more tricep (back arm) into your routine by keeping your elbows by your side.

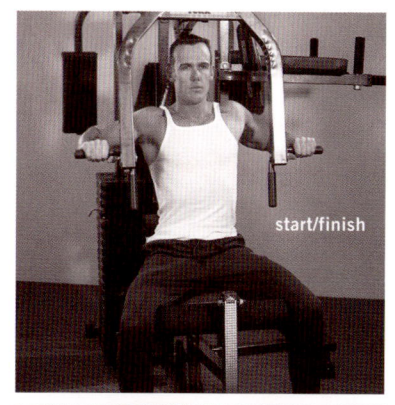

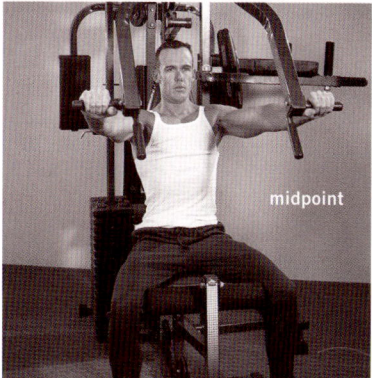

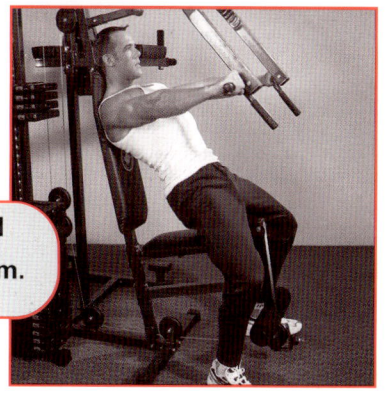

> **Try to avoid lifting your hips off the bench as you press and don't allow the weights to either bounce or rest at the bottom.**

incline barbell bench press

muscles working: **Pectorals (front of chest)**

                                  Deltoids (front shoulder)

                                  Triceps (back arm)

The start/finish position: Lie on the bench set at approximately 30 – 45 degrees incline with the barbell positioned in front of your eyes. Position your feet flat on the floor and your lower back hard against the bench. Grasp the bar slightly wider than shoulder width with an overhand grip and press the bar out of the racks to a held position right over the upper portion of your chest.

The movement: With your eyes fixed on a spot on the ceiling, slowly lower the bar down to just touch your chest somewhere close to your collarbone. Pause for a count of one then press the weight back to the start/finish position Hold again for a count of one and repeat.

Tip As the weight you are lifting increases, try to have someone assist you as a 'spotter' just in case you get into trouble.

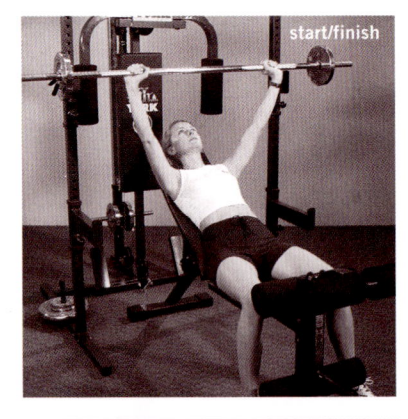

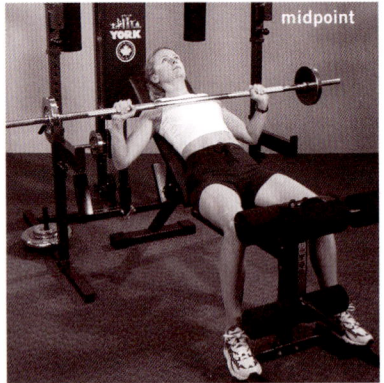

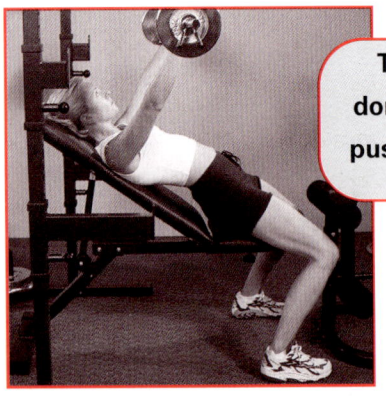

Try to avoid lifting your hips off the bench as you press and don't allow the barbell to bounce off your chest. Make sure you push the weight vertically up and not out away from your body.

incline dumbell bench press

muscles working: Pectorals (front of chest)
Deltoids (front shoulder)
Triceps (back arm)

The start/finish position: Sit on the incline bench set at approximately 30 - 45 degrees incline with a dumbell in each hand resting on your knees. Position your feet flat on the floor or resting in a comfortable position on the bench. Your lower back should be hard against the bench. Lift the dumbells to your shoulders as you lean back. The dumbells should be held in a position right over the upper portion of your chest.

The movement: With your eyes fixed on a spot on the ceiling, slowly press the dumbells away to a point above your upper chest. Hold the top position for a count of one then slowly lower the dumbbells back towards the points of your shoulders. Hold again for a count of one and repeat.

Tip As you press the weight back to the start/finish position make sure you push the dumbells vertically up and not out away from your body.

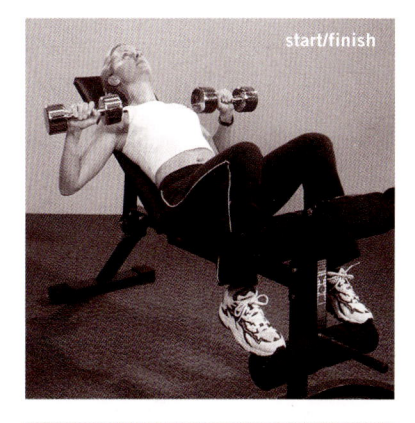

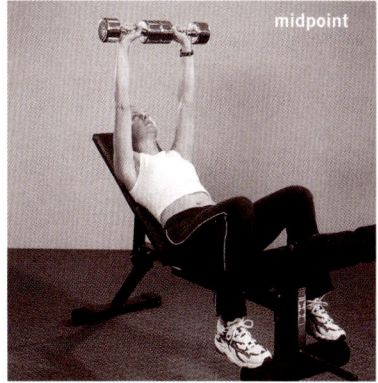

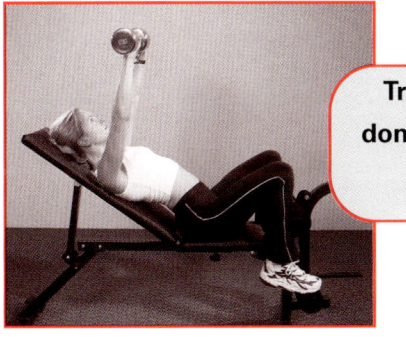

Try to avoid lifting your hips off the bench as you press and don't allow your elbows to go too deep, your elbows should at all times stay directly beneath your wrists.

lying machine bench press

muscles working: Pectorals (front of chest)

Deltoids (front shoulder)

Triceps (back arm)

The start/finish position: Lie on the flat bench press machine with the handles positioned across the middle of your chest and your head supported on the bench. Position your feet anywhere that enables your back to have permanent contact with the bench, either flat on the floor or flat on the bench. Grasp the handles with an overhand grip and find a focal point on the roof

The movement: Press the handles away from you until your arms are fully extended and hold for a count of one. Slowly lower the weight back to the start/finish position being careful not to let the weight stack touch down, this will decrease the intensity and increase the chance of injury. Hold again for a count of one and repeat.

Tip Try not to allow the weights to either bounce or rest at the bottom.

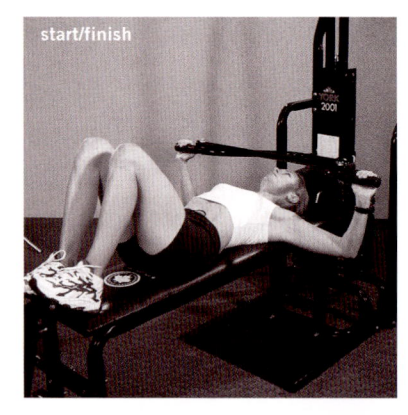

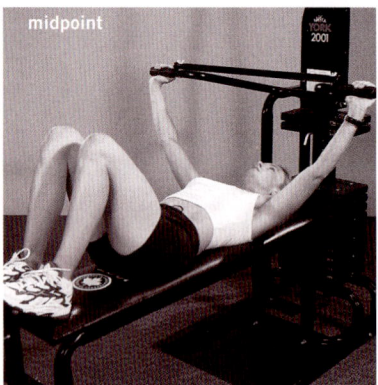

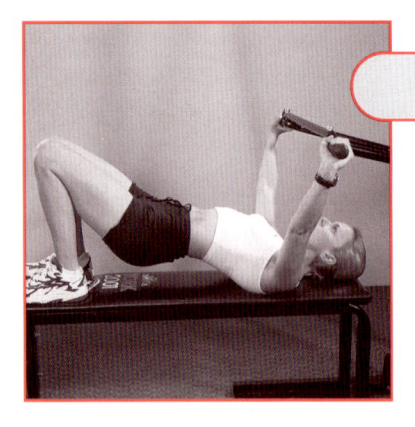

Try to avoid lifting your hips off the bench as you press.

straight arm pec deck

muscles working: Pectorals (front of chest)

The start/finish position: Sit on the pec deck seat with your back firmly against the back support. Slide both arms in behind the pec deck arm pads so that your arms are parallel with the floor and your thumbs are pointing towards the roof as you make a fist. Position your feet flat against the floor slightly wider than shoulder width.

The movement: With your eyes fixed on a spot straight ahead, slowly and smoothly draw your hands together in front in a hugging action until your knuckles and the pec deck pads touch in front of your eyes. Hold for a count of one then slowly return to the start/finish position ensuring a comfortable stretch. Hold again for a count of one and repeat.

Tip Make sure you always keep control of the weight as it travels and that you don't let the weight drop on the return.

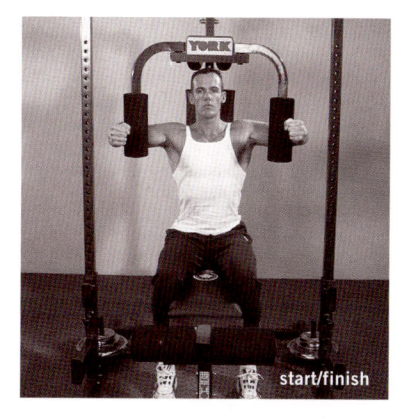

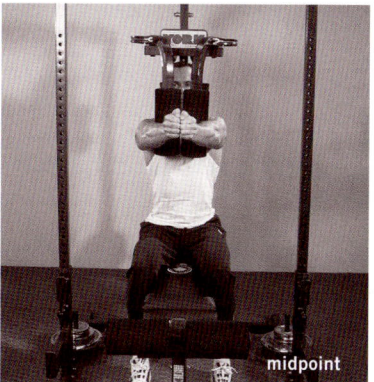

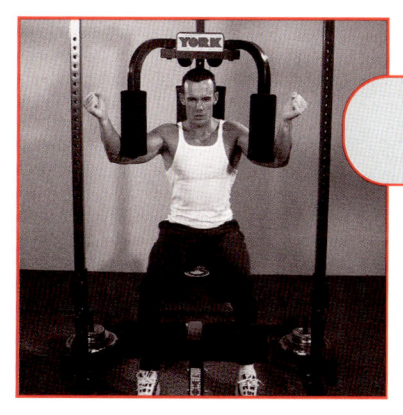

Try not to let your elbows drop as you "hug" in, and keep your head back against the headrest.

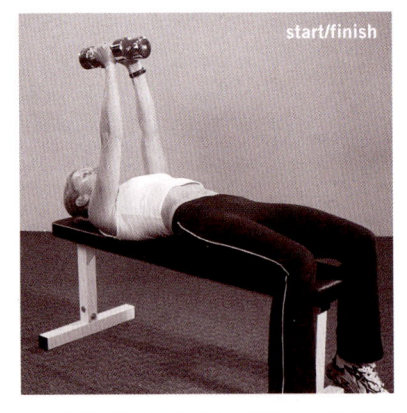

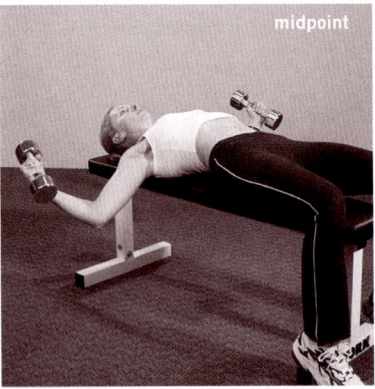

flat bench dumbell flyes

muscles working: **Pectorals (front of chest)**

The start/finish position: Sit on the flat bench with a dumbell in each hand. Lie back and press the dumbells directly above your shoulders as you would for a dumbell press. At the top position, rotate both hands by 90 degrees so that your palms face each other. Position your feet anywhere that enables your back to have permanent contact with the bench, either flat on the floor or flat on the bench.

The movement: With your eyes fixed on a spot on the roof and your elbows slightly bent, slowly lower the dumbells out to the sides drawing an imaginary half circle with the dumbells ensuring that you do not go any deeper than level with your shoulders. At a comfortable full stretch position, hold for a count of one then with your elbows still slightly bent, commence following the same half circle to return with a big "bear hug" action. Reach the start/finish position with straight arms. Hold again for a count of one and repeat.

Tip Make sure you always keep control of the dumbells as they travel.

> **Try not to let the dumbells travel too deep to the sides and avoid letting your elbows straighten as this will place too much stress on the joints.**

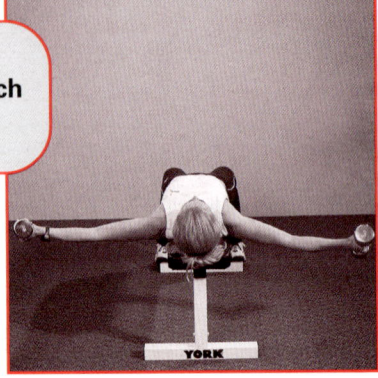

incline bench dumbell flyes

muscles working: Pectorals (front of chest)

The start/finish position: Sit on the incline bench set at approximately 30 – 45 degrees with a dumbell in each hand. Lie back and press the dumbells directly above your shoulders as you would for a dumbell press. At the top position, rotate both hands by 90 degrees so that your palms face each other. Position your feet anywhere that enables your back to have permanent contact with the bench, either flat on the floor or flat on the bench.

The movement: With your eyes fixed on a spot on the ceiling and your elbows slightly bent, slowly lower the dumbells out to the sides drawing an imaginary half circle with the dumbells ensuring that you do not go any deeper than level with your shoulders. At a comfortable full stretch position, hold for a count of one then with your elbows still slightly bent, commence following the same half circle to return with a big "bear hug" action. Reach the start/finish position with straight arms. Hold again for a count of one and repeat.

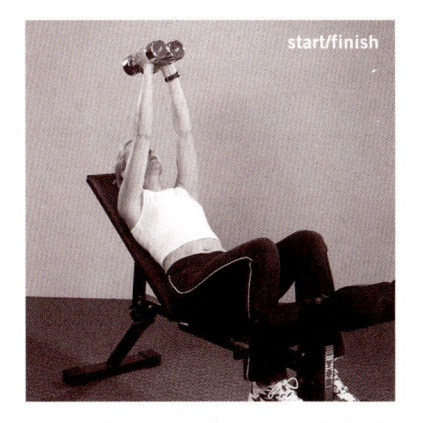

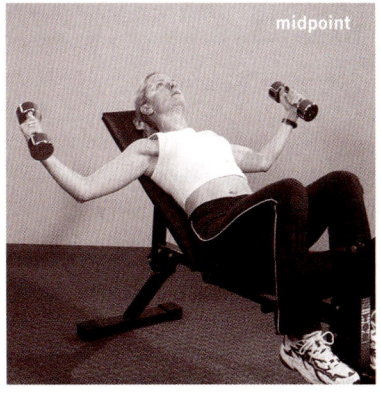

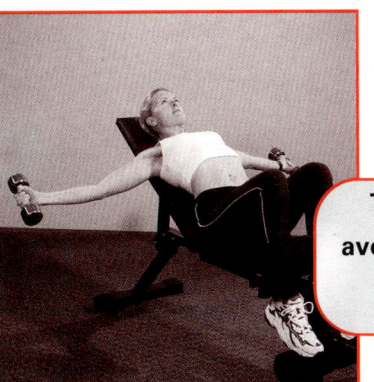

Tip Make sure you always keep control of the dumbbells as they travel.

Try not to let the dumbells travel too deep to the sides and avoid letting your elbows straighten as this will place too much stress on the joints.

pec deck

muscles working: Pectorals (front of chest)

The start/finish position: Sit on the pec deck seat with your back firmly against the back support. Slide both arms in behind the pec deck arm pads so that your upper arm is parallel with the floor (approx. 90 degrees at your elbows). Position your feet flat against the floor slightly wider than shoulder width.

The movement: With your eyes fixed on a spot across the room, slowly and smoothly draw the elbows together so the pads touch in front of your eyes. Hold for a count of one then slowly return to the start/finish position ensuring a comfortable stretch. Hold again for a count of one and repeat.

Tip Make sure you always keep control of the weight as it travels and that you don't let the weight drop on the return.

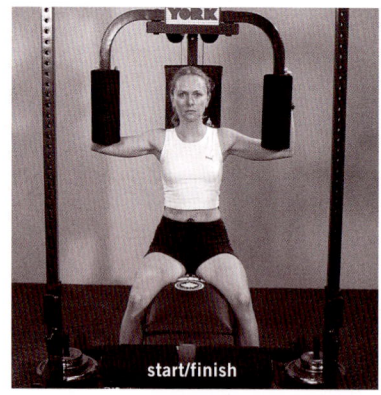

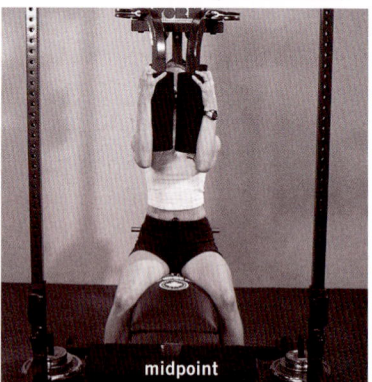

Try to make sure that your elbows stay firmly against the pads and you avoid pushing with your hands and forearms. Keep your head back against the bench.

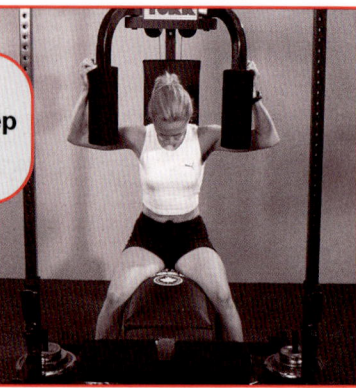

UPPER BODY

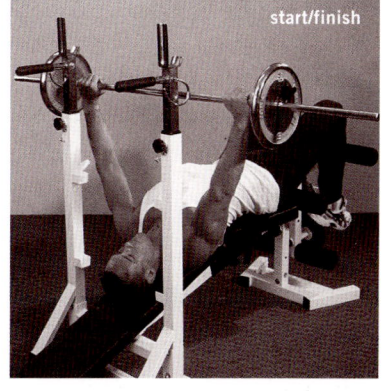

decline barbell bench press

muscles working: Pectorals (front of chest)
Deltoids (front shoulder)
Triceps (back arm)

The start/finish position: Lie on the decline bench so that your head is lower than your hips, and with the barbell positioned in front of your eyes. Position yourself so that your lower back is hard against the bench. Grasp the bar slightly wider than shoulder width with an overhand grip (palms facing away from you) and press the bar out of the racks to a held position right over the lower portion of your chest.

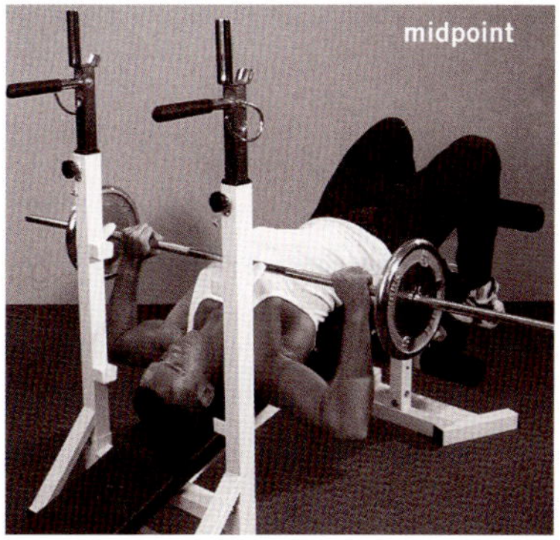

The movement: With your eyes fixed on a spot on the ceiling, slowly lower the bar to just touch the lower part of your chest. Pause for a count of one then press the weight back to the start/finish position. Hold again for a count of one and repeat.

FOR ADVANCED LIFTERS ONLY

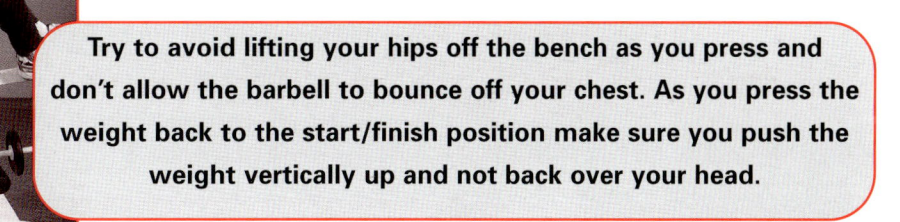

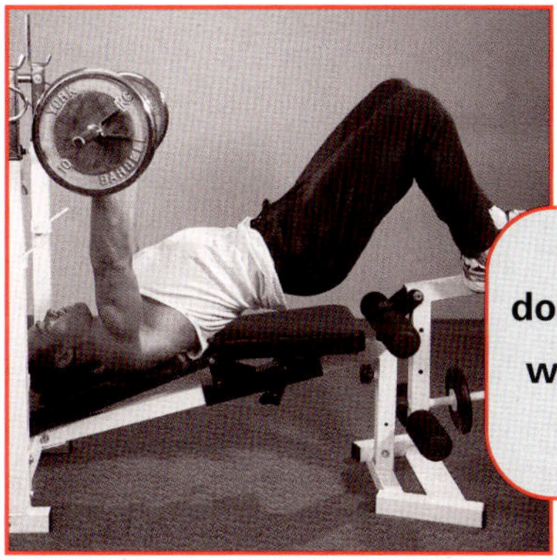

Tip As the weight you are lifting increases, try to have someone assist you as a 'spotter' just in case you get into trouble.

Try to avoid lifting your hips off the bench as you press and don't allow the barbell to bounce off your chest. As you press the weight back to the start/finish position make sure you push the weight vertically up and not back over your head.

decline dumbell bench press

muscles working: Pectorals (front of chest)

Deltoids (front shoulder)

Triceps (back arm)

The start/finish position: Sit on the decline bench with a dumbell in each hand resting on your knees. Secure your feet and roll back on the bench with the dumbells held close to your chest. Position the dumbells to sit close to your shoulders with your palms facing away from you.

The movement: With your eyes fixed on a spot on the ceiling, slowly press the dumbells away to a point above your lower chest. Hold the top position for a count of one then slowly lower the dumbells back towards the points of your shoulders. Hold again for a count of one and repeat.

FOR ADVANCED LIFTERS ONLY

Tip Your elbows should at all times stay directly beneath your wrists.

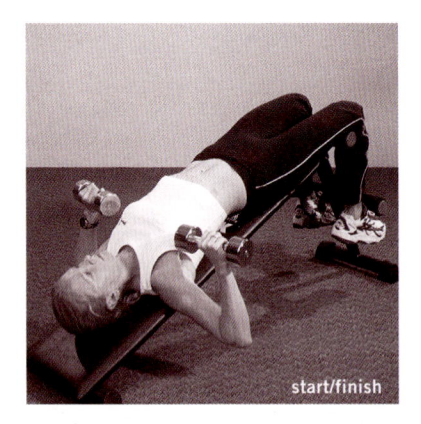

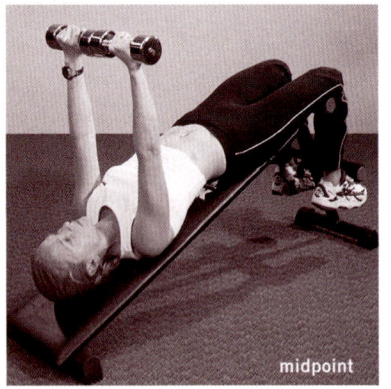

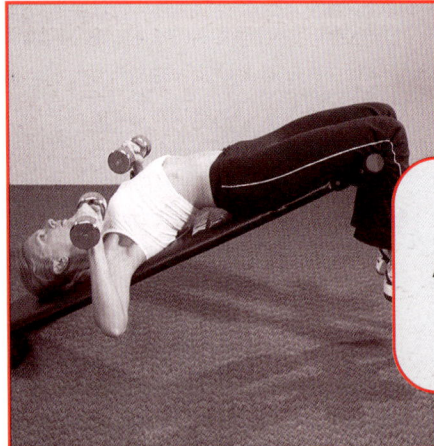

Try to avoid lifting your hips off the bench as you press and don't allow your elbows to go too deep. As you press the weight back to the start/finish position make sure you push the dumbells vertically up and not back over your head.

UPPER BODY

decline bench dumbell flyes

muscles working: Pectorals (front of chest)

The start/finish position: Sit on the decline bench with a dumbell in each hand resting on your knees. Secure your feet and roll back on the bench with the dumbells held close to your chest. Position the dumbells to sit close to your shoulders with your palms facing away from you. Press the dumbells directly above your shoulders as you would for a dumbell press. At the top position, rotate both hands by 90 degrees so that your palms face each other.

The movement: With your eyes fixed on a spot on the ceiling and your elbows slightly bent, slowly lower the dumbells out to the sides drawing an imaginary half circle with the dumbells ensuring that you do not go any deeper than level with your shoulders. At a comfortable full stretch position, hold for a count of one then with your elbows still slightly bent, commence following the same half circle to return with a big "bear hug" action. Reach the start/finish position with straight arms. Hold again for a count of one and repeat.

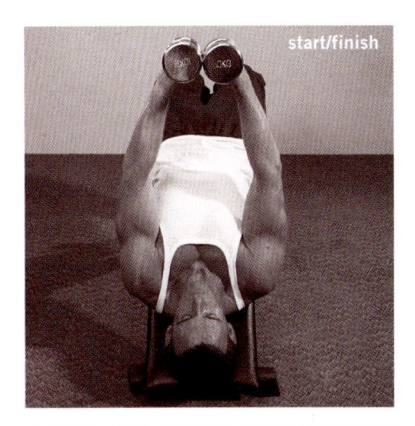

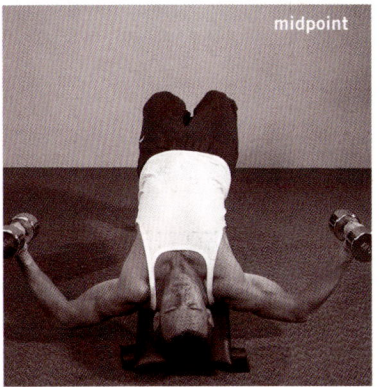

FOR ADVANCED LIFTERS ONLY

Tip Make sure you always keep control of the dumbbells as they travel.

Try not to let the dumbell's travel too deep to the sides and avoid letting your elbows straighten as this will place too much stress on the joints.

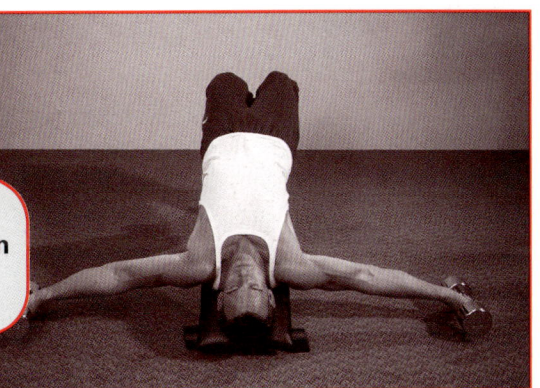

page 127

www.yorkfitness.co.uk

shoulders - deltoids

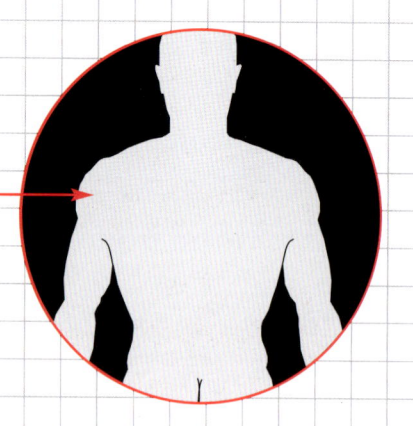

s-t-r-e-t-c-h Don't forget to stretch. Every muscle you strengthen, you should also stretch. Hold this stretch for at least 10 seconds between each set. See page 257

REMEMBER Keep your abdominal and lower back muscles tight through out the movement and remember to exhale during the lifting phase.

Tips The weight should always be under your control and if you need to cheat, you're probably trying to lift too much weight.

A lifting belt may also be of assistance to you in some overhead pressing exercises when the weights you are lifting become more challenging (see accessories).

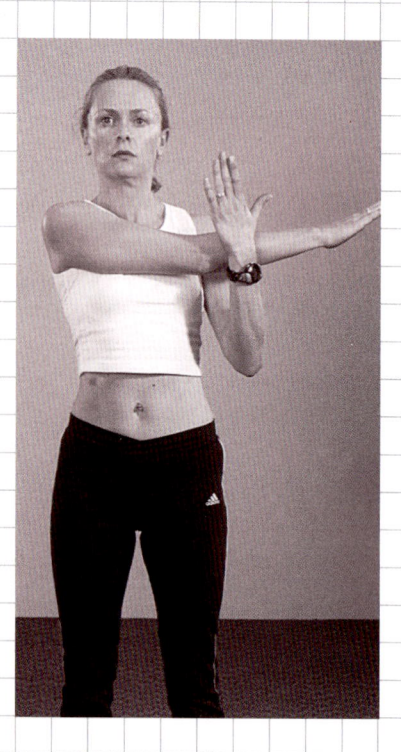

page 128

barbell overhead press seated

muscles working: Deltoids (shoulder)

Triceps (back arm)

The start/finish position: Sit on the flat bench with the barbell resting across your knees. Grasp the barbell with a slightly wider than shoulder width, overhand grip. Lift the barbell to rest across the front of your shoulders. Position your feet flat against the floor at about shoulder width. Keep your eyes up and your back straight.

The movement: With your eyes fixed on a spot across the room and while keeping your back straight, press the barbell straight up above your head with your arms fully extended. Pause for a count of one then slowly control the weight back to the start / finish position. Hold again for a count of one and repeat.

Tip As the weight you are lifting increases, try to have someone assist you as a 'spotter' just in case you get into trouble.

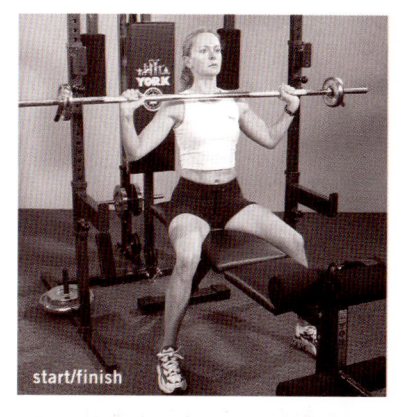

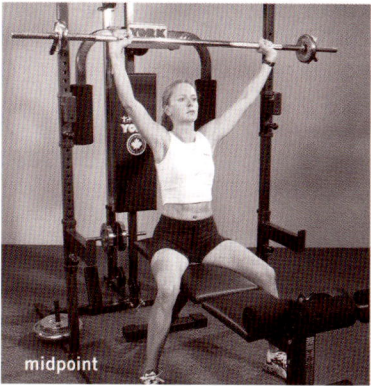

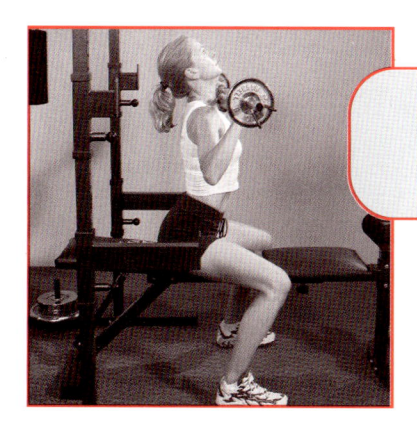

Try to avoid leaning back and arching your back as you press the weight as this can place undue stress on your lower back.

dumbell overhead press seated

muscles working: Deltoids (shoulder)

Triceps (back arm)

The start/finish position: Sit on the flat bench with a dumbell in each hand. Lift the dumbells to shoulder height with your elbows out and your palms facing forward. Position your feet flat against the floor at about shoulder width. Keep your eyes up and your back straight.

The movement: With your eyes fixed on a spot straight ahead and while keeping your back straight, press the dumbells straight up above your head to touch end to end, with your arms fully extended. Pause for a count of one then slowly control the weight back to the start/finish position. Hold again for count of one.and repeat

Tip Try to keep the weights steady as you press and don't allow them to sway in the air.

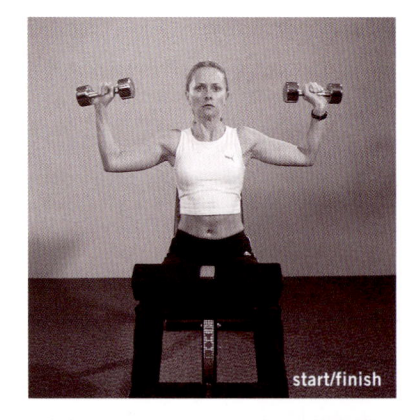

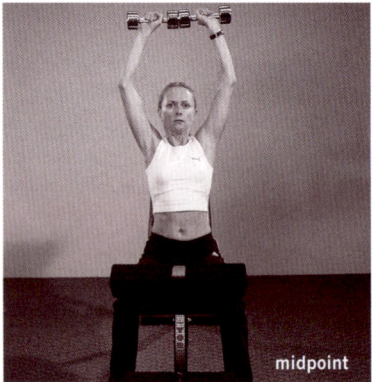

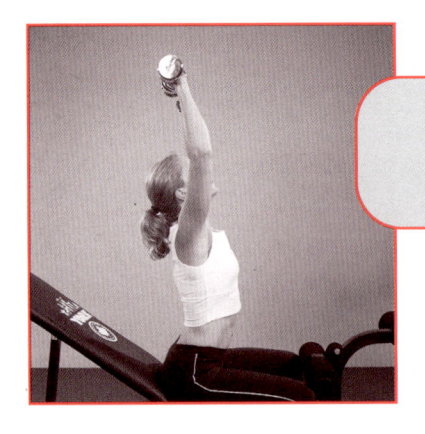

start/finish

midpoint

Try to avoid leaning back and arching your back as you press the weight as this can place undue stress on you lower back.

UPPER BODY

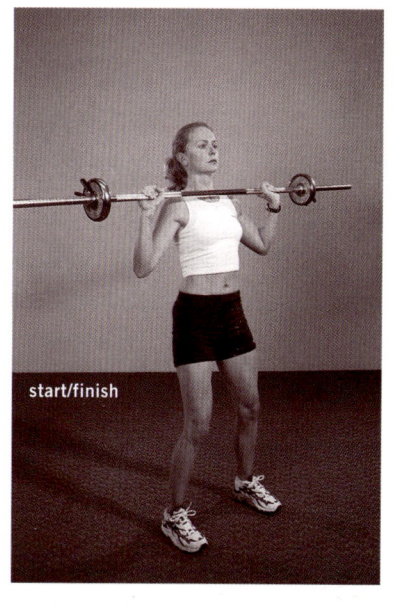

barbell overhead press standing

muscles working: Deltoids (shoulder)

Triceps (back arm)

The start/finish position: Grasp a barbell on the floor with a slightly wider than shoulder width, overhand grip (palms facing you). With your head up and your back straight, lift the weight to a standing position and then onto a shoulder height position, right above your collarbone. Your feet should be shoulder width apart with your knees slightly bent and your back straight.

The movement: With your eyes fixed on a spot straight ahead and keeping your back straight, press the barbell straight up above your head with your arms fully extended. Pause for a count of one then slowly control the weight back to the start/finish position. Hold again for a count of one.and repeat

Tip Try not to get any "driving bounce" from your legs as you press the weight above your head.

Try to avoid leaning back and arching your back as you press the weight as this can place undue stress on your lower back.

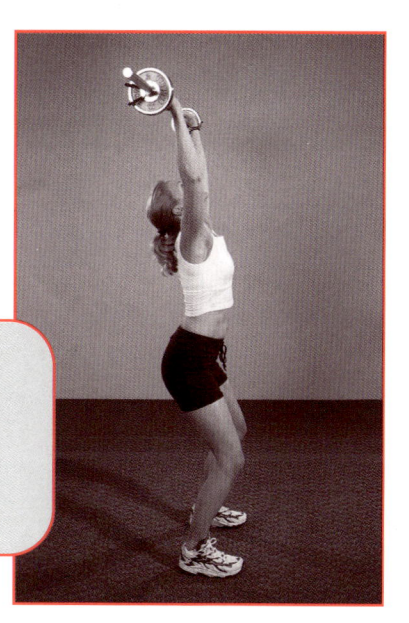

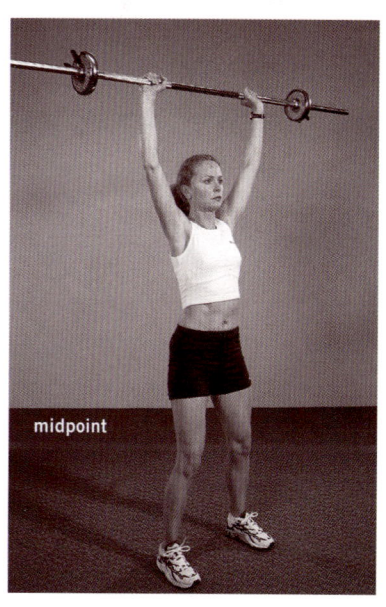

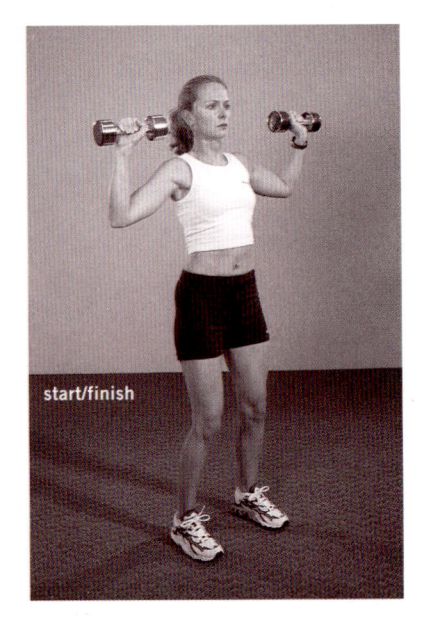

dumbell overhead press standing

muscles working: Deltoids (shoulder)

Triceps (back arm)

The start/finish position: Grasp a dumbell in each hand and with your head up and your back straight. Lift the dumbells to a standing position and then onto a shoulder height position, with your elbows out and your palms facing forward. Your feet should be shoulder width apart with your knees slightly bent and your back straight.

The movement: With your eyes fixed on a spot across the room and while keeping your back straight, press the dumbells straight up above your head to touch end to end with your arms fully extended. Pause for a count of one then slowly control the weight back to the start/finish position. Hold again for a count of one and repeat.

Tip Try not to get any "driving bounce" from your legs as you press the dumbells above your head and keep the weights steady as you press, don't allow them to sway in the air.

Try to avoid leaning back and arching your back as you press the dumbells as this can place undue stress on your lower back.

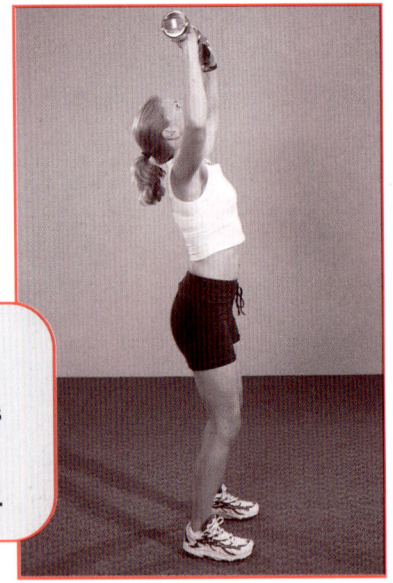

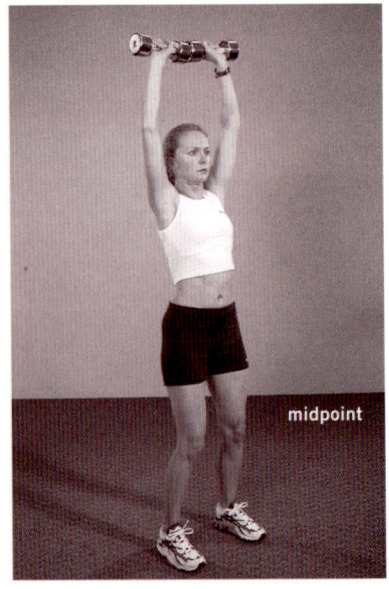

machine overhead press seated

muscles working: Deltoids (shoulder)

Triceps (back arm)

The start/finish position: Sit on the press machine bench and grasp the handles with a 'palms facing away' grip. Position your feet flat against the floor at about shoulder width. Keep your head up and your back straight.

The movement: With your eyes fixed on a spot across the room and while keeping your back straight, press the bar straight up above your head with your arms fully extended. Pause for a count of one then slowly control the weight back to the start/finish position being careful not to allow the weights to touch down on each other at the bottom. Hold again for a count of one and repeat.

Tip Try to make sure you keep your elbows directly below the press bar.

> **Try to avoid leaning back and arching your back as you press the weight as this can place undue stress on your lower back**

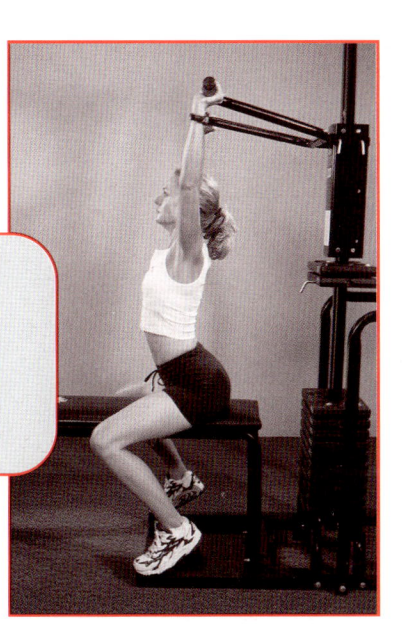

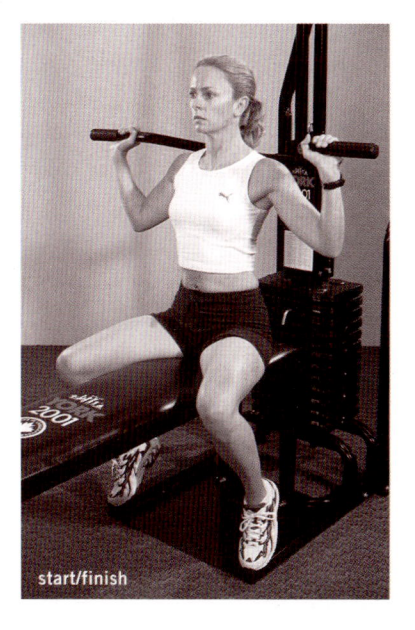

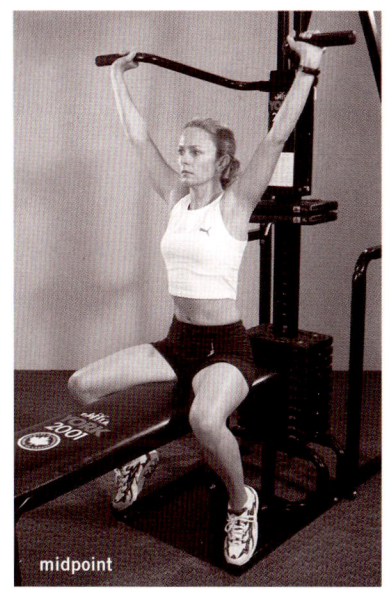

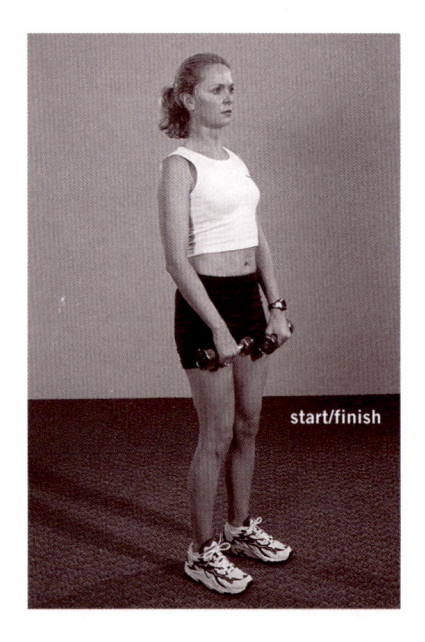

dumbell raises front

muscles working: Deltoids (shoulder)

The start/finish position: Grasp a dumbell in each hand and hold them with a knuckles forward grip, hanging at arms length. Place your feet at shoulder width with your head up and your back straight and slightly bend your knees to better support your lower back.

The movement: With your eyes fixed on a spot across the room and while keeping your back straight, raise the right dumbell out in front of you to approximately shoulder height, being sure to keep your knuckles pointing straight ahead. Pause for a count of one then slowly control the dumbell back to the start/finish position. Hold again for a count of one and then follow the same procedure for the left arm. Continue alternating until the desired number of repetitions has been completed for each arm.

Tip Try not to swing the weights with momentum and therefore rob the muscles of their true workload.

> **Try to avoid leaning back and arching your back as you raise the dumbells as this can place undue stress on your lower back.**

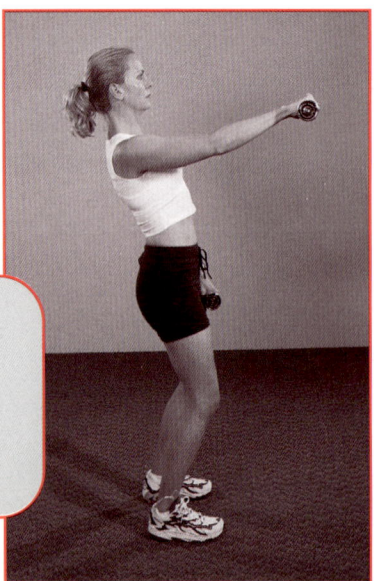

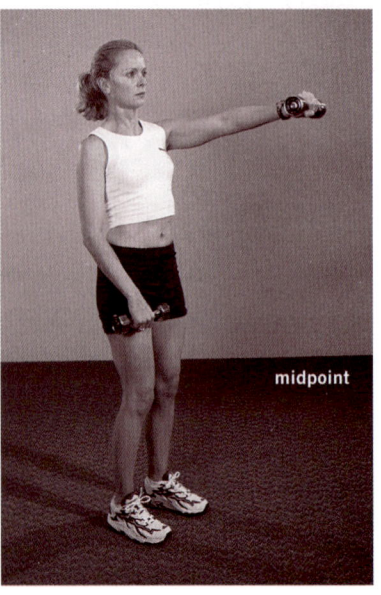

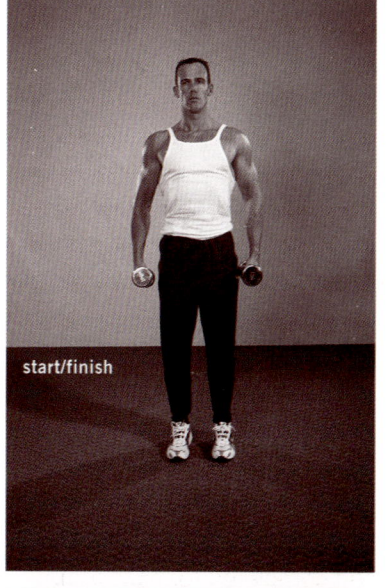

dumbell raise side

muscles working: Deltoids (shoulder)

The start/finish position: Grasp a dumbell in each hand and hold them with your palms facing the sides of your thighs and hanging at arms length. Place your feet at shoulder width with your eyes up and your back straight and slightly bend your knees to better support your lower back.

The movement: With your eyes fixed on a spot across the room and while keeping your back straight, raise both dumbells up and out to your sides to finish at approximately shoulder height. Try to make sure that your wrists, elbows and shoulders finish in a straight line. Pause for a count of one then slowly control the dumbells back to the start/finish position. Hold again for a count of one and repeat.

Tip Try to visualise your elbows being pulled toward the ceiling by puppet strings.

> **Try to not let the dumbells swing in front of your body. Avoid leaning backward and arching your back as you raise the dumbells as this can place undue stress on your lower back.**

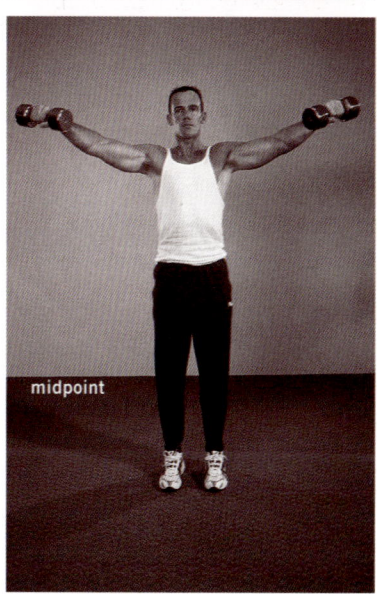

dumbell raise rear

muscles working: Deltoids (shoulder)

The start/finish position: Grasp a dumbell in each hand and position your feet at shoulder width as you bend from the waist to bring your upper body parallel with the floor. Let the dumbells hang at arms length and hold them with your palms facing each other. Slightly bend your knees to better support your lower back and keep your eyes focused on the floor a couple of meters in front.

The movement: Raise both dumbells up, leading with your elbows and following a half circle pattern while keeping your upper body parallel with the floor. Finish the movement at approximately shoulder height with your shoulders, elbows and wrists in line. Pause for a count of one then slowly lower the dumbells back to the start/finish position.

Tip Try not to swing the weights and try to visualise your elbows being pulled toward the ceiling by puppet strings.

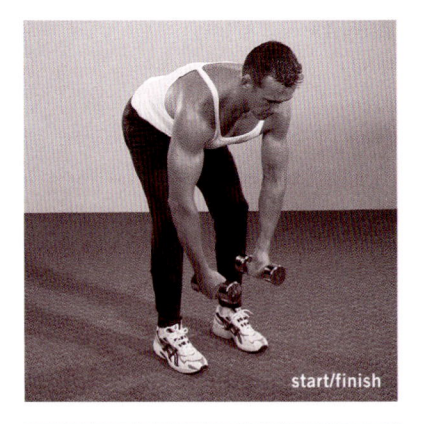

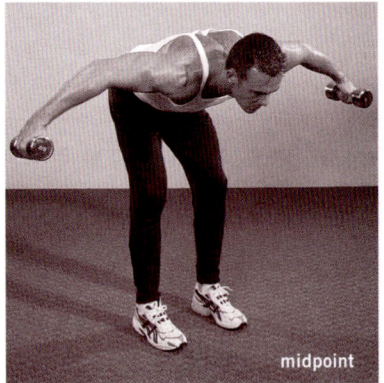

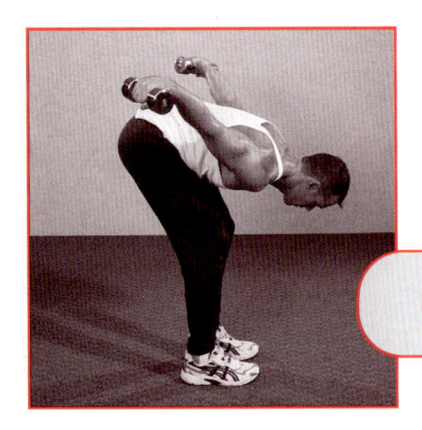

Try to not let your head drop or let the dumbells travel behind you back towards your hips.

cable raise front

muscles working: Deltoids (shoulder)

The start/finish position: Grasp the low pulley handle (with the chain extension attached) in your right hand and stand upright with your right arm hanging by your side, knuckles forward grip, and grasping the machine for stability with your left hand. Position your feet shoulder width apart with your head up and your back straight. Slightly bend your knees to better support your lower back.

The movement: With your eyes fixed on a spot across the room and while keeping your back straight, raise your right hand out in front of you to approximately shoulder height, being sure to keep your knuckles pointing straight ahead. Pause for a count of one then slowly control the handle back to the start/finish position. Hold again for a count of one and then repeat. Complete the desired number of repetitions for the right side and do the same for the left.

Tip Try not to 'heave' the weight from the bottom with momentum and therefore rob the muscles of their true work load.

Try to avoid leaning and twisting your back as you raise the handle as this can place undue stress on your lower back.

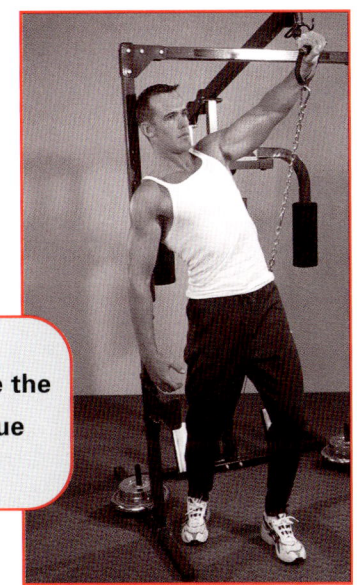

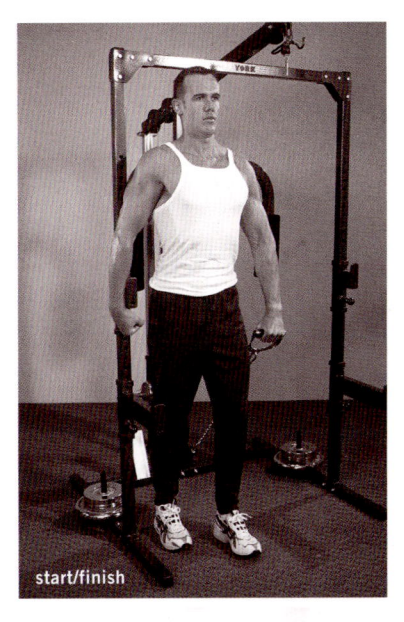

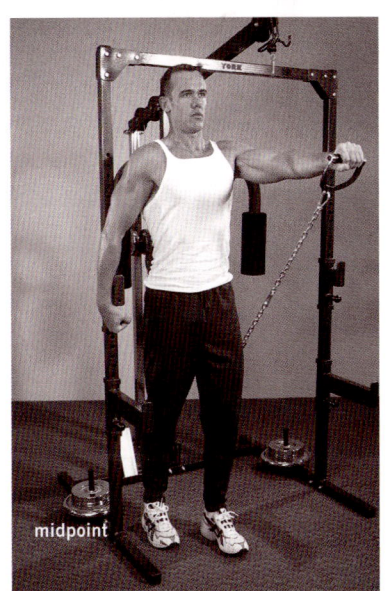

cable raise side

muscles working: Deltoids (shoulder)

The start/finish position: Grasp the low pulley handle (with the chain extension attached) in your right hand and stand upright, left side to the pulley with your right arm hanging at full extension in front of your right thigh allowing the chain to pass in front of your body with your knuckles facing up to the side. Place your left hand on your hip for stability and position your feet shoulder width apart with your head up and your back straight, slightly bend your knees to better support your lower back.

The movement: With your eyes fixed on a spot across the room and while keeping your back straight, raise your right hand out to the side to approximately shoulder height, being sure to keep your knuckles pointing up. Pause for a count of one then slowly control the handle back to the start / finish position. Hold again for a count of one and then repeat. Complete the desired number of reps for the right side and do the same for the left.

Tip Try not to let the handle swing through past your body to lift with momentum and therefore rob the muscles of their true workload.

> **Try to avoid leaning and twisting your back as you raise the handle as this can place undue stress on your lower back.**

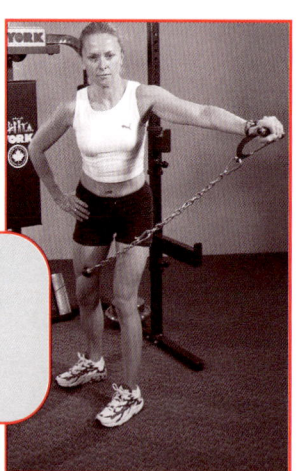

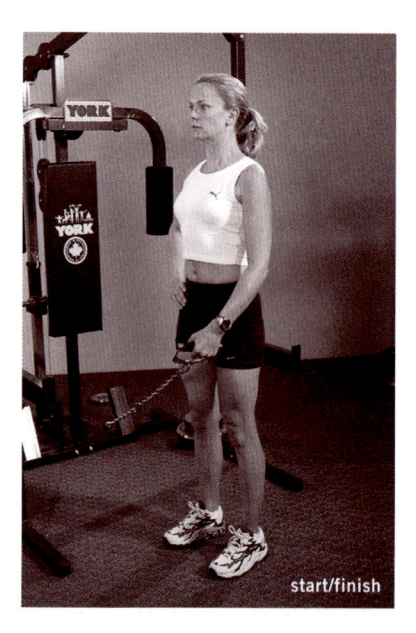

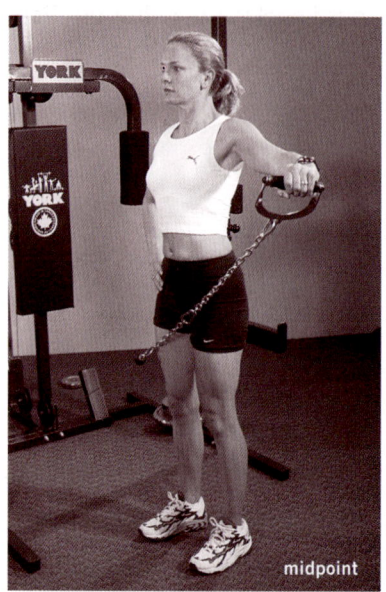

cable raise rear

muscles working: Deltoids (shoulder)

The start/finish position: Grasp the low pulley handle (with the chain extension attached) in your right hand and position your feet shoulder width apart as you bend from the waist to bring your upper body parallel to the floor with your left side to the pulley and your right arm hanging toward the floor, palm facing the pulley. Grasp the machine for stability with your left hand while slightly bending your knees to better support your lower back and keeping your eyes focused on the floor a couple of meters in front.

The movement: Raise your right hand out to the side following a half circle pattern while keeping your upper body parallel with the floor. Finish the movement at approximately shoulder height with your shoulders, elbows and wrists in line and being sure to keep your knuckles pointing up. Pause for a count of one then slowly control the weight back to the start/finish position. Hold again for a count of one and repeat. Complete the desired number of reps for the right side and do the same for the left.

Tip Try not to let the handle swing through past your body to lift with momentum and therefore rob the muscles of their true workload.

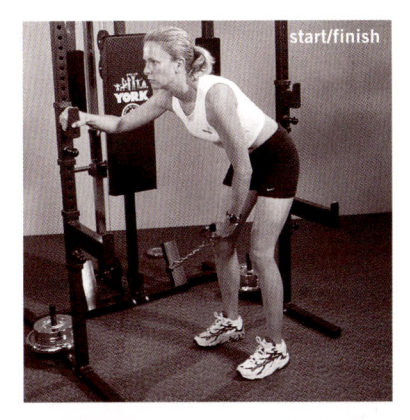

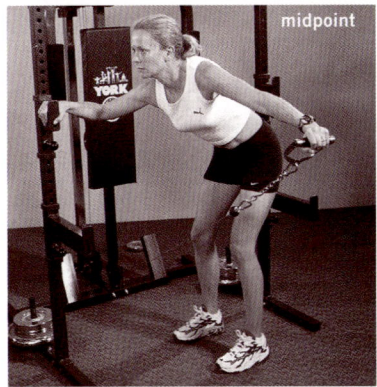

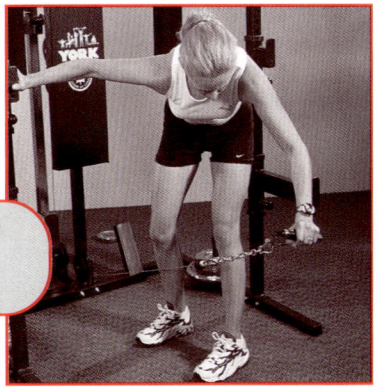

> **Try to avoid leaning and twisting your back as you raise the handle as this can place undue stress on your lower back.**

rear pec deck

muscles working: Deltoids (shoulder)

Rhomboids (mid back)

The start/finish position: Sit on the pec deck machine with the reverse approach to the conventional way, facing the back support. Place the back of your elbows against the pec deck arms at shoulder height with your elbows at a 90-degree angle and forearms parallel to the floor. Keep your back straight and your feet flat against the floor.

The movement: Slowly draw the pec deck arms together as you squeeze your elbows towards each other behind you. Finish the movement at a point where you can hold the weight for a count of one then slowly control the weight back to the start/finish position. Hold again for a count of one and repeat.

FOR ADVANCED LIFTERS ONLY

Tip Try not to let the weights touch down on each other at the completion of each repetition as this will jolt you and the machine and decrease the effectiveness of the exercise.

Try to avoid letting your elbows drop towards your waist and your head dropping down as the exercise will become less effective.

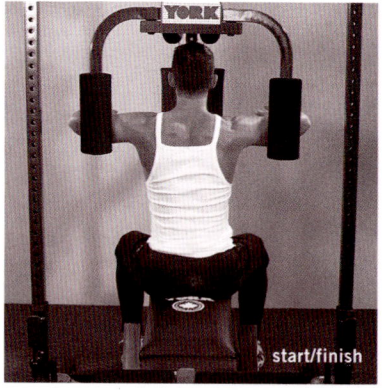

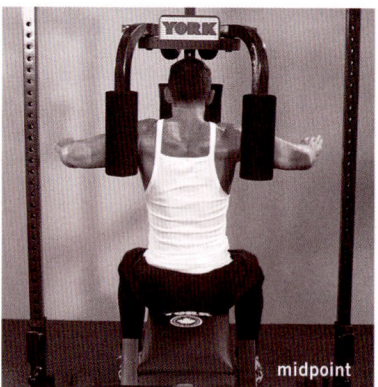

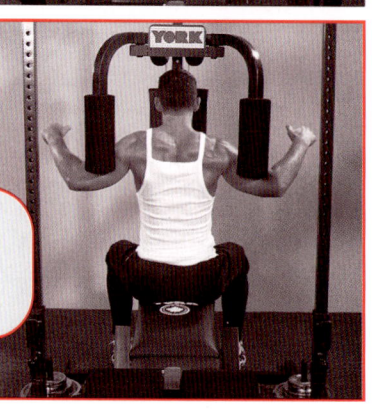

SECTION NINE arms

front arms - biceps

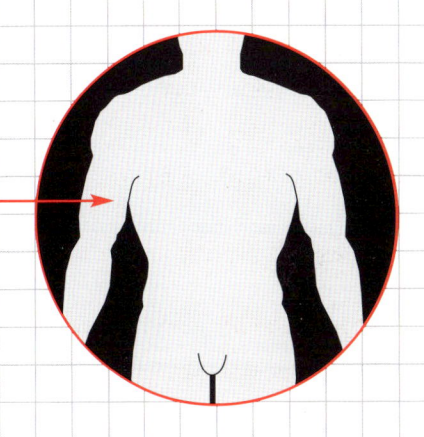

s-t-r-e-t-c-h Don't forget to stretch. Every muscle you strengthen, you should also stretch. Hold this stretch for at least 10 seconds between each set. See page 260

REMEMBER keep your abdominal and lower back muscles tight through out the movement and remember to exhale during the lifting phase.

Tips The weight should always be under your control and if you need to cheat, you are probably trying to lift too much weight.

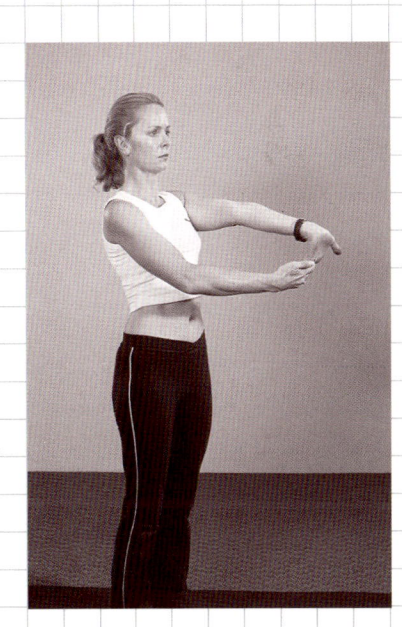

barbell curls standing

muscles working: Biceps (front arms)

Forearms (wrists)

The start/finish position: Approach the barbell on the floor and with feet at shoulder width apart grasp the barbell with a shoulder width grip, palms facing up. Lifting with your legs, stand to an upright position with your arms held straight down in front of you. Keep your chest up and your shoulders back with your eyes focused ahead.

The movement: Slowly curl the barbell towards your shoulders without leaning back and 'heaving' the weight up. Be sure to keep your elbows tight by your side. Hold the weight at the top position for a count of one and then slowly control the weight back to the start/finish position.

Tip This exercise can also be done with an ez curl (bent) bar.

start/finish

> **Try to avoid letting your back arch as you curl the weight. This usually means you are trying to lift too much weight.**

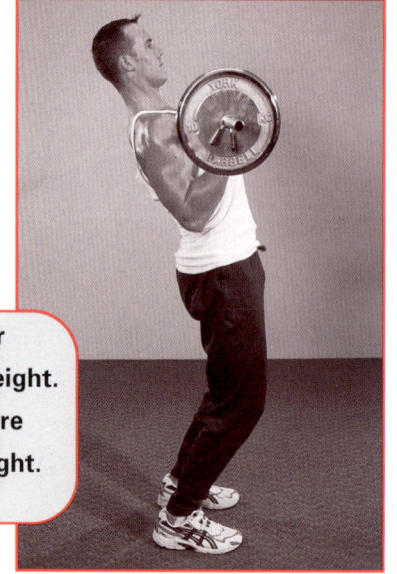

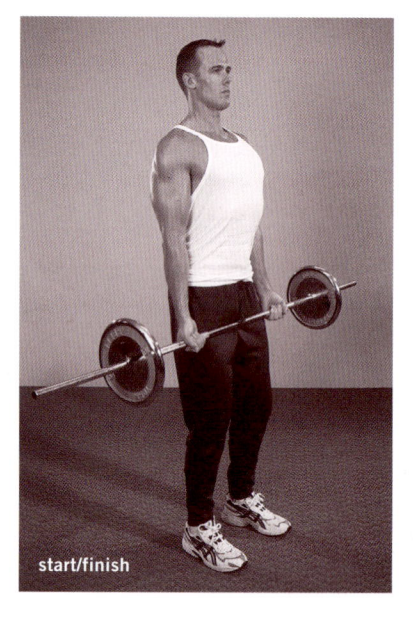

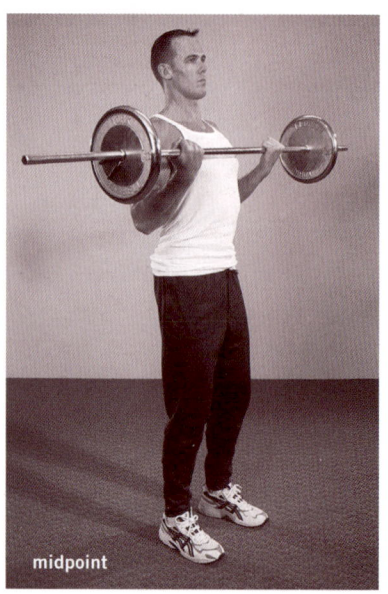

midpoint

low cable curl standing

muscles working: Biceps (front arms)

Forearms (wrists)

The start/finish position: Approach the low pulley bar on the floor. Position feet shoulder width apart and grasp the bar with a shoulder width grip, palms facing up. Lifting with your legs, stand to an upright position with your arms held straight down in front of you. The weight should just hover above the top of the stack. Keep your chest up and your shoulders back with your eyes focused ahead.

The movement: Slowly curl the bar towards your shoulders without leaning back and 'heaving' the weight up. Be sure to keep your elbows tight by your side. Hold the weight at the top position for a count of one and then slowly control the weight back to the start/finish position without letting the weight rest on the stack. Hold again for a count of one and repeat.

Tip You may need to lengthen the low pulley cable with chain to ensure correct travel range of the weights.

Try to avoid letting your back arch as you curl the weight. This usually means you are trying to lift too much weight.

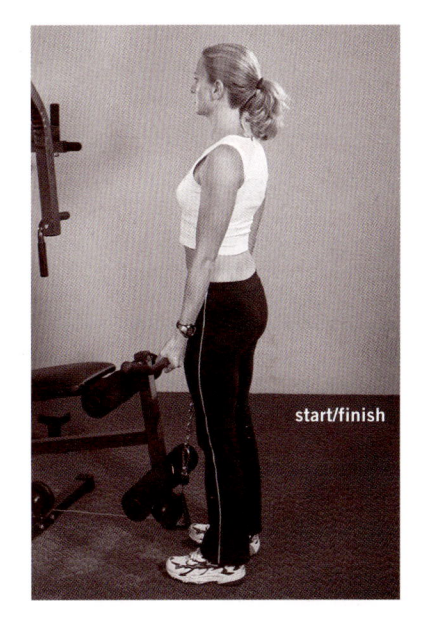

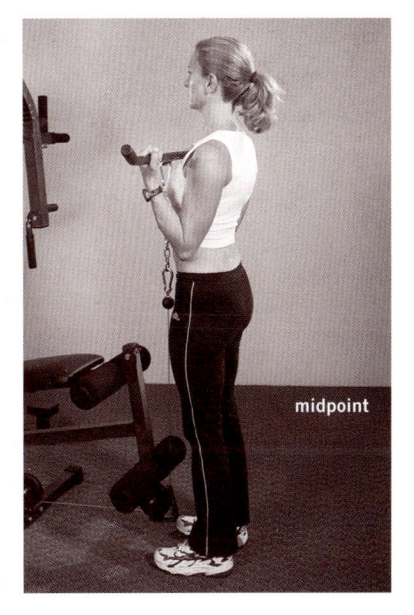

dumbell curl seated

muscles working: Biceps (front arms)

Forearms (wrists)

The start/finish position: While seated on the flat bench, position your feet close together and flat against the floor. Grasp a dumbell in each hand, palms facing up. Allow your arms to hang straight down beside you as you roll your shoulders back and keep your chest high and eyes focused straight ahead.

The movement: Slowly curl both the dumbells towards your shoulders without leaning back and 'heaving' the weight up. Be sure to keep your elbows tight by your side. Hold the weight at the top position for a count of one and then slowly control the weight back to the start/finish position.

Tip This exercise can also be done standing and for variation you could curl one arm up at a time.

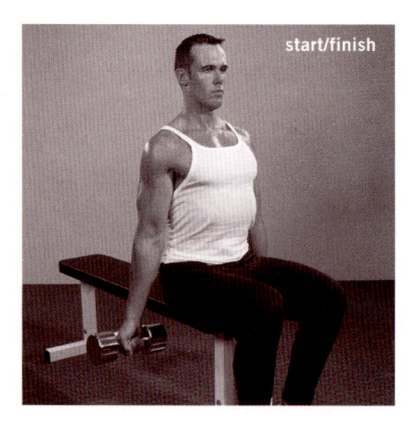

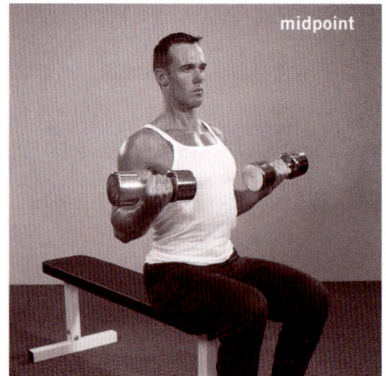

Try to avoid letting your back arch as you curl the weight. This usually means you are trying to lift too much weight.

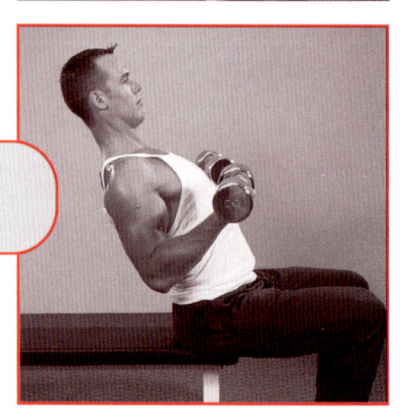

dumbell curl incline

muscles working: Biceps (front arms)

Forearms (wrists)

The start/finish position: With a dumbell in each hand, sit down on an incline bench set at about 45 degrees and position your feet flat against the floor. Hold the dumbells with your palms facing up. Allow your arms to hang straight down beside you as you roll your shoulders back and keep your chest high and eyes focused straight ahead.

The movement: Slowly curl both the dumbells towards your shoulders without letting your back leave the bench or 'heaving' the weight up and being sure to keep your elbows tight by your side. Hold the weight at the top position for a count of one and then slowly control the weight back to the start/finish position. You will feel a greater stretch in the bicep than you do with normal vertical curls because of the angle.

Tip This exercise can also be done curling one arm up at a time.

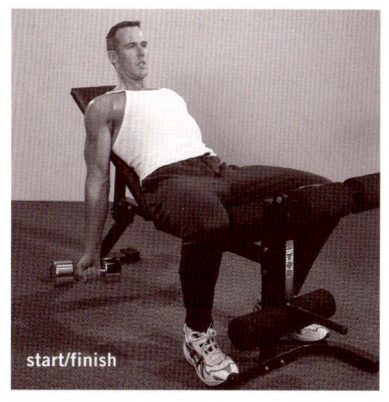

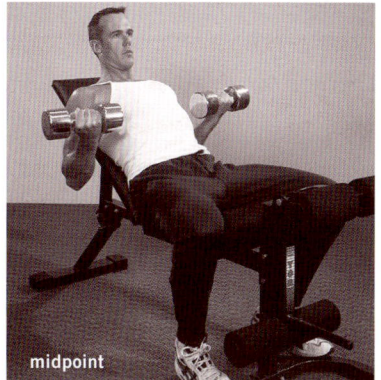

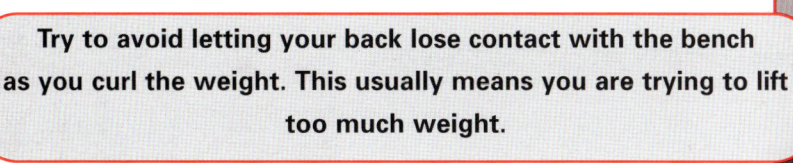

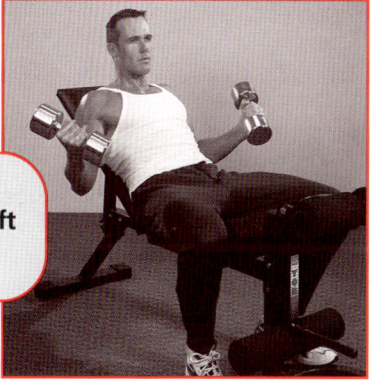

> **Try to avoid letting your back lose contact with the bench as you curl the weight. This usually means you are trying to lift too much weight.**

dumbell hammer curl

muscles working: Biceps (front arms)

Forearms (wrists)

The start/finish position: While seated on a flat bench, position your feet close together and flat against the floor. Grasp a dumbell in each hand, palms facing in. Allow your arms to hang straight down beside you as you roll your shoulders back and keep your chest high and eyes focused straight ahead.

The movement: Slowly curl both the dumbells towards your shoulders with your thumbs up in a hammer holding grip without 'heaving' the weight up and being sure to keep your elbows tight by your side. Hold the weight at the top position for a count of one and then slowly control the weight back to the start/finish position. Hold again for a count of one and repeat.

Tip This exercise can also be done curling one arm up at a time.

> **Try to avoid letting your back arch as you curl the weight. This usually means you are trying to lift too much weight.**

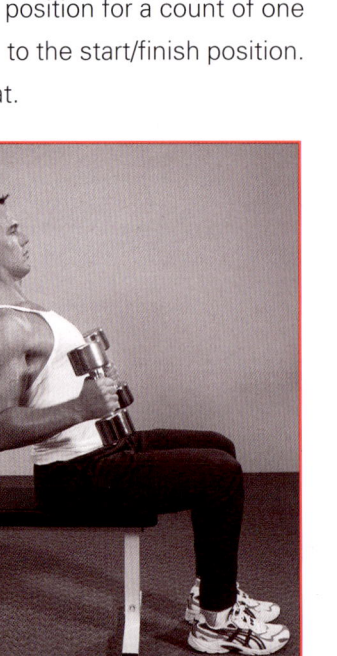

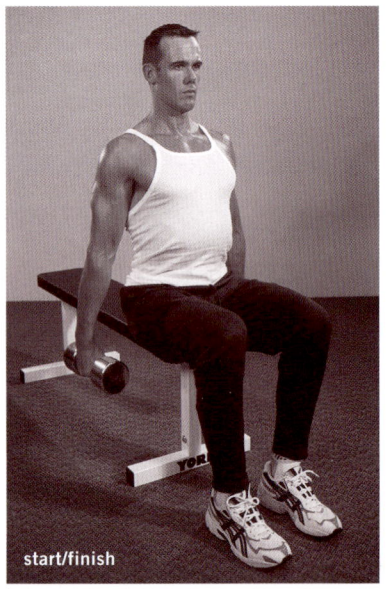

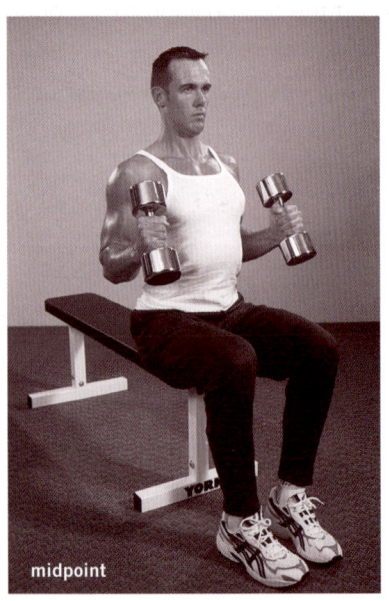

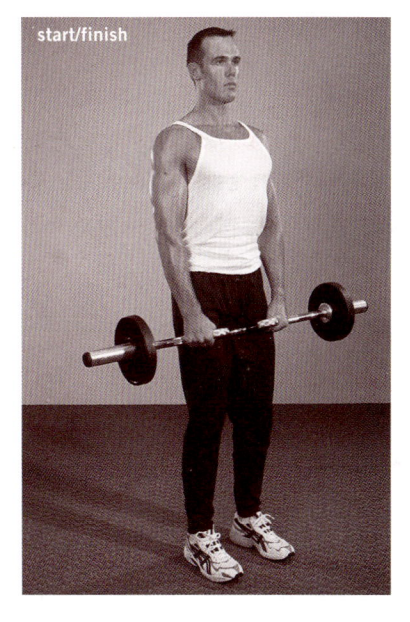

reverse curls standing

muscles working: Biceps (front arms)

Forearms (wrists)

The start/finish position: Approach the ez bar on the floor and with feet at shoulder width, grasp the barbell with a shoulder width overhand grip, palms facing down. Lifting with your legs, stand to an upright position with your arms held straight down in front of you. Keep your chest up and your shoulders back with your eyes focused ahead.

The movement: Slowly curl the ez bar towards your shoulders without leaning back and 'heaving' the weight up and being sure to keep your elbows tight by your side. You will feel the muscles on the top of your forearms do more work than you do in any other curl as well as a different part of your upper arms. Hold the weight at the top position for a count of one and then slowly control the weight back to the start/finish position. Hold again for a count of one and repeat.

FOR ADVANCED LIFTERS ONLY

Tip This exercise can also be done with a normal barbell however the grip is a little more difficult.

> Try to avoid letting your back arch as you curl the weight. This usually means you are trying to lift too much weight.

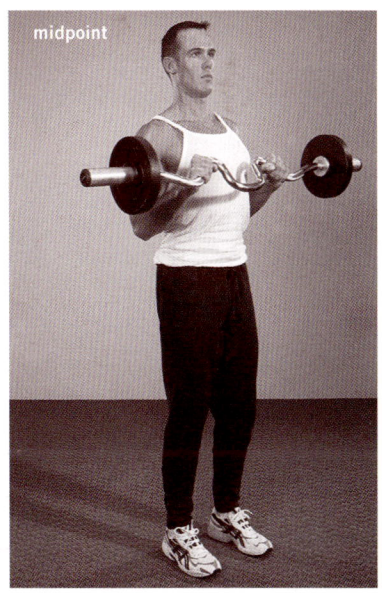

cable reverse curls

muscles working: Biceps (front arms)

Forearms (wrists)

The start/finish position: Approach the low cable bar on the floor and with feet at shoulder width, grasp the bar with a shoulder width overhand grip, palms facing down. Lifting with your legs, stand to an upright position with your arms held straight down in front of you. The weight should just hover above the top of the stack. Keep your chest up and your shoulders back with your eyes focused ahead.

The movement: Slowly curl the bar towards your shoulders without leaning back and 'heaving' the weight up and being sure to keep your elbows tight by your side. You will feel the muscles on the top of your forearms do more work than you do in any other curl as well as a different part of your upper arms. Hold the weight at the top position for a count of one and then slowly control the weight back to the start/finish position without letting the weight rest on the stack.

FOR ADVANCED LIFTERS ONLY

Tip You may need to lengthen the low pulley cable with chain to ensure correct travel range of the weights.

> **Try to avoid letting your back arch as you curl the weight. This usually means you are trying to lift too much weight.**

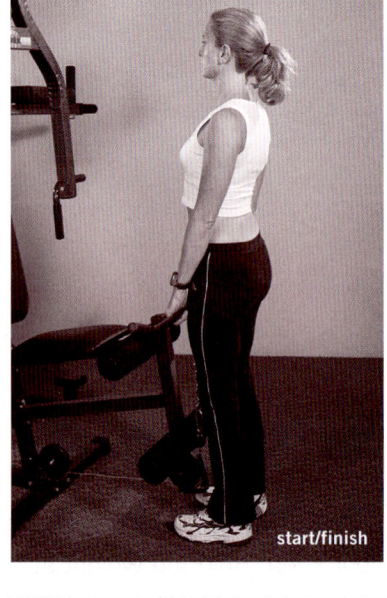

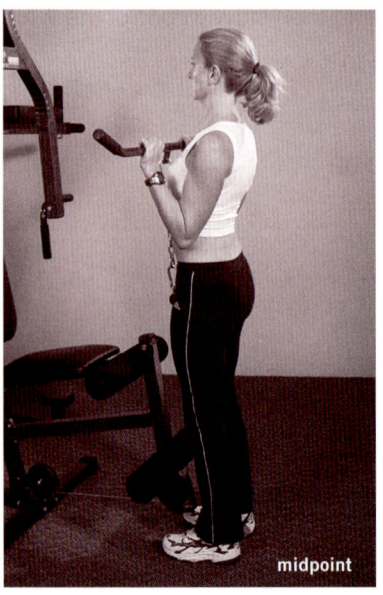

concentration curls

muscles working: Biceps (front arms)

Forearms (wrists)

The start/finish position: While seated on the flat bench, position your feet wide apart and flat against the floor. Grasp a dumbell in your right hand with your palm facing your left leg and brace your right elbow against your right knee. Allow your right arm to hang straight down to form a vertical straight line from your shoulder through your elbow to your wrist. Keep your chin over your right shoulder and support your left hand on your left knee.

The movement: Slowly curl the dumbell towards your right shoulder without leaning back and 'heaving' the weight up and twisting your shoulders. Be sure to keep your elbow tight against your knee. Hold the weight at the top position for a count of one and then slowly control the weight back to the start/finish position. Hold again for a count of one and repeat. Complete the desired number of repetitions for the right side and repeat for the left

FOR ADVANCED LIFTERS ONLY

Tip You could use your non-working hand to give you a small amount of assistance if required to force your way through the last few repetitions.

> **Try to avoid letting your body twist as you curl the weight and keep your chin over your shoulder.**

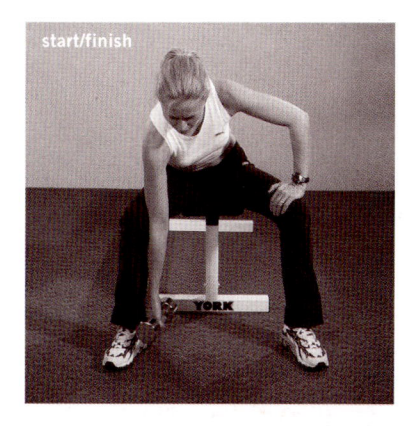

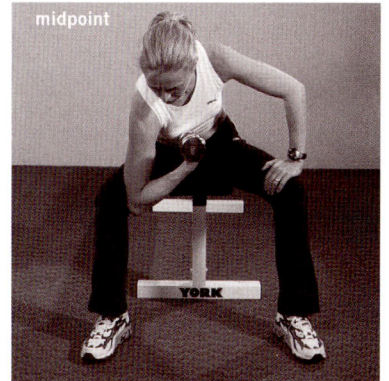

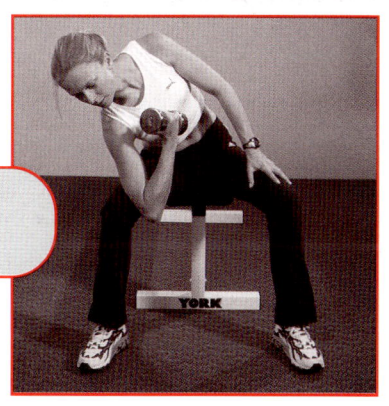

barbell preacher curls

muscles working: Biceps (front arms)

Forearms (wrists)

The start/finish position: Lean over the preacher attachment on your bench and grasp the barbell at about shoulder width with an underhand grip. Sit back down on the bench and position your elbows about shoulder width apart against the padding and keep your feet flat against the floor and your eyes focused straight ahead. Be sure to keep tension on your biceps and not let the weight place excess stress on your elbow joints.

The movement: Slowly curl the barbell towards your shoulders without leaning back and 'heaving' the weight up. Hold the weight at the top position for a count of one and then slowly control the weight back to the start/finish position. Hold again for a count of one and repeat. Be careful not to bounce the weight out of the bottom phase or let your bottom lift off the seat.

FOR ADVANCED LIFTERS ONLY

Tip This exercise can also be done with an ez curl bar or dumbells. If using dumbells, the exercise can also be done one arm at a time. If you don't have a preacher attachment, standing behind an incline bench doing single arm dumbell preacher curls can be just as effective.

> **Try to avoid letting your body weight lift away from the seat as you control the weight back to the start/finish position.**

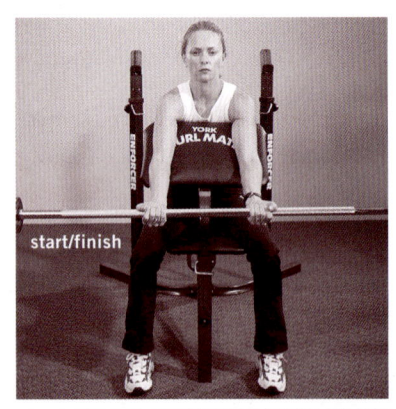

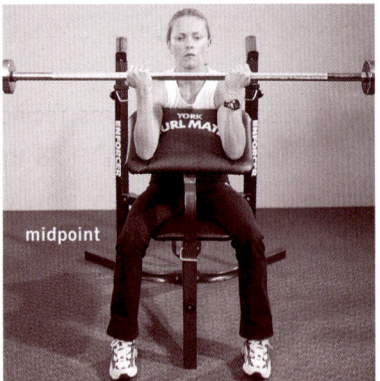

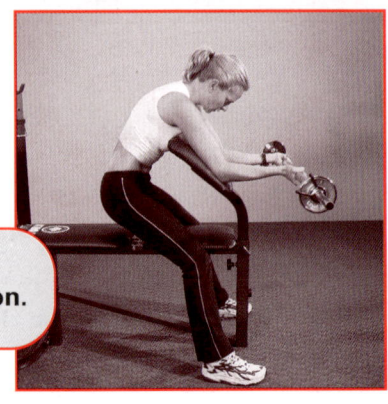

twisting dumbell curl

muscles working: Biceps (front arms)

Forearms (wrists)

The start/finish position: While seated on a flat bench, position your feet close together and flat against the floor. Grasp a dumbell in each hand, palms facing in. Allow your arms to hang straight down beside you as you roll your shoulders back and keep your chest high and eyes focused straight ahead.

The movement: Slowly curl both the dumbells toward your shoulders with your thumbs up in a hammer holding grip without 'heaving' the weight up and being sure to keep your elbows tight by your side. As the dumbells pass the sides of your legs, twist your wrists from a palms facing in grip to a palms facing up grip and squeeze the bicep. Hold the weight at the top position for a count of one and then slowly control the weight back to the start/finish position twisting the wrists back to their original grip.

FOR ADVANCED LIFTERS ONLY

Tip This exercise can also be done curling one arm up at a time or standing if you prefer.

Try to avoid letting your back arch as you curl the weight. You will also need to do this one slowly to get the timing right.

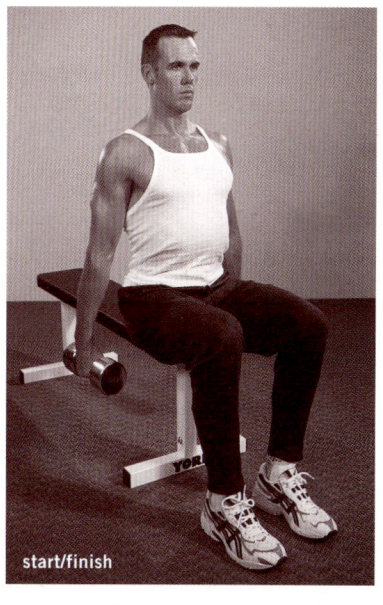

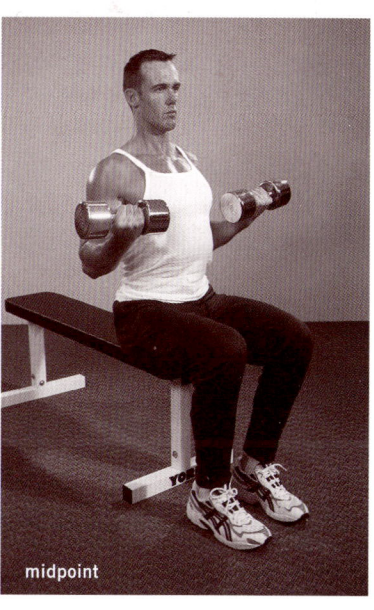

www.yorkfitness.co.uk

back arms - triceps

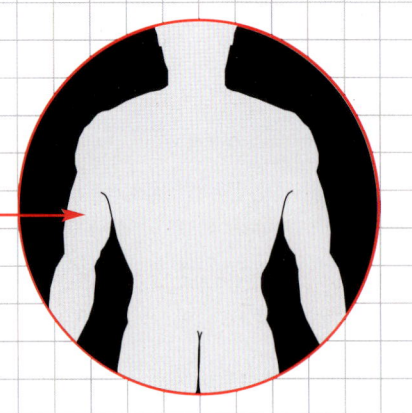

s-t-r-e-t-c-h Don't forget to stretch. Every muscle you strengthen, you should also stretch. Hold this stretch for at least 10 seconds between each set. See page 258

REMEMBER Keep your abdominal and lower back muscles tight through out the movement and remember to exhale during the lifting phase.

Tips The weight should always be under your control and if you need to cheat, you are probably trying to lift too much weight.

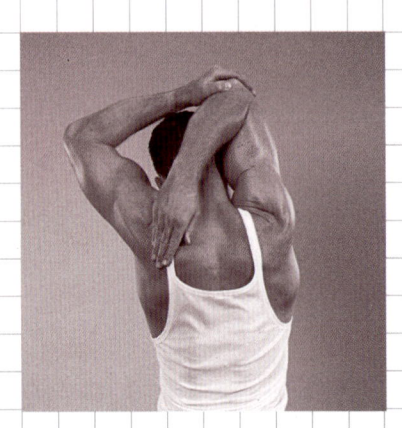

lying ez bar extensions

muscles working: Triceps (back arms)

Forearms (wrists)

The start/finish position: While sitting on a flat bench, reach down to grasp the ez curl bar with an overhand grip at about shoulder width. Lift the bar towards you and roll back onto the bench holding the weight at arms length above your eyes. Make sure your head is fully supported by the bench and both feet are either flat against the floor or flat against the bench.

The movement: Slowly lower the bar towards yourself bending at the elbows and finishing slightly behind your head while being sure to keep your elbows pointing in. Hold the weight at the bottom position for a count of one and then slowly push the weight, extending through the elbows and without bouncing, back to the start/finish position.

Tip This exercise can also be done with a straight barbell.

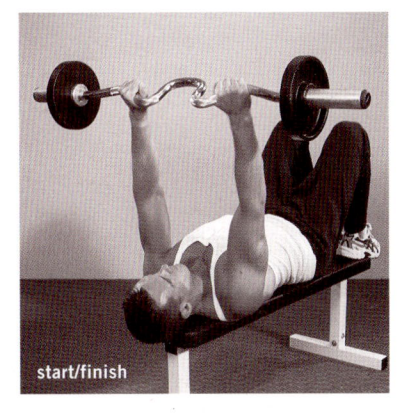

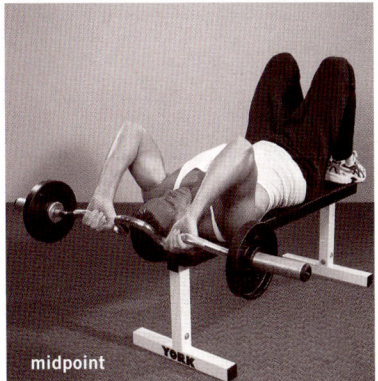

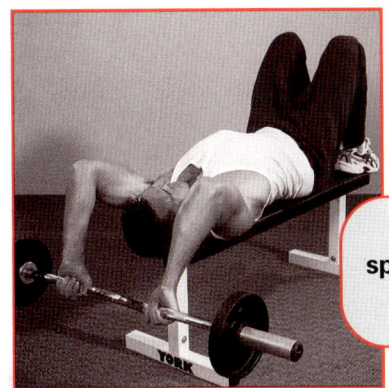

Try to avoid going too deep and your elbows splaying out to the sides as you push the weight to the top.

lying dumbell extensions

muscles working: Triceps (back arms)

Forearms (wrists)

The start/finish position: While sitting on a flat bench, grasp a dumbell in each hand, palms facing in. Lift the dumbells towards you and roll back onto the bench holding the dumbells at arms length above your chest, palms facing each other. Make sure your head is fully supported by the bench and both feet are either flat against the floor or flat against the bench.

The movement: Slowly lower the dumbells towards your shoulders bending at the elbows and finishing with the dumbells beside your ears while being sure to keep your elbows pointing in. Hold the weight at the bottom position for a count of one and then slowly push the weight, extending through the elbows and without bouncing, back to the start/finish position.

Tip Try to limit any movement through your shoulders, only the elbow joint should move. This exercise can also be done one arm at a time.

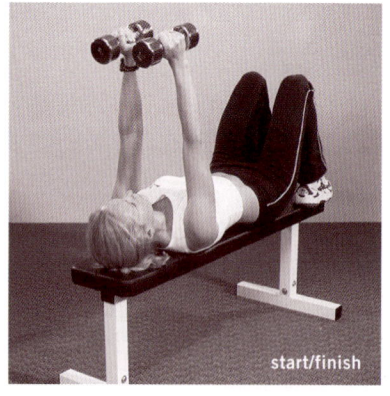

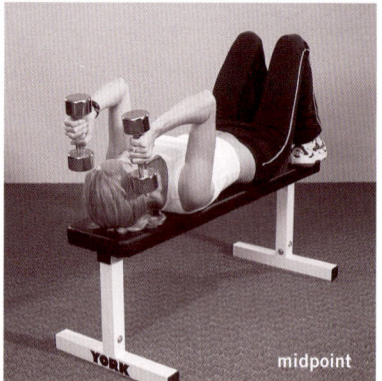

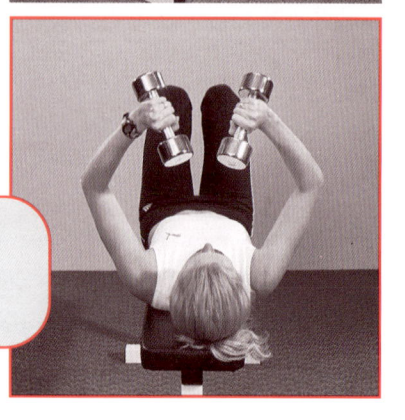

Try to avoid letting your elbows stick out to the side and always have control over the dumbells to avoid hitting your head.

single dumbell seated extension

muscles working: Triceps (back arms)

Forearms (wrists)

The start/finish position: While sitting on a flat bench with both feet flat against the floor, grasp a single dumbell, lift it above your head and hold with both hands flat against the plate, palms facing up. Keep your back straight and eyes focused ahead and elbows close by your forehead. Note: You must only use a dumbell that has securely fastened collars and weights.

The movement: Slowly lower the dumbell behind your head bending from the elbows and keeping your elbows close by your head. Lower the dumbell as far as you comfortably can with no movement through your shoulders. Hold the weight at the bottom position for a count of one and then slowly push the weight, extending through the elbows and without bouncing, back to the start/finish position being careful to clear the back of your head.

Tip Try to limit any movement through your shoulders, only the elbow joint should move and try not to let your back arch. This exercise can also be done standing.

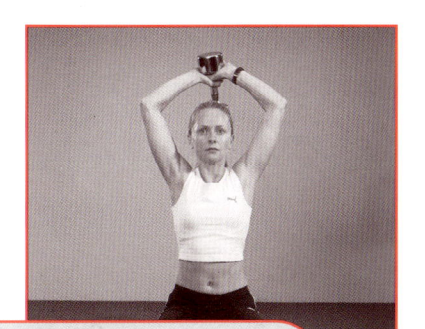

> Try to avoid letting your elbows stick out to the side and always have control over the dumbell to avoid hitting the back of your head.

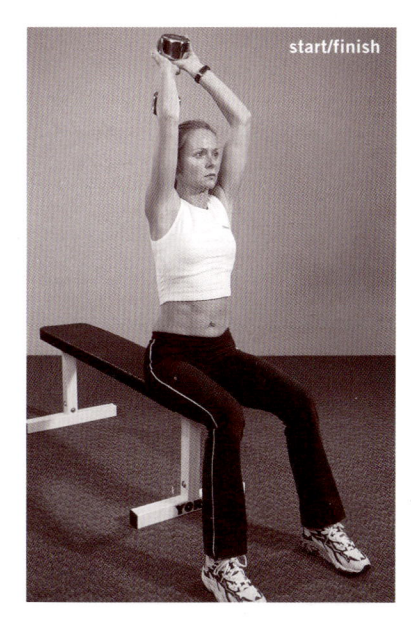

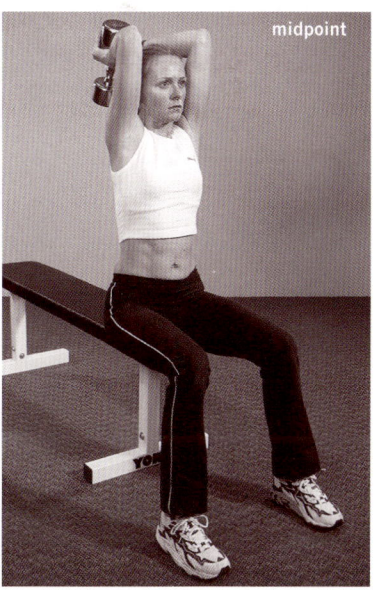

single dumbell kickbacks

muscles working: Triceps (back arms)

Forearms (wrists)

The start/finish position: Using a flat bench, place your left knee on the bench and your left hand on the bench directly below your left shoulder. Place your right foot flat against the floor and grasp a single dumbell in your right hand, palms facing in. Bring your right elbow back until it is locked in tight by your side forming a 90 degree angle at your elbow joint. Focus your eyes straight ahead on the floor in front of you and keep your shoulders square.

The movement: Slowly push the dumbell back behind you until you form a straight line from your shoulder, through your elbow and to your wrist. Make sure the line you form is parallel with the floor. Hold the weight at the back position for a count of one feeling the tricep muscle squeeze like you are trying to wring water out of a sponge and then slowly lower the weight back to the start/finish position. Complete the desired number of repetitions for the right side and repeat for the left.

Tip Try to keep your working arm elbow high to achieve a straight line parallel with the floor and keep your elbows tucked in.

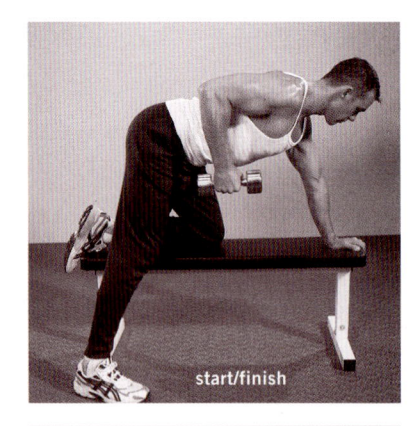

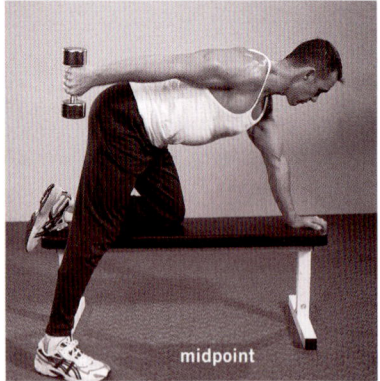

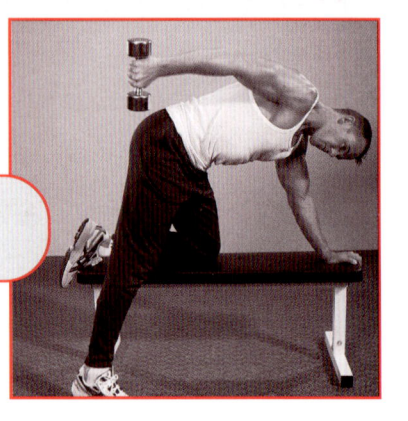

> **Try to avoid letting your body twist through the movement and keep your shoulders square.**

high cable pushdowns

muscles working: Triceps (back arms)

Forearms (wrists)

The start/finish position: Approach the high cable and grasp the pushdown bar with a slightly closer than shoulder width, overhand grip. Lock your elbows in tight by your sides and bring the handle down until your forearms are parallel with the floor. Keep your feet flat against the floor with your knees slightly bent. Your wrists should be solid, not allowing any movement up or down. Keep your head up and your shoulders back with your eyes focused straight ahead.

The movement: Slowly push the bar down until it reaches the top of your legs and your arms are forming a straight line from your shoulder, through your elbow and to your wrist. Hold the weight at the bottom position for a count of one feeling the tricep muscle squeeze and then slowly return the weight back to the start/finish position.

Tip Try to place the pushdown bar closer to your wrists on the hard part of your hand rather than in the fingers as this may cause movement thru your wrists.

> **Try to keep your body straight and avoid letting your shoulders hunch forward as you push the bar down.**

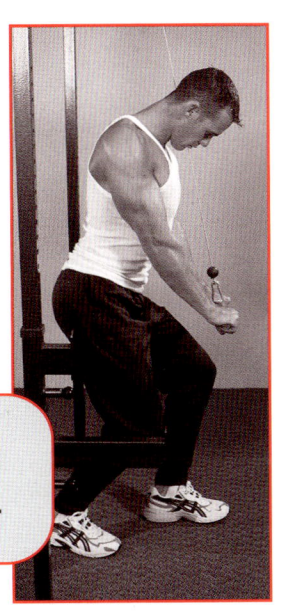

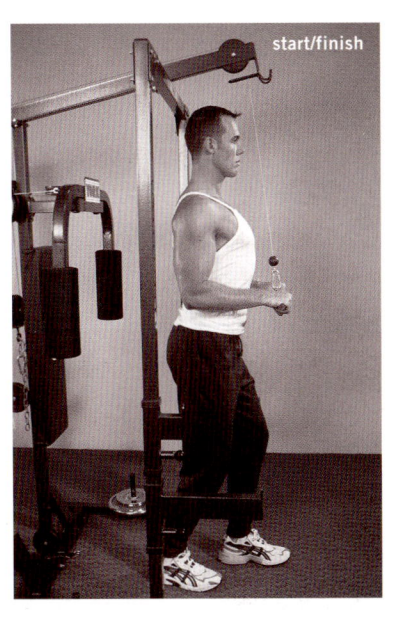

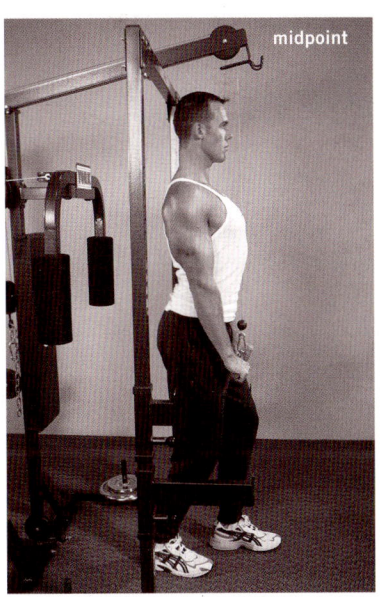

flat bench dips

muscles working **Triceps (back arms)**

Forearms (wrists)

The start/finish position: Sit on the side of a flat bench with your hands grasping the edge of the bench, fingers over the front edge. Make sure your hands are as close to your sides as possible and your feet are positioned close together at a distance away that allows a 90 degree angle in your knees when you take your weight on your hands. Keep your head up and your shoulders back with your eyes focused straight ahead.

The movement: With your body weight supported by your arms, slowly lower your body until your upper arms are parallel with the floor. As you drop, your back should almost brush the bench and your elbows should be pointing straight behind. Hold the bottom position for a count of one and then slowly straighten your arms to return to the start/finish position. Note: You should not sit back down onto the bench between each repetition.

Tip The further away from the bench that you place your feet, the harder the exercise becomes, until you eventually reach straight legs. To increase the intensity further you can also elevate your extended straight legs.

> **Try not to allow your body to drop too far to the floor as this can place undue stress on your shoulders.**

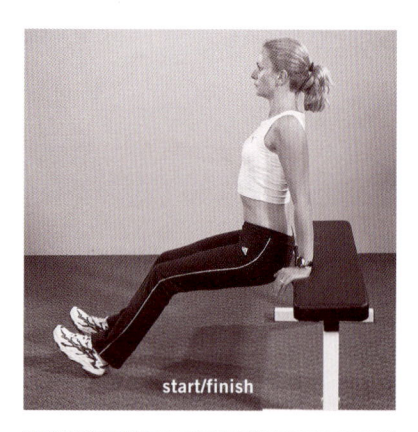

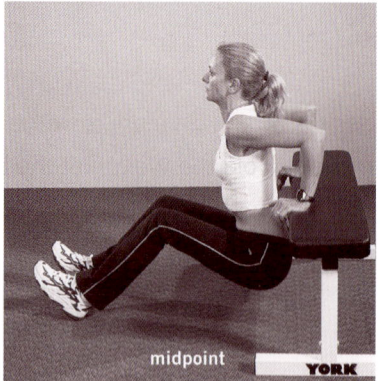

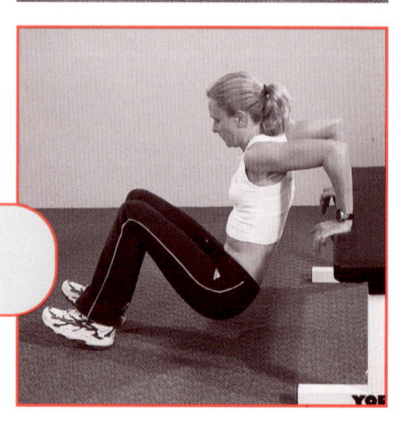

rope pushdowns

muscles working: Triceps (back arms)

                                    Forearms (wrists)

The start/finish position: Approach the high cable and grasp the double ended rope section with a thumbs up grip, palms facing each other. Lock your elbows in tight by your sides and bring the rope down until your forearms are parallel with the floor. Keep your feet flat against the floor with your knees slightly bent. Keep your head up and your shoulders back with your eyes focused straight ahead.

The movement: Slowly push the rope down until it almost reaches the top of your legs, at which point the rope handles separate and continue on past the sides of your thighs to form a straight line in each arm and give an extremely strong contraction in the tricep muscle. Hold the weight at the bottom position for a count of one feeling the tricep muscle squeeze and then slowly return the weight back to the start/finish position. Hold again for a count of one and repeat.

FOR ADVANCED LIFTERS ONLY

Tip Try to keep the rope handles from touching each other through out the full range of the exercise and keep your elbows tight by your side.

> **Try to keep your body straight and avoid letting your shoulders hunch forward as you push the rope down.**

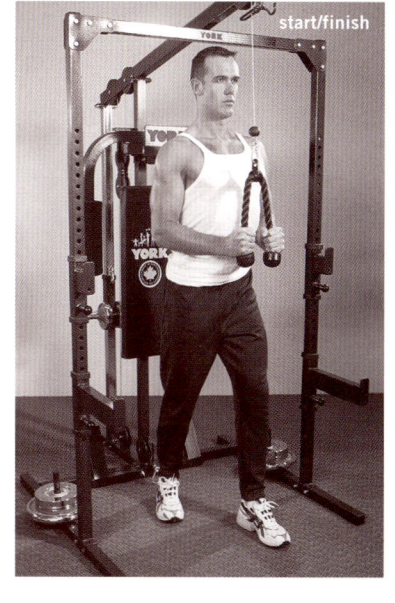

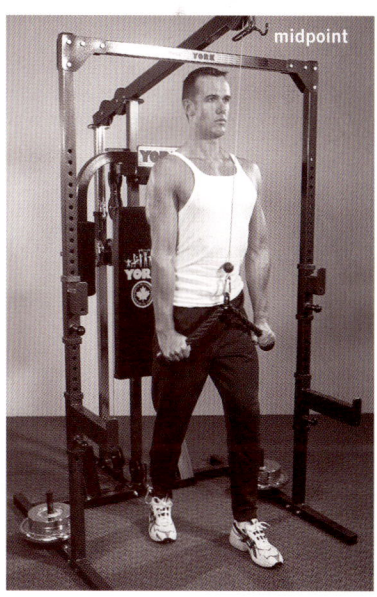

underhand pushdowns

muscles working: Triceps (back arms)

Forearms (wrists)

The start/finish position: Approach the high cable and grasp the pushdown bar with an underhand, slightly closer than shoulder width grip. Lock your elbows in tight by your sides and bring the bar down until your forearms are parallel with the floor. Keep your feet flat against the floor with your knees slightly bent and your wrists should be solid not allowing any movement up or down. Keep your head up and your shoulders back with your eyes focused straight ahead.

The movement: Slowly push the bar down until it reaches the top of your legs and your arms are forming a straight line from your shoulder, thru your elbow and to your wrist. Hold the weight at the bottom position for a count of one feeling the tricep muscle squeeze and then slowly return the weight back to the start/finish position. Hold again for a count of one and repeat.

FOR ADVANCED LIFTERS ONLY

Tip Try not to let your elbows splay out to the sides as they will want to do in this particular exercise.

> **Try to keep your body straight and avoid letting your shoulders hunch forward as you push the bar down.**

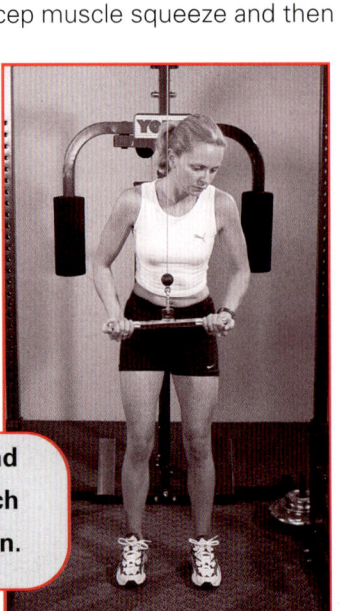

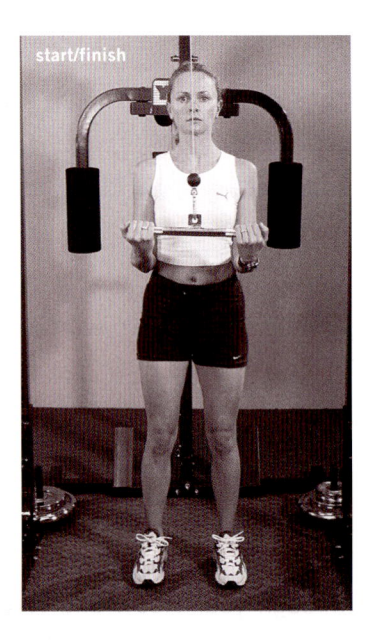

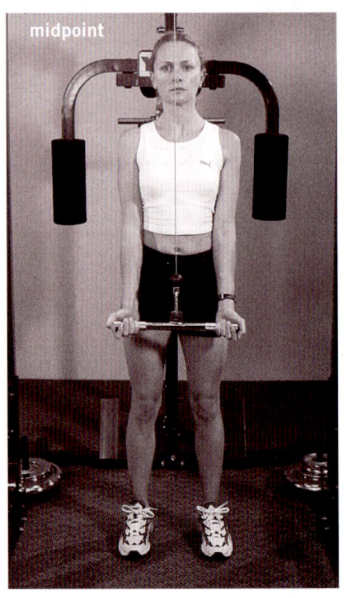

single handle pushdowns

muscles working: Triceps (back arms)

Forearms (wrists)

The start/finish position: Approach the high cable with the single handle attachment fitted and grasp the handle with your right hand with an overhand, palms facing down grip. Lock your right elbow in tight by your side and support your left hand against your body. Bring the handle down until your forearm is parallel with the floor. Keep your feet flat against the floor with your knees slightly bent. Your right wrist should be solid not allowing any movement up or down. Keep your head up and your shoulders back with your eyes focused straight ahead.

The movement: Slowly push the handle down until it reaches the top of your legs and your arm is forming a straight line from your shoulder, through your elbow and to your wrist. Hold the weight at the bottom position for a count of one feeling the tricep muscle squeeze and then slowly return the weight back to the start/finish position. Complete the desired number of repetitions for the right side and repeat for the left.

FOR ADVANCED LIFTERS ONLY

Tip You can also do this exercise with an underhand grip. Try not to let your elbow leave your side.

> **Try to keep your body straight and avoid letting your shoulders hunch forward or your body to twist as you push the handle down.**

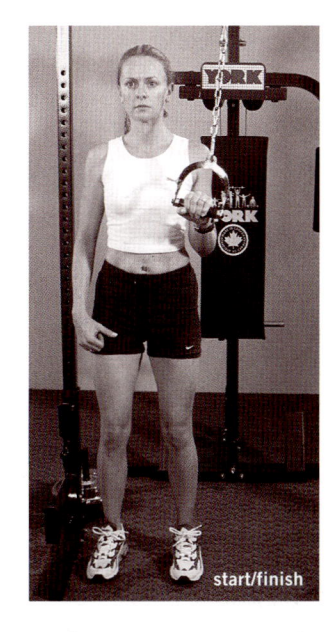

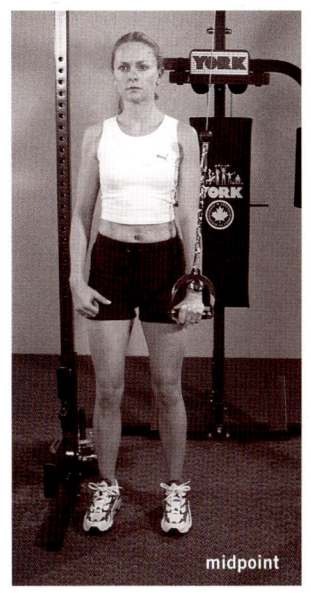

parallel bar dips

muscles working   Triceps (back arms)

　　　　　　　　　　　Forearms (wrists)

The start/finish position: Approach the vertical knee raise station of your home gym and grasp the parallel bars. Use the foot step to lift yourself up and get yourself to an arms straight position holding your bodyweight. Cross your ankles and bend your knees to a 90 degree angle so your knees point straight to the floor. Keep your head up and your shoulders back with your eyes focused straight ahead.

The movement: With your body weight supported by your arms, slowly lower your body until your upper arms are parallel with the floor. As you drop, be sure to keep your balance and avoid swinging. Your back should not arch and your elbows should be pointing directly behind you. Hold the bottom position for a count of one and then slowly straighten your arms to return to the start/finish position.

FOR ADVANCED LIFTERS ONLY

Tip You may want to start with half repetitions until you get used to holding your own full body weight.

> **Try not to allow your body to drop too far as this can place undue stress on your shoulders.**

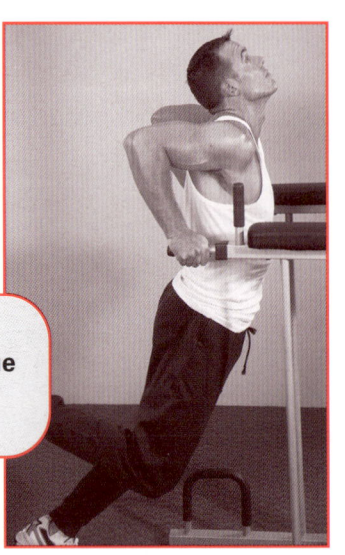

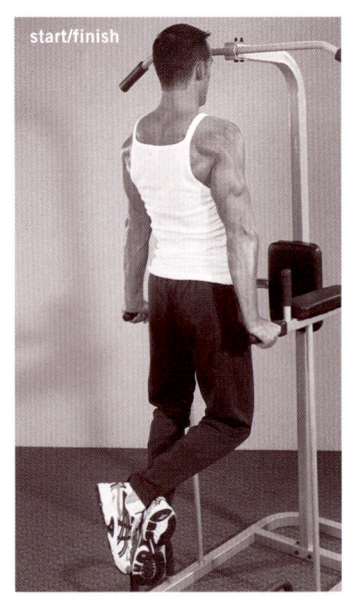

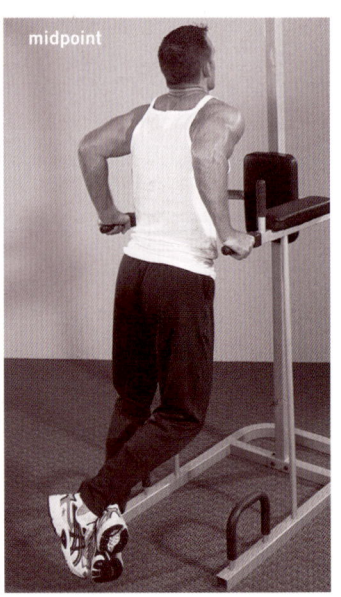

single hand dumbell extension

muscles working: Triceps (back arms)
Forearms (wrists)

The start/finish position: While sitting on a flat bench with both feet flat against the floor, grasp a single dumbell in your right hand and lift it above your head and hold with a palm facing away grip. Keep your back straight and eyes focused ahead and your right bicep close by your right ear. Support your left hand against your body.

The movement: Slowly lower the dumbell behind your head bending from the elbow and keeping your bicep close to your ear. Lower the dumbell as far as you comfortably can with no movement through your shoulders. Hold the weight at the bottom position for a count of one and then slowly push the weight, extending through the elbow and without bouncing, back to the start/finish position being careful to clear the back of your head. Complete the desired number of repetitions for the right side and repeat for the left.

FOR ADVANCED LIFTERS ONLY

Tip Try to limit any movement thru your shoulders, only the elbow joint should move and try not to let your back arch. This exercise can also be done standing.

> **Try to avoid letting your body twist and your bicep straying too far from your ear and always have control over the dumbell to avoid hitting the back of your head.**

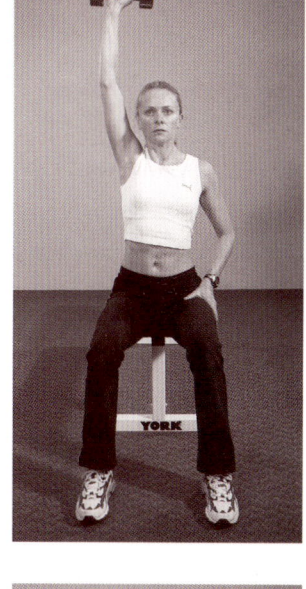

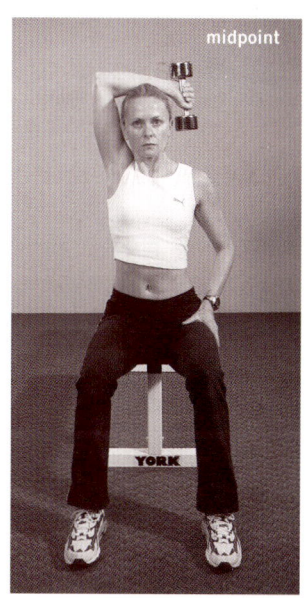

www.yorkfitness.co.uk

wrists - forearms

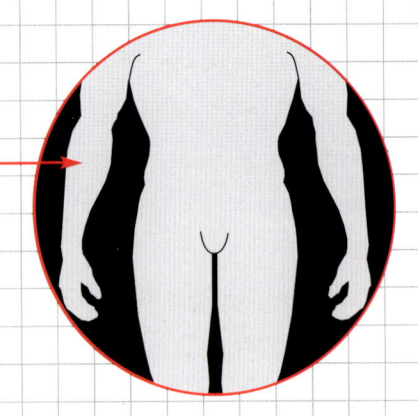

s-t-r-e-t-c-h Don't forget to stretch. Every muscle you strengthen, you should also stretch. Hold this stretch for at least 10 seconds between each set. You will also need to stretch with your palms facing down for forearm extensions. See page 260

REMEMBER Keep your abdominal and lower back muscles tight through out the movement and remember to exhale during the lifting phase.

Tips The weight should always be under your control and if you need to cheat, you are probably trying to lift too much weight.

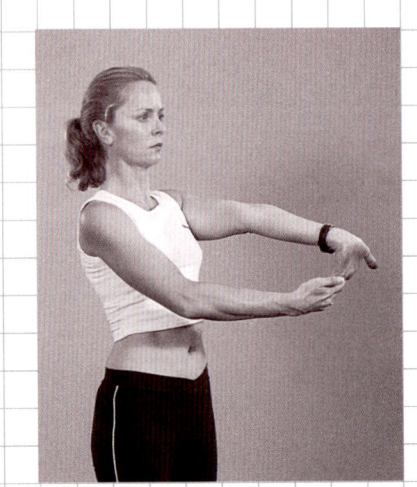

dumbell double wrist flexion

muscles working: **Forearms (wrists)**

The start/finish position: Kneel down behind a flat bench and grasp a dumbell in each hand. Place your forearms on the bench, palms up, at shoulder width and forward enough to allow your hands to drop over the edge. With the dumbell bars gripped in your fingers, keep your head up, shoulders back and your eyes focused ahead.

The movement: Slowly pull the weights back up over the edge of the bench using the muscles of the forearms. Hold the weight at the top position for a count of one and then slowly lower the weight back to the start/finish position.

Tip You will not need very heavy dumbells to do this exercise if you do it correctly. You can also do this one with a barbell or one dumbell at a time.

Try to avoid leaning back and lifting your forearms off the bench and bringing bicep work into the exercise.

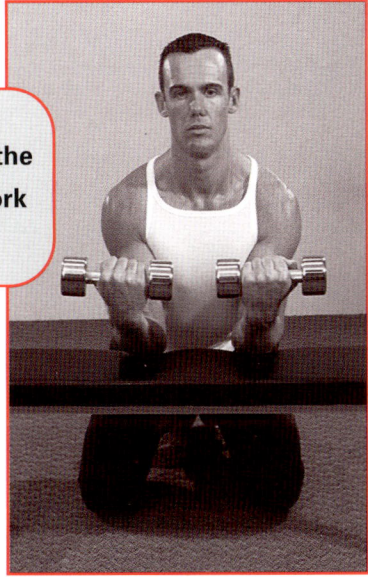

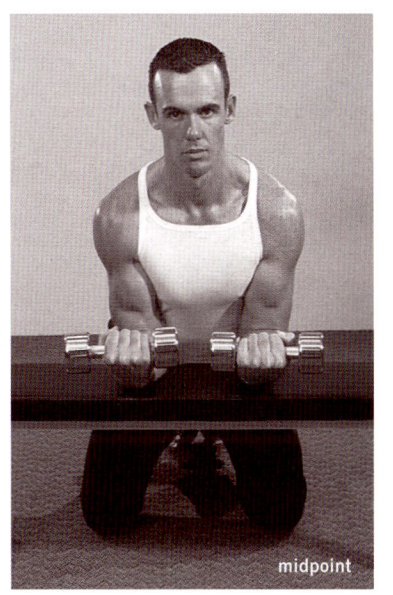

dumbell double wrist extension

muscles working: **Forearms (wrists)**

The start/finish position: Kneel down behind a flat bench and grasp a dumbell in each hand. Place your forearms on the bench, palms down, at shoulder width and forward enough to allow your hands to drop over the edge. With the dumbbell bars gripped in your fingers, keep your head up, shoulders back and your eyes focused ahead.

The movement: Slowly pull the weights back up over the edge of the bench using the muscles of the forearms. Hold the weight at the top position for a count of one and then slowly lower the weight back to the start/finish position.

Tip You will not need very heavy dumbells to do this exercise if you do it correctly. You can also do this one with a barbell or one dumbell at a time.

Try to avoid leaning back and lifting your forearms off the bench and bringing bicep work into the exercise.

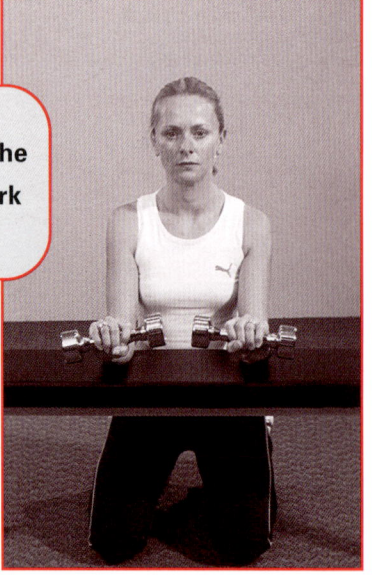

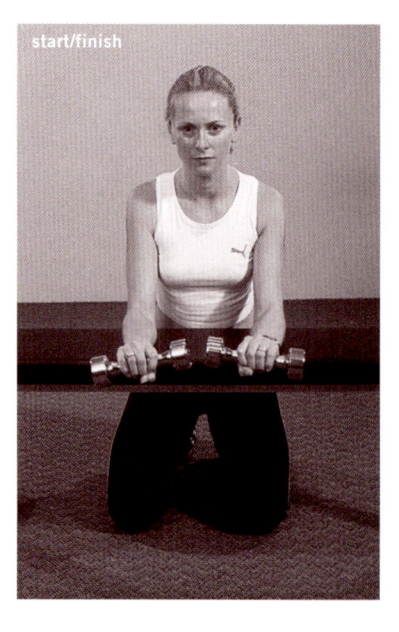

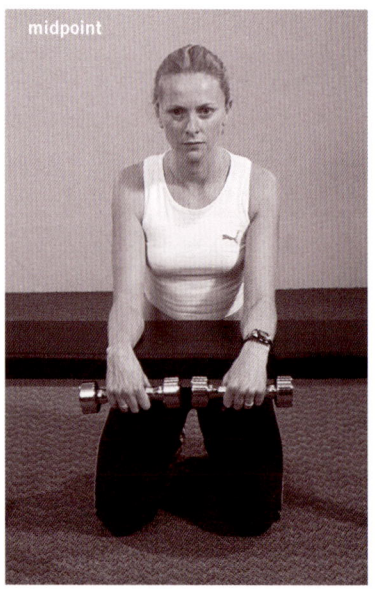

SECTION TEN torso

torso abdominals

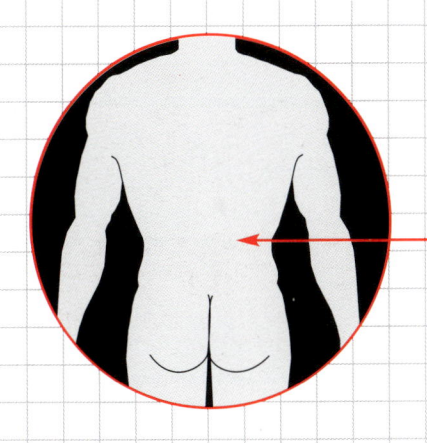

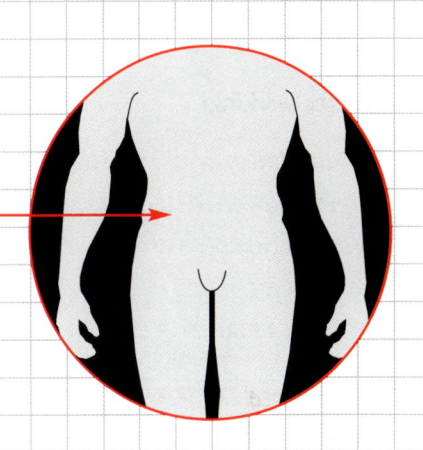

torso lower back

s-t-r-e-t-c-h Don't forget to stretch. Every muscle you strengthen, you should also stretch. Hold these stretches for at least 10 seconds between each set. See page 260

REMEMBER Keep your abdominal and lower back muscles tight through out the movement and remember to exhale during the lifting phase.

Tip There are many more additional exercises for the abdominals and lower back that can be performed on a gym ball. Consult your gym ball instruction manual for more detailed coverage.

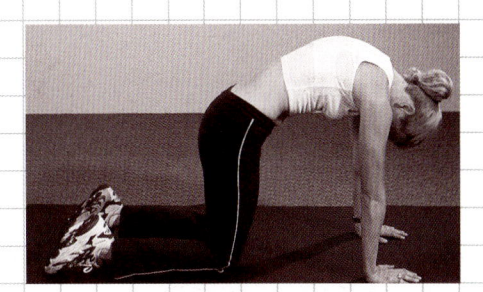

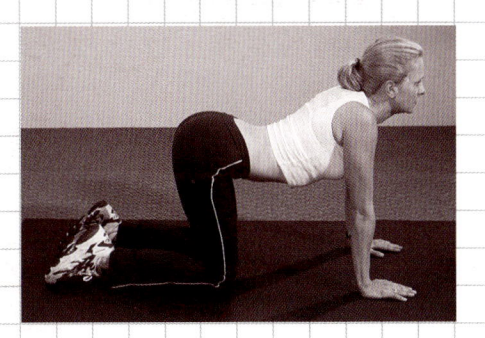

crunches feet on floor

muscles working: Abdominals (tummy)

The start/finish position: Lie flat on the floor with your arms crossed over your chest and your hands on your shoulders. Try to keep a gap between your chin and your chest about the size of a tennis ball. This will help to keep your eyes up and avoid discomfort in your neck. Your feet should be placed flat against the floor about 12 inches away from your bottom while your knees and ankles are kept together.

The movement: With your eyes high and keeping your tennis ball gap, slowly force your lower back down into the floor. When you have felt your abdominal muscles fully tighten, then start to lift your shoulders off the floor while at the same time focusing on drawing your belly button towards your spine. You should start to exhale as soon as you begin to tense your abdominal muscles and keep exhaling until you reach the midpoint where all the air should now be exhaled. Hold the top position for a count of one and then slowly lower your shoulders back towards the floor where you should not allow your body weight to fully rest on the floor and give the abdominals a break but rather keep tension at the start/finish position for a count of one then repeat.

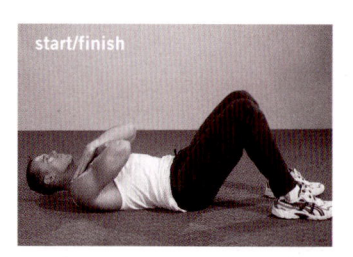

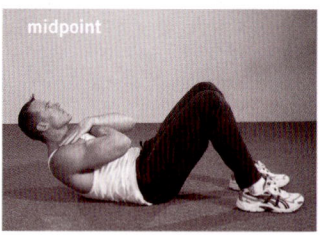

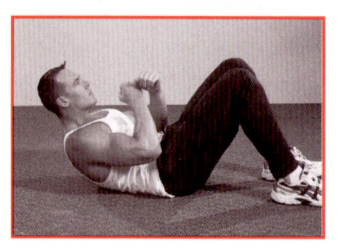

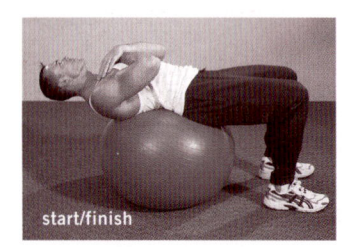

Tip A similar exercise can also be performed on a gym ball but requires a lot more balance and stability and you must be careful not to let too much body weight drop over the back of the ball.

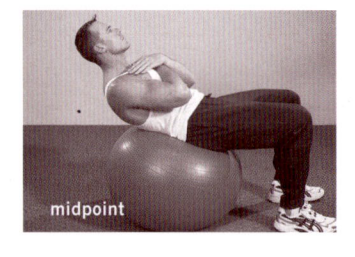

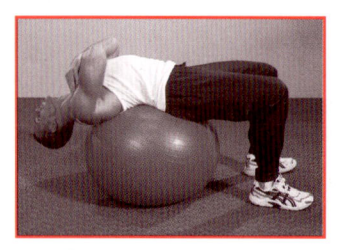

Try to avoid letting your hands lift away from your body and your chin dropping into your chest

page 168

crunches feet on bench

muscles working: Abdominals (tummy)

The start/finish position: Lie flat on the floor close to a flat bench with your hands held beside your head. Try to keep a gap between your chin and your chest about the size of a tennis ball. This will help to keep your eyes up and avoid discomfort in your neck. Place your lower legs on top of the bench creating a 90-degree angle at your hips and your knees while your knees and ankles are kept together.

The movement: With your eyes high and keeping your tennis ball gap, slowly force your lower back down into the floor. When you have felt your abdominal muscles fully tighten, then start to lift your shoulders off the floor while at the same time focusing on drawing your belly button towards your spine. You should start to exhale as soon as you begin to tense your abdominal muscles and keep exhaling until you reach the midpoint where all the air should now be exhaled. Hold the top position for a count of one and then slowly lower your shoulders back towards the floor where you should not allow your body weight to fully rest on the floor and give the abdominals a break but rather keep tension at the start/finish position for a count of one then repeat.

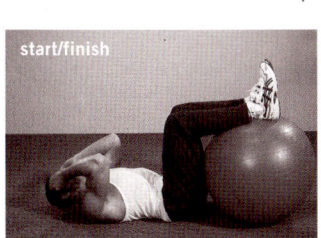

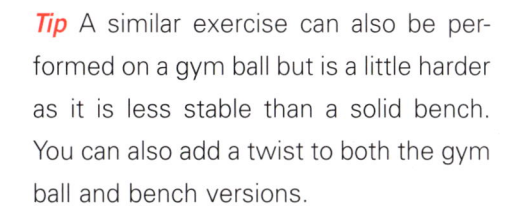

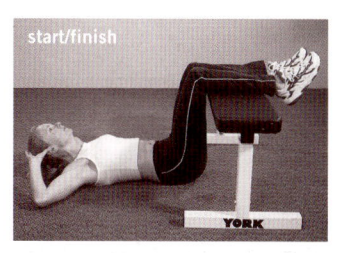

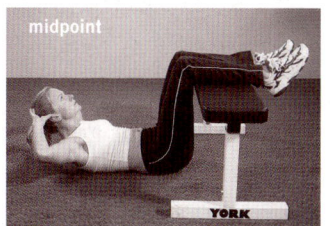

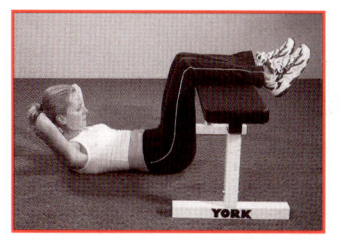

Tip A similar exercise can also be performed on a gym ball but is a little harder as it is less stable than a solid bench. You can also add a twist to both the gym ball and bench versions.

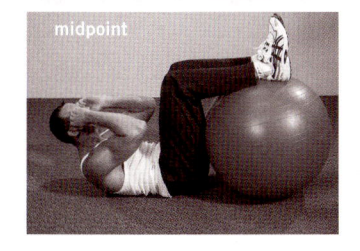

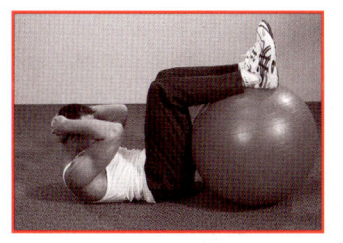

Try to avoid pulling your head forward with your hands as you begin to fatigue.

crunches feet elevated

muscles working: Abdominals (tummy)

The start/finish position: Lie flat on the floor with your hands supporting your neck and your forearms cradling your head. Try to keep a gap between your chin and your chest of about the size of a tennis ball. This will help to keep your eyes up and avoid discomfort in your neck. Raise your feet out in front creating a 90-degree angle at your hips and your knees while your knees are together and your ankles are crossed.

The movement: With your eyes high and keeping your tennis ball gap, slowly force your lower back down into the floor. When you have felt your abdominal muscles fully tighten, then start to lift your shoulders off the floor while at the same time focusing on drawing your belly button towards your spine. You should start to exhale as soon as you begin to tense your abdominal muscles and keep exhaling until you reach the midpoint where all the air should now be exhaled. Hold the top position for a count of one and then slowly lower your shoulders back towards the floor where you should not allow your body weight to fully rest on the floor and give the abdominals a break but rather keep tension at the start/finish position for a count of one then repeat.

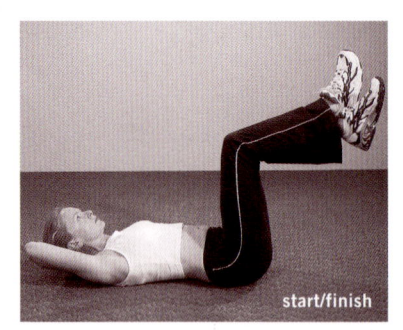

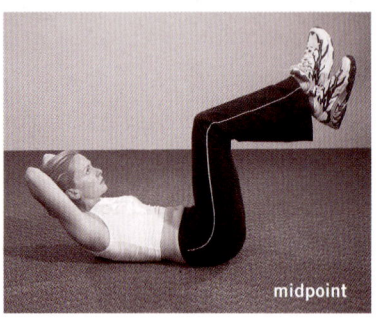

Tip You could also do this exercise with your feet up against a wall.

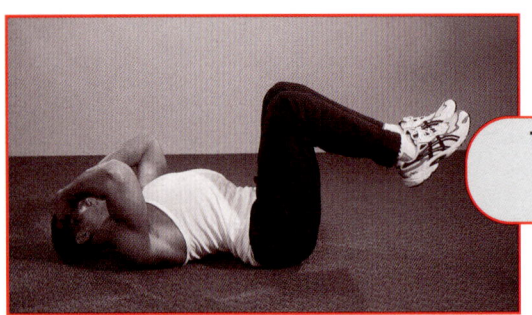

Try to avoid your lower back arching away from the floor by letting your feet drop.

crunches with knee raise

muscles working: Abdominals (tummy)

The start/finish position: Lie flat on the floor with your hands held beside your head. Try to keep a gap between your chin and your chest of about the size of a tennis ball. This will help to keep your eyes up and avoid discomfort in your neck. Raise your feet out in front creating a 90-degree angle at your hips and your knees while you keep your knees and ankles together.

The movement: With your eyes high and keeping your tennis ball gap, slowly force your lower back down into the floor. When you have felt your abdominal muscles fully tighten, then start to lift your shoulders off the floor while at the same time focusing on drawing your belly button towards your spine. As you crunch your upper body off the floor, raise your lower body to meet your upper body at the midpoint. You should start to exhale as soon as you begin to tense your abdominal muscles and keep exhaling until you reach the midpoint where all the air should be exhaled. Hold the top position for a count of one and then slowly lower your shoulders back towards the floor and your legs back to their start position. Do not allow your body weight to fully rest on the floor to give the abdominals a break but rather keep tension at the start/finish position for a count of one then repeat.

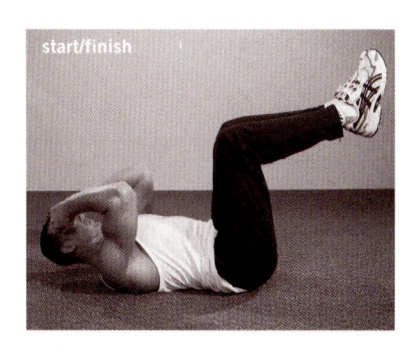

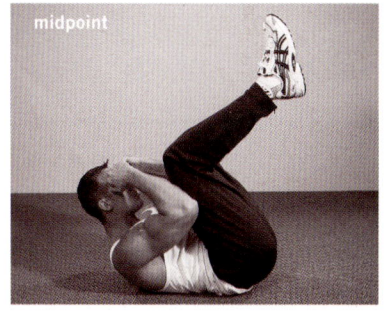

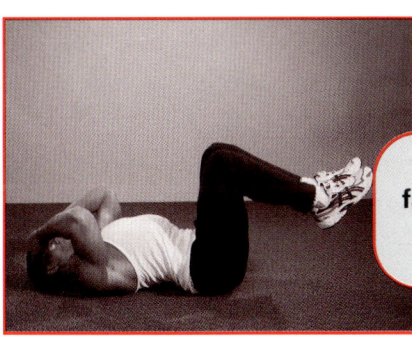

Tip You will need to do this one slowly and with purpose to avoid rolling about all over the floor.

Try to avoid letting your lower body drop too far towards the floor between each repetition so as to not place excess stress on your lower back.

floor knee raises

muscles working: **Abdominals (tummy)**

The start/finish position: Lie flat on the floor with your hands down by your side, flat against the floor at about 45 degrees from your side. Keep your head against the floor and your eyes focused on the ceiling. Raise your feet out in front creating a 90-degree angle at your hips and your knees while you keep your knees and ankles together.

The movement: With your eye high and keeping your keeping your head against the floor, slowly force your lower back down into the floor. When you have felt your abdominal muscles fully tighten, then start to raise your legs in towards your chest as you tuck into a ball. Your bottom will lift slightly off the floor as you focus on drawing your belly button towards your spine. Your knees only need to reach your chest, you are not trying to touch your toes on the floor behind you. You should start to exhale as soon as you begin to tense your abdominal muscles and keep exhaling until you reach the midpoint where all the air should now be exhaled. Hold the top position for a count of one and then slowly lower your legs back to their start position not allowing your abdominals a break but rather keeping tension at the start/finish position for a count of one then repeat.

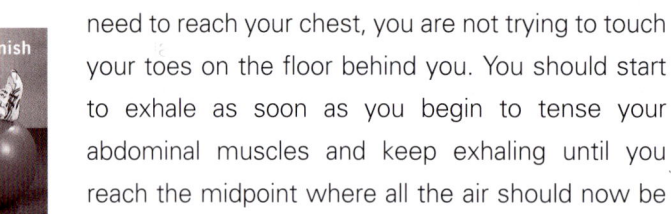

Tip A similar exercise can also be performed on a gym ball by locking the ball under your legs and raising the ball, this ensures a 90-degree angle remains at all times

> **Try to avoid 'kicking' your feet up, the 90 degree angle at your knees should not change and avoid letting your lower body drop too far towards the floor between each repetition so as to not place excess stress on your lower back.**

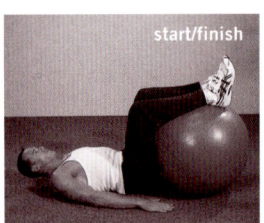

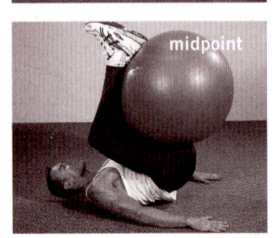

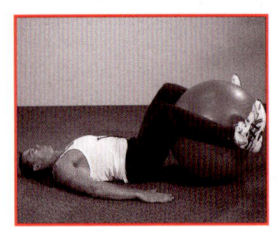

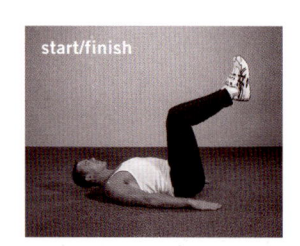

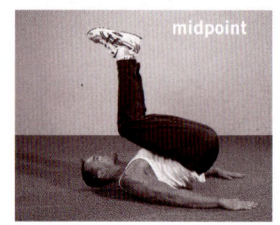

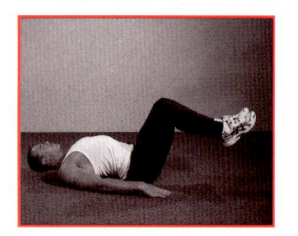

TORSO

crunches knees over

muscles working: **Abdominals (tummy)**

Obliques (side tummy)

The start/finish position: Lie flat on the floor with your arms beside your head. Try to keep a gap between your chin and your chest of about the size of a tennis ball. This will help to keep your eyes up and avoid discomfort in your neck. Your feet should be placed flat against the floor about 12 inches away from your bottom while your knees and ankles are kept together. Drop both knees over towards the floor to your right and make sure your left leg stays hard against your right.

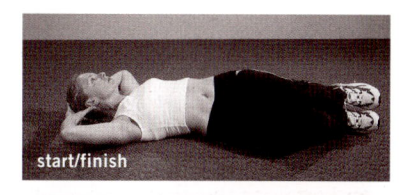

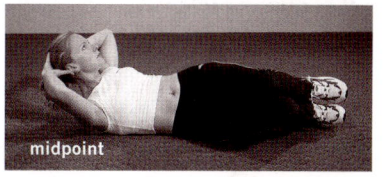

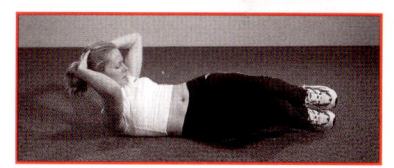

The movement: With your eyes high and keeping your tennis ball gap, slowly force your lower back down into the floor. When you have felt your abdominal muscles fully tighten, then start to lift your shoulders off the floor crunching straight ahead even though your legs are over to one side, while at the same time focusing on drawing your belly button towards your spine. You should start to exhale as soon as you begin to tense your abdominal muscles and keep exhaling until you reach the midpoint where all the air should now be exhaled. Hold the top position for a count of one and then slowly lower your shoulders back towards the floor where you should not allow your body weight to fully rest on the floor and give the abdominals a break but rather keep tension at the start/finish position for a count of one then repeat. Continue until the desired number of repetitions are completed and repeat for the other side.

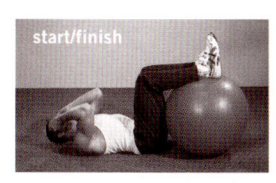

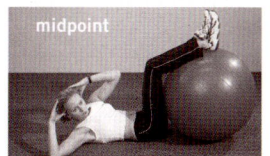

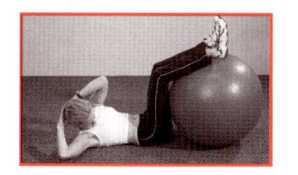

Tip A similar exercise can also be performed on a gym ball only the legs stay square over the ball and the body twists so the right elbow aims toward the left knee and vice versa.

> **Try to avoid letting your hands pull against your head and pull your chin into your chest.**

vertical knee raise

muscles working: Abdominals (tummy)

Hip flexor (upper legs)

The start/finish position: Approach the vertical knee raise section of your home gym and use the foot steps to step up. Place your back against the padded section while supporting your body weight on the elbow pads. Make sure that your elbows are positioned directly below your shoulders. Keep your shoulders back, chest high and your eyes focused straight ahead as you remove your feet from the foot steps and take your full body weight, with your legs hanging directly to the floor, knees and ankles together.

The movement: With your eyes high, slowly force your lower back into the back support pad. When you feel your abdominal muscles fully tighten, start to raise your knees toward your hand grips creating a 90 degree angle at your hip and knee joint, while at the same time focusing on drawing your belly button towards your spine. You should start to exhale as soon as you begin to tense your abdominal muscles and keep exhaling until you reach the midpoint where all the air should now be exhaled. Hold the top position for a count of one and then slowly lower your feet back down towards the floor where you should not allow your body weight to fully rest and give the abdominals a break but rather keep tension at the start/finish position for a count of one then repeat.

FOR ADVANCED LIFTERS ONLY

Tip This exercise can also be done by keeping the legs straight, making the body form an 'L' shape.

Try to avoid letting your lower back arch away from the back support pad and try not to allow your legs any swing through momentum at the bottom end of the range.

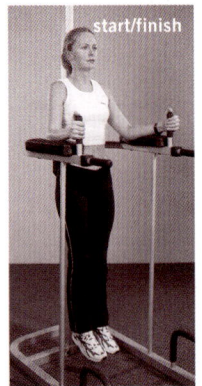

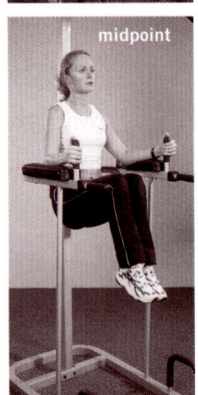

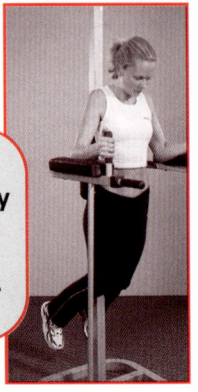

decline bench sit-ups

muscles working: Abdominals (tummy)

The start/finish position: Sit on the top of a decline sit up bench and hook your ankles under the roller pads closest to the floor. Fold your arms across your chest with your hands touching each shoulder. Try to keep a gap between your chin and your chest of about the size of a tennis ball. This will help to keep your eyes up and avoid discomfort in your neck. Brace your abdominal muscles and slightly roll back until you form a 90-degree angle at your hip joint as well as your knees. This will keep constant tension on your abdominals before you even go anywhere.

The movement: With your eyes high and keeping your tennis ball gap, slowly lower your upper body toward the bench but only travel about half way down while focusing on drawing your belly button towards your spine. When you reach the midpoint, squeeze your abdominals hard and hold for a count of one and then slowly sit back up to the start/finish position being careful not to let your back arch. Remember to sit up no further than the same 90-degree angle start position to keep the abdominals under tension.

FOR ADVANCED LIFTERS ONLY

Tip As your strength increases, try placing a small weight plate on your chest, beneath your crossed arms, to increase the intensity.

> Try to avoid going back too far and placing too much stress on your lower back by forcing an arch.

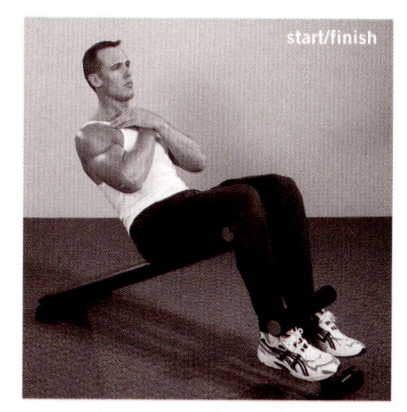

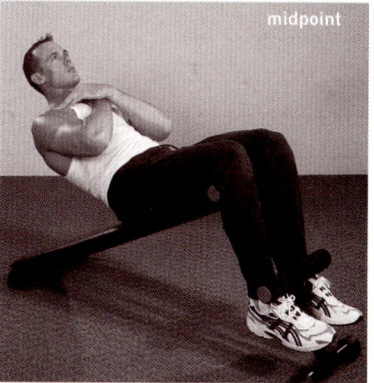

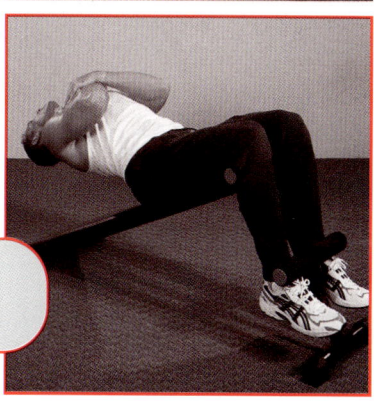

horizontal hold - knees

muscles working: Abdominals (tummy)

The action: Lie face down on the floor with your upper body weight supported on your forearms. Your eyes should be focused down on the floor in front of you and your feet and knees kept close together. Begin to squeeze your abdominals tight as you prepare to lift to the working position. Raise your hips off the floor to form a straight line from your knees to your shoulders while at the same time keeping a 90-degree angle at your elbows. While in this held position try to keep focused on squeezing your belly button towards your spine and making your waist line as narrow as possible. Hold this position for as long as you can keep tight with no wobble and then rest. You may only start with as little as 10 seconds and then try to build up to 1 minute in 10 second increases.

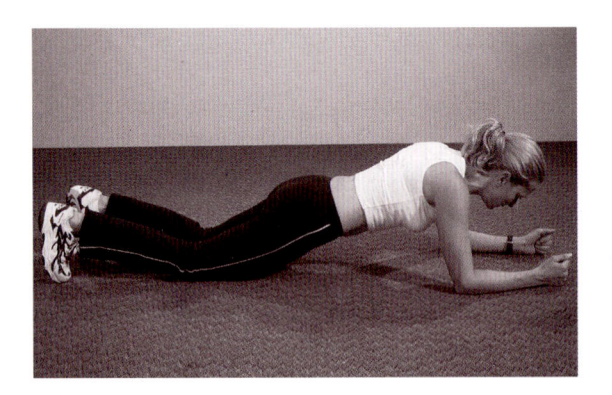

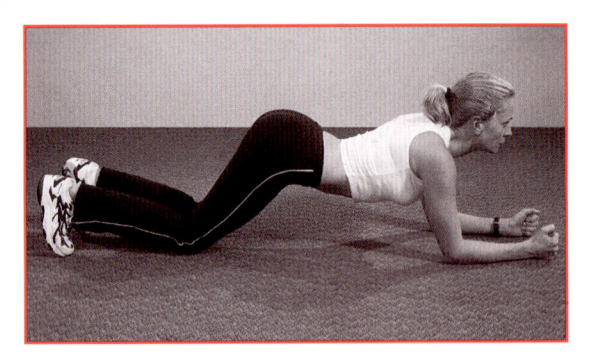

FOR ADVANCED LIFTERS ONLY

Tip A similar exercise can also be performed on a gym ball but requires a lot more balance and stability as the ball will wobble around beneath your forearms.

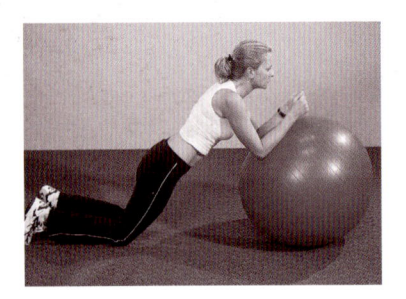

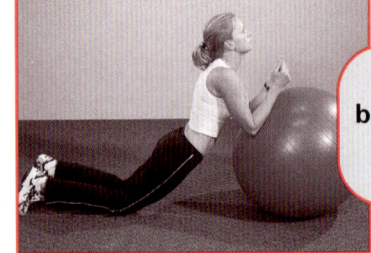

Try to avoid arching your back and lifting your head. Focus on keeping that straight line.

horizontal hold - toes

muscles working: Abdominals (tummy)

The action: Lie face down on the floor with your upper body weight supported on your forearms. Your eyes should be focused down on the floor in front of you and your feet and knees kept close together. Begin to squeeze your abdominals tight as you prepare to lift to the working position. Raise your hips off the floor to form a straight line from your toes to your shoulders while at the same time keeping a 90- degree angle at your elbows. While in this held position try to keep focused on squeezing your belly button towards your spine and making your waist line as narrow as possible. Hold this position for as long as you can keep tight with no wobble and then rest. You may only start with as little as 10 seconds and then try to build up to 1 minute in 10-second increases.

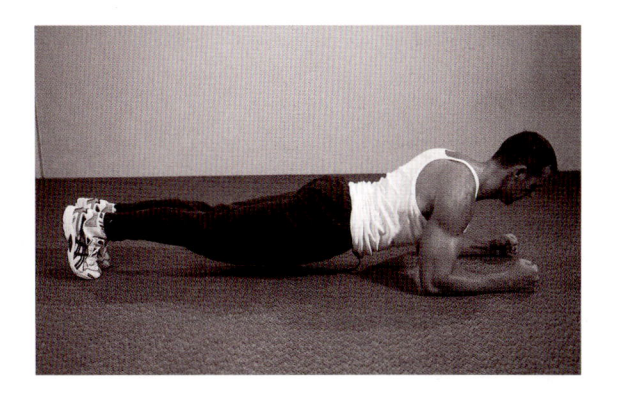

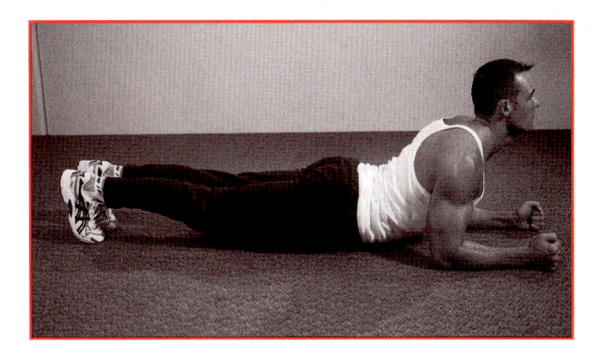

FOR ADVANCED LIFTERS ONLY

Tip A similar exercise can also be performed on a gym ball. It involves supporting your upper body on your hands at shoulder width while your ankles rest on top of the ball.

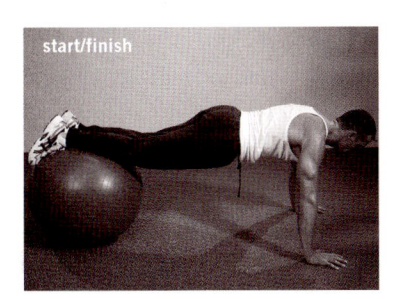

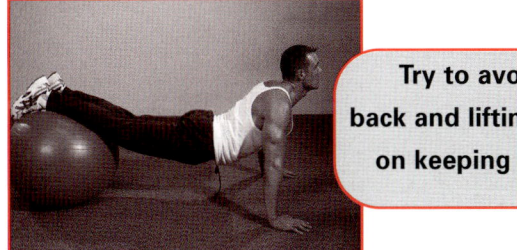

start/finish

Try to avoid arching your back and lifting your head. Focus on keeping that straight line.

hanging knee raise

muscles working: Abdominals (tummy)

Hip flexor (upper legs)

The start/finish position: Approach the chin up section of your home gym and use the footsteps to step up and grasp the bar with an overhand, shoulder width grip. Step off the footsteps and allow your body to hang directly toward the floor with your knees and ankles together as you keep your chest high and your eyes focused straight ahead.

The movement: With your eyes high, begin to tighten your abdominal muscles. When you have felt your abdominal muscles fully tighten, start to raise your knees toward your chest creating a 90-degree angle at your hip and knee joint, while at the same time focusing on drawing your belly button towards your spine. You should start to exhale as soon as you begin to tense your abdominal muscles and keep exhaling until you reach the midpoint where all the air should now be exhaled. Hold the top position for a count of one and then slowly lower your feet back down towards the floor where you should not allow your body weight to fully rest and give the abdominals a break but rather keep tension at the start/finish position for a count of one then repeat.

FOR ADVANCED LIFTERS ONLY

Tip This exercise can also be done by keeping the legs straight, and making the body form an 'L' shape.

> Try to avoid letting your body arch and your head to swing away and try not to allow your legs any swing-through momentum at the bottom end of the range.

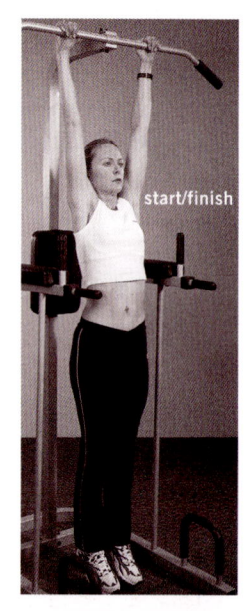

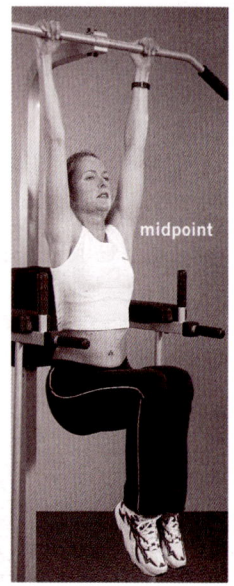

lower back hyperextension

muscles working: Erectors (lower back)

The start/finish position: Lie face down on the floor with your fingertips overlapped and placed beneath your chin. Your elbows should be out by your side. Focus your eyes down on the floor directly in front of you as your keep your ankles and knees together.

The movement: With your eyes remaining down, begin to lift your chest off the floor while at the same time raising your elbows in the same fashion as you keep both feet hard against the floor. When you reach the midpoint, squeeze your lower back muscles hard and hold for a count of one before slowly lowering back towards the floor where you should not allow your body weight to fully rest and give the lower back muscles a break but rather keep tension at the start/finish position for a count of one then repeat.

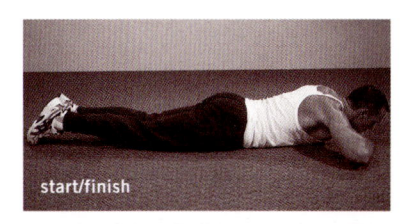

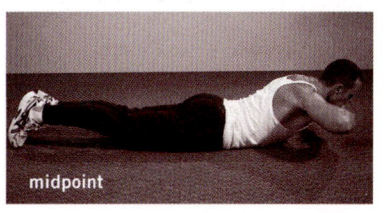

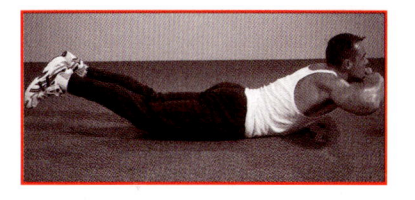

THOSE WITH LOWER BACK PROBLEMS SHOULD TAKE EXTREME CARE WITH THIS EXERCISE

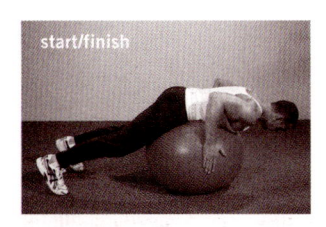

Tip Try to do this exercise slowly while keeping the abdominal muscles tight. A similar exercise can also be performed on a gym ball but requires a lot more balance and stability as the ball will wobble around beneath you, so you may need your hands for stability.

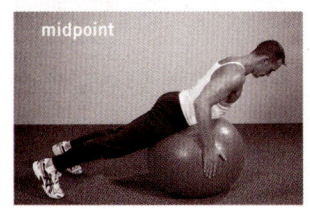

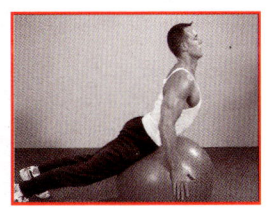

> Try to avoid going up too high and lifting your head. This will place too much stress on your lower back by forcing an arch. Try to also keep both feet on the floor.

single arm and leg raise

muscles working: Erectors (lower back)

The action: Lie face down with your forehead on the floor and your arms outstretched in front of you. Focus your eyes down as your keep your ankles and knees together. With your eyes remaining down, slowly begin to lift your left arm at the same time as you lift your right leg. When you reach the midpoint position, squeeze your lower back muscles hard and hold for a count of one before slowly lowering back towards the floor where you will need to pause for a brief moment as you swap to lift your right arm and left leg. However you should not allow your body weight to fully rest and give the lower back muscles a break but rather keep tension at the start/finish position for a count of one then repeat.

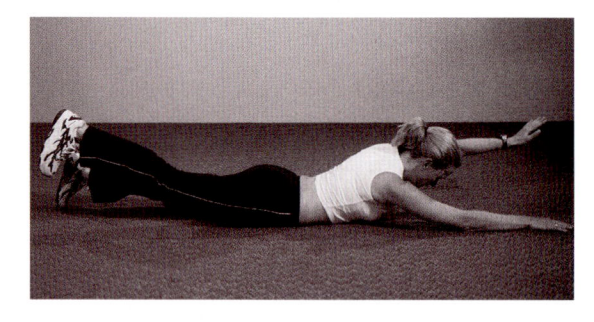

THOSE WITH LOWER BACK PROBLEMS SHOULD TAKE EXTREME CARE WITH THIS EXERCISE

Tip Try to do this exercise slowly while keeping the abdominal muscles tight. Try to make sure you pull your toes towards your shins, ensuring your heel is the leading point of your leg travel.

> **Try to avoid going up too high and lifting your head. This will place too much stress on your lower back by forcing an arch.**

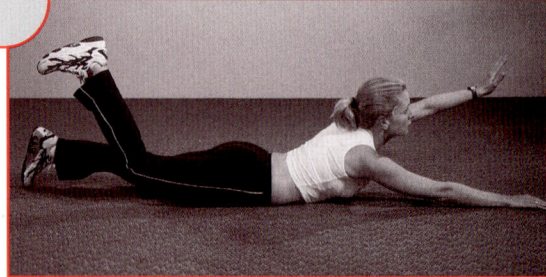

SECTION ELEVEN cardio training

Everybody needs to do some cardio training. Put simply, and aside from anything else, it keeps you healthy. Maintaining an elevated heart rate for an extended period of time has numerous benefits, these include:

- Increased fitness levels
- Increased blood flow to muscles and organs
- Body fat reduction
- Increased energy and vitality

Sounds good doesn't it? No huffing and puffing when walking up stairs, more energy to chase the kids around, and the real possibility of taking up a sport of some kind. These are the sorts of things that people look to achieve from regular cardio training, other than the obvious and most popular goal – to burn body fat.

Cardio machines these days are also built for comfort and ease of use, they come with detailed computers that tell you everything you need to know, they are aesthetically attractive, and are designed to suit all budgets. They're not subject to seasonal weather either; you can jump on your bike at any time of the day or night that suits you. That's the beauty of having these things set up at home, it's there to be used at your convenience.

Cardio machines, when used correctly are a brilliant way to stay fit and healthy at home without spending a cent on gym memberships that run out and often don't get used to their full value anyway. All you have to do is use them.

Of course we know what you are saying right now, how many people buy these machines and use them as expensive clothes hangers? And our answer yes, it does happen. But remember all that stuff you read at the start about staying motivated? That's the key, its simple; you just need to want to do it. There are also lots of people out there with cardio machines in their homes that get used all the time. Those people all have one common asset, motivation. So no more talk about clothes hangers, just get in there and do it.

It does get a little more technical than just getting on the treadmill for a run though. There are different types of cardio training for different goals. That isn't to say that if you did jump on the treadmill and go for it that you wouldn't get results, you just might not get the desired result and in the desired time frame. That's what we're here for, to help you get the most out of every training session and to educate and inform you of just what your body is capable of, so read on.

There are also other ways to elevate the heart rate while utilising all of your home studio equipment – it's called circuit training, something you may or may not have heard of. These classes are popular in gyms because they require a lot less co-ordination than an ordinary aerobic class. They can also be a good deal more interesting for those who like to use the machines.

Circuit training involves timed periods of exercise on a range of machines that are designed and laid out to keep your heart rate elevated through use of major muscle groups of the body. Each station will involve somewhere between one and five minutes of work with a rest time of 15 to 60 seconds between stations. The idea is to keep moving from station to station while following the nominated work and rest periods. The number of laps of the circuit performed will depend on the amount of stations per lap, the goals of the participant/s and the abilities of the participant/s.

It will be easy for you to set up a small circuit in your home studio. Your only criteria will be available space. If you have assigned your spare garage to a training facility, then you will be able to set up a fairly elaborate circuit. If you have managed to squeeze a bench and free weights into the other end of your living room, you can still set up an effective circuit, just use a few less stations. We will talk more about circuits in 'cardio for fitness'

cardio for good health

There are a lot of people out there who are not out to break any land speed records, they don't want to look like Mr. or Mrs. Universe and they don't want to spend hours in their home studio burning off every gram of fat on their bodies. They just want to look and feel a bit healthier.

Does this sound like you?

Don't tell us, you work long hours, don't do any exercise at the moment and know you should be. You feel sluggish and tired most of the time and you know that some gentle training a few times a week will make you feel a whole lot better, or that's what you've heard anyway.

Hitting the cardio gear to keep you healthy inside and out is a great idea. Many adults train for this reason, it keeps them active, strong and flexible and in great shape. But this type of training is not just for older adults, it's user-friendly, so just about anyone can do it, from kids through to the elderly.

When using good quality machines, there is little or no impact, the machine can be adjusted to your size requirements, and your progress is easily monitored via heart rate monitors and pre-set programs.

Gentle cardio training will increase your fitness level, helping you get through day-to-day tasks easier and with more energy. Your flexibility will improve too, through increased range of motion with the muscles of the upper and lower body and you will more than likely burn off some excess body fat.

the guidelines

how often? This form of training is gentle. At this level you should not be stressing joints or muscles to any extent, which means that there is no need for a recovery period after each session. This training can be done every day. We suggest five to six times per week.

how long? 30 to 60 minutes duration, including warm up and cool down.

how hard? You should be able to comfortably hold a conversation without struggling for breath. The exercise should not be so easy that you do not feel like you are doing anything though. By the end of your training session, you should be feeling sufficiently tired, the muscles should be warm and should feel as though they have 'done some work'.

warm up. Start at a pace that is 3/4 of the total workload that you will perform e.g. if you will walk on a treadmill at 6kph, your warm up pace will be 4.5kph. Maintain this pace for 5 minutes, and then increase it to your total workload.

cool down. Use the same guideline for cooling down as for warming up only reversed. Don't forget to stretch before you begin and after you finish your training session.

heart rate. Heart rate monitoring is handy with this form of training but not essential. Follow the guidelines for health training for your age on our heart rate chart if you will be using a heart rate monitor, this will keep you in a training zone that is 50% - 60% of your maximum heart rate.

The chart will keep you inside a zone that will have you relying on both body-fat and sugars for energy, and at a level that will provide you with enough exertion to maintain your fitness level while also slowly and steadily burning fat.

Regardless of your goals, heart rate monitors are a great tool and will help you to better understand your body's functions during a training session. It will also take the guesswork out of whether you are training in your optimum range.

how does it work?

Your body was designed for regular exercise; ok not the type that we do on treadmills and resistance machines, but the manual stuff. Once upon a time when there was no such thing as washing machines, remote controls and automatic garage doors, we were a much more active bunch.

These days, things have changed and we are not using our bodies the way we are supposed to, so we now rely on machines to help us. Muscles have to be worked with resistance exercises and the heart, which is also a muscle, has to be worked as well. Hence the name cardio-training, designed to give your heart a work out by making it pump faster to get blood around the body.

Training the heart to be more efficient at pumping blood around the body is important. Your improvements in cardio vascular fitness can be marked by checking your resting heart rate. Someone who does no exercise will have a reasonably high resting heart beat (genetic differences aside). If this person then undertakes a program of regular exercise designed to specifically increase their fitness levels, they will more than likely see a decrease in their resting heart rate. We have seen it happen with just about all clients during our years as personal trainers.

What this means is that through putting the heart under load, just like we do with any other muscle to make it stronger, the heart becomes more efficient at it's job and therefore doesn't have to work as hard, hence a lower resting heart rate.

Tip Check your resting heart rate first thing in the morning, preferably before you even get out of bed, this will give you the most accurate indication. This is the best time because you have done no exercise and have had no stimulation of any kind e.g. music, television, caffeine etc. These things will all increase your heart rate.

Two fingers placed on the side of the neck, below the jaw and forward of the ear should pick up a beat. Hold this and then count the number of beats in ten seconds and times it by six to get your total beats per minute. Or if you prefer, count the number of beats in a 30 second period and then times it by two.

Bear in mind that this form of monitoring will produce a different result to that of a heart rate monitor. Holding the fingers to the neck will provide a manipulative or vascular reading because of the pressure applied to find the beat. A heart rate monitor will give you a true indication, but it is not essential. Either will be fine, just don't use one method the first time and the other method the next, stick with the same routine each time to ensure accurate comparisons.

Compare your resting heart rate as often as you want, don't expect to see results in a few days though. Our advice is to perform this test about once a month. As long as you have been a good little exerciser and done all your training sessions for the month, you should see a decrease in your resting heart rate.

cardio for weight loss

If you are doing cardio training for the purpose of losing body fat, it is important for you to regularly monitor your heart rate to ensure that you are within the zone that will have you burning the most amount of body-fat for energy.

The bottom line here is that you need to burn off that excess fat, and there are two approaches you can take. The first is slow and steady. The good news here is that this form of training is easy, you won't feel like you are going to drop from exhaustion or lack of air to the lungs. You will have to be patient though, because to get results from this kind of training, you need to be doing it for about an hour at a time, most days of the week.

The second approach is the faster, more intense one. This involves high-level cardio training performed for 30 minutes or so. At this level your body is working quite hard and so we recommend you train every second day and allow yourself some time to recover between sessions.

Which approach you take will depend on your preferences, the time you have available for exercising and your physical abilities. If all this stuff is new to you and you are starting out from the beginning, we suggest you take the slow and steady approach. You can be assured that it won't be long before your strength, stamina and confidence increase and you will be able to push yourself just that little bit harder each session. This will be the time to increase the intensity and look at modifying your routine to be more in line with the fast, intense approach.

However, if you continue to get results from your hour-long cardio sessions each day and you are still enjoying your training 12 months down the track, then don't change. This slow and constant form of training is great for those with old sports injuries or legacies that will continue to cause pain and discomfort during high-level training. In this case it's just not worth thrashing yourself and then paying for it for weeks afterward because your knee joints ache from all those years of netball or soccer.

On the other hand, you may be approaching an age where you lack the aggression and drive to work at such an intense pace even though you are relatively fit and healthy. In this case perhaps a combination of the two would be suitable.

The downfall of sticking with a slow and steady routine is that you are not constantly supplying your mind and body with a new challenge. For your mind this means getting bored with what you are doing and possibly dropping out altogether. For your body the lack of new challenges will see your results plateau. The body is a clever machine and will adapt to a constant form of strain quite quickly, therefore if your routine is not assessed regularly and the intensity increased, you will stop achieving results. You will maintain what you have achieved so far; you just won't see any further changes.

The fast, intense approach will be better suited to those who are familiar with cardio training. If you have an understanding of what it feels like to push your body close to its limits, then you may want to adapt the principles of the fast, intense approach. This form of training isn't easy, that's for sure, but it has been suggested in recent times, and we tend to agree, that elevating your heart rate to a high level for shorter periods of time is more effective in the quest for body fat reduction. Basically because of the number of calories you will burn.

On a long, slow distance workout your body will draw a greater percentage of its energy from fat storage and a lesser percentage from sugar storage.

On a high intensity session, the opposite occurs, however total calories burned are far greater and although in percentage terms it would seem that you burn more fat on long slow distance exercise, your total calories burnt are far less than high intensity which means that in simple terms a greater percentage of fewer calories is not as beneficial to fat loss as a lesser percentage of calories burnt. The amount of fuel drawn from fat can be just as high if not higher from high intensity effort as well as the greater benefits of raising the metabolic rate to ensure your body continues to burn up calories throughout your day.

Now we are not discounting the slow and steady approach altogether, there is no doubt that you will burn body fat by following this method. We are simply saying that the fast, intense approach is a more efficient way of doing it.

As suggested earlier, there are plenty of good reasons to stick with a gentle training format, so make up your mind which will be best for you based on your own sound principles and ability. Remember that every body is different, what works for one will not work for another, and after all, nothing is set in concrete, if you don't like what you are doing, change it.

The bottom line is, burn as many calories as you can during your training session and the stored body fat will begin to disappear. There are no secrets and there is a time for each form of training, however for maximum results it stands to reason that the harder you work, the greater the benefits.

Tip Make sure you set the television or stereo up before you start so that you have an enjoyable distraction. Reading a book can also help to pass the time, although this will not be possible at a high intensity or on machines such as a rower.

Tip You also don't have to spend all of your time on the one machine, if you have more than one piece of cardio equipment at home, try dividing your time between them, this will cut down on the boredom factor. If you only have one piece of equipment and you do find this form of training boring, a distraction such as television will help, try taping your favourite show and watching it while you train.

We also highly recommend that you include at least one, preferably two, resistance sessions each week as well as your cardio training. Weight training is extremely useful in the quest for body-fat loss because it will increase your overall lean muscle mass; that is it makes your muscles bigger. Carrying more muscle means that you will burn more calories overall as muscle requires more energy to perform day-to-day tasks, so the more muscle tissue you have, the more body-fat you will burn.

the guidelines

how often? Slow and Steady - For maximum results, this training needs to be performed most days of the week. Aim for five to six sessions per week and include one 'training-free' day each week as well. This form of training is gentle and will not require any recovery time between sessions. It can also be backed up with your resistance session on the same day if you wish (one in the morning, one in the afternoon).

Fast and furious – Give yourself at least 48 hours recovery time between these sessions, and also take into account your resistance sessions for the week. Aim for three sessions each.

how long? Slow and Steady - Minimum of 45 minutes, you can keep going for as long as you like!

Fast and furious – 30 to 40 minutes per session, including warm-up and cool-down.

how hard? Slow and Steady - As with health training, you should be able to comfortably hold a conversation without struggling for breath. The exercise should not be so easy that you do not feel like you are doing anything though. By the end of your training session, you should be feeling sufficiently tired, the muscles should be warm and should feel as though they have 'done some work'.

Fast and furious – Your body will be working close to its maximum capabilities here, so you can expect to be a little uncomfortable during your session. You will be able to talk but not to hold a conversation. Concentrate on your breathing and get as much air as you can in through your nose and out through your mouth. It is not unusual to feel a little light-headed or nauseous, but stop if these symptoms continue to occur and seek a medical check up.

warm up. Slow and Steady - Start at a pace that is 3/4 of the total workload that you will perform e.g. if you will walk on a treadmill at 6kph, your warm up pace will be 4.5kph. Maintain this pace for 5 minutes, and then increase it to your total workload.

Fast and furious – Choose a comfortable pace that is roughly half that of your total workload. Maintain this pace for 5 minutes, stop and stretch, and then move into your work phase.

cool down. Slow and Steady - Use the same guideline for cooling down as for warming up, only reversed. Don't forget to stretch before you begin and after you finish your training session.

Fast and furious – Use the same guideline for cooling down as for warming up, only reversed. And stretch again at the completion of your cool-down.

heart rate. Slow and Steady - Follow the guidelines for fat burning for your age on our heart rate chart if you will be using a heart rate monitor. This will keep you inside a training zone that is 60% - 70% of your maximum heart rate.

Fast and furious – Follow the guidelines for intense fat burning for your age on our heart rate chart if you will be using a heart rate monitor. This will keep you inside a training zone that is 70% - 80% of your maximum heart rate.

Stop to take your pulse periodically if you are training without a heart rate monitor and adjust your workload accordingly. For example if your pulse rate is lower than the guidelines, increase the intensity, if it is higher, decrease the intensity.

Remember that a pulse rate is different to heart rate and should serve as a guideline only. Although the figures will be similar, a heart rate monitor will always provide a more accurate reading.

how does it work?

Your body draws energy from two different sources to function, fat and sugar. Both sources of energy are readily available at all times but will be utilised differently depending upon what type of activity your body is performing at the time. Sugar is mostly relied upon for short bursts of explosive energy, e.g. running for the bus. Fat is your long, slow distance fuel.

Your body stores excess fat and sugar for use as fuel later on, and that is the unsightly stuff that none of us like, the stuff you need to burn off. If you are expending more energy on a daily basis than you are eating, that is keeping active, training regularly and following a low-fat healthy diet, your body will be utilising all calories that are taken in, and there will be little or no excess for storage. Once you are in this position, your body will be constantly tapping into stored energy for fuel, and your body fat levels will be reduced.

cardio for fitness

If you are training for fitness, then you may have a specific goal, like completing a fun run or walk, or may be something more serious like a mini-marathon. You may be going snow skiing and so you want to improve your fitness level to get more out of your trip. On the otherhand you may want increased stamina for your Saturday afternoon football or netball match, or maybe you just want to tackle day-to-day tasks easier and with more gusto.

First of all, you need to be aware that any form of training will increase your 'fitness level', that is your body's tolerance to exercise, the more strain you put your body under, the more resilient it will become. When training with the specific goal of increasing your fitness and becoming more efficient at exercising, you need to have a clear-cut idea of what you want to achieve and how you want to achieve it.

If you have a specific goal like the ones mentioned above e.g. a fun run or ski trip, then your program and form of training should be different to that of someone who just wishes to feel better. Your goals should be set out three to six months before the event and you will need to do some 'sports specific' training as well as fitness work to improve your cardio vascular system. Sports specific training for skiing for example would involve lots of leg work to strengthen muscles and prepare them for six or so hours of constant exercise. Sports specific training for a fun run would involve plenty of endurance work for the legs and so on. So give some thought as to what your goals are and design a program based on those goals.

Ok once you have worked out what your fitness goals are, its time to get into it. The bottom line for everyone here is that you want to elevate your heart rate to a level which will have you working quite hard and therefore train the heart to be more efficient at working both at rest and during exercise, thus increasing your level of fitness.

This form of training will be the hardest of the three because of the level you will push yourself to during your sessions. However, unlike the fast and furious method for fat loss, you will get small breaks during your session when your heart rate should be lowered and you will get a chance to recover.

Fitness training involves elevating your heart rate to a very high level – around 90% of your maximum heart rate, to maintain this level, you will need to be training fairly rigorously. Staying at this level for 30 or 40 minutes though is extremely taxing and so you will need to take small intervals of rest between, hence the name interval training.

A fitness program would typically involve one to two minute bouts of intense exercise followed by a recovery period of 30 to 60 seconds and so on. If your cardio machine has pre-set programs, you will probably find one called interval training – that's the one to follow. Programs should also have different user levels, so make sure you chose the one that will have you working inside your heart rate training zone. Alternatively you could follow your own format for fitness training based on your preferences for duration of workloads and your current fitness level.

It stands to reason that you will need to closely monitor your heart rate if you wish to improve your fitness since this whole routine is based around cardio vascular health. Follow the designated zone for your age and remember that your heart rate will drop during the recovery phase of your program. Don't worry too much about this unless it is taking a long time for your heart rate to elevate to your training zone once you begin the work phase again, if so you may want to increase the intensity or decrease your rest time.

Tip If you have a heart rate monitor and it has the feature that allows you to set training zones, then take advantage of it. This will prevent you looking at the monitor all the time to find out what your heart rate is doing. Most monitors with this feature will be silent whilst you are in your training zone, but if you go above or below, a steady alarm will sound to let you know.

Tip If you do not have a heart rate monitor, check your heart rate at the end of every second work phase. You wont have to do this all the time, just until you get a feel for what your heart rate is doing and how you should feel when you are inside your training zone. Check it periodically from then on to make sure you are not slacking off!

the guidelines

how often? Like the fast and furious method for fat burning, you will require some recovery time between sessions; we recommend at least 48 hours. Aim for three to four sessions each week.

how long? 30 minutes per session, including warm-up and cool-down.

how hard? Follow the guidelines for your training zone. Your body will be working close its maximum capabilities in short bursts, so you can expect to be a little uncomfortable during your session. Carrying on a conversation during these sessions will be difficult, and is not recommended. Focus more on your training and breathing techniques and save the chitchat for cool down time. It is not unusual to feel a little light-headed or nauseous, but stop if these symptoms continue to occur and seek a medical check up.

warm up. Choose a comfortable pace that is roughly half that of your work phase, this will probably be similar to that of the recovery pace you will follow between work phases. Maintain this pace for 5 minutes, stop and stretch, and then move into your work phase.

cool down. Use the same guideline for cooling down as for warming up. And stretch again at the completion of your cool-down.

heart rate. Follow the guidelines for fitness training for your age on our heart rate chart if you will be using a heart rate monitor. This will keep you inside a training zone that is 80% - 90% of your maximum heart rate.

Stop to take your pulse after every couple of work phases if you are training without a heart rate monitor and adjust your workload accordingly. For example if your pulse rate is lower than the guidelines, increase the intensity, if it is higher, decrease the intensity.

Remember that a pulse rate is different to heart rate and should serve as a guideline only. Although the figures will be similar, a heart rate monitor will always provide a more accurate reading.

how does it work?

Your heart is muscle, not unlike the other muscles of your body. It is a muscle who's job it is to pump blood around the body. Your heart can be developed and conditioned using the same principals that you would use to develop any muscle.

Anaerobic, or high-level fitness conditioning will improve the efficiency of your heart; it can actually grow in size, thus making it stronger and more able to shunt blood around your body. A bigger, stronger heart won't have to work as hard to do its job, and so it will beat slower and be more efficient.

This is where the term 'improved fitness' comes in. You will be fitter and better able to run the same distance across the park but with less effort and a lower heart rate at the end.

the four training techniques in review

Training Format	Zone %Max HR	Session Duration	System Trained	Maximum Pace	Training Term
Moderate Activity	50% -60%	30 - 60+ minutes	Fuel Burning	Walking	Cardio for Health
Weight Management	60% - 70%	45+ minutes	Fuel Burning	Walking/ Striding	Fat burning Slow/steady
Weight Management	70% - 80%	30 – 40 minutes	Aerobic	Interval Sprints	Fat burning Fast/furious
Improved Fitness	80% - 90%	30 minutes	Anaerobic	Interval Sprints	Cardio for Fitness

target heart rates

There is a simple method for working out your target heart rate or training zone. Calculate this by first determining your maximum heart rate:

220 minus your age equals your maximum heart rate (MHR).

For example 220 – 35 = 185bpm

Now to calculate your target heart rate zone, simply multiply your MHR by the applicable percentage:

185bpm x 60% = 111bpm

If your aim is to keep your heart rate between 60% and 70% calculate a rate for both percentages and then maintain a heart rate somewhere between the two. If your heart rate goes below 60% you can increase the intensity and if it goes above 70% you can ease off a little.

Below is a chart that shows percentages of maximum heart rate. This will save you constantly calculating where your heart rate should be. Photocopy this chart and put it on your wall for easy reference.

We have included a 'red-line zone' on this chart. There are legitimate uses for training at such an intense level. However we suggest this zone only be used by those with a high level of training experience or under the supervision of a fitness professional.

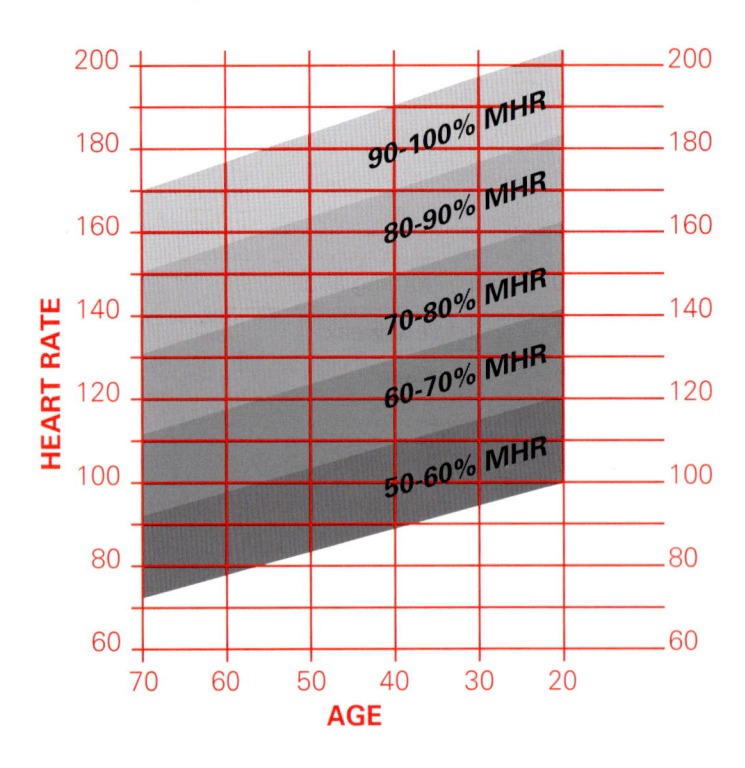

Max Heart Rate (MHR) = 220 − AGE

perceived rate of exertion

Other than heart rate monitoring, the 'Perceived Rate of Exertion Scale' or PRE can also determine your training intensity. This scale can be especially useful for those people who have an unusually high or low heart rate, and also those on medication that affects the working heart rate such as those used to lower blood pressure.

Be honest with yourself when using this scale, otherwise it will not be accurate. Keep the scale in easy view while you are exercising and regularly assess your perceived level of exertion on the scale. In this way you will be able to determine your workload and know what intensity to set your cardio machine at.

Score	Intensity level
0	Nothing at all
1	Very weak
2	Weak
3	
4	Moderate
5	
6	Somewhat hard
7	
8	Very hard
9	
10	Extremely hard

cardio machines

Now that you have worked out which form of cardio training is right for you, it is time to decide on which machine is right for you. We have reviewed the most favourite machines and the ones that we would most recommend. Your fitness level, strength, expertise, sense of balance and injury list should all be considered when choosing a machine.

treadmills

Baseline treadmills will suit those who wish to walk and not run, top pace for a smaller treadmill is around 6.5kph – 7kph. These machines will usually have some kind of manual incline which isn't difficult to use. Incline is an important feature, as it will easily increase the intensity of your workout by simulating hill climbing. This is good for building core strength in the lower body and elevating your heart rate.

Mid range treadmills will offer a slightly larger and more robust motor, which will be capable of speeds of around 9kph – 10kph, a comfortable jogging pace for most.

If you are planning on doing some interval work, or a constant jog, this treadmill will be fine. It will also come with a manually adjustable incline.

If you intend on doing a serious amount of fitness work, then we highly recommend a high range treadmill. These machines will offer a greater speed range of up to 16kph and a heavy-duty motor to provide constant power to keep you going. High range machines will also include an automatic incline feature of 0% - 10%. This means that you push a button on your treadmill and the machine automatically inclines to your desired height, a handy feature if you intend doing some interval training.

All machines come with computers to record time, speed, distance and calories. Many will also include a heart rate monitor pick up, and most will fold away to save on space when not in use, both are great features.

Treadmills tend to be the favourite because of their versatility to provide a format for any type of cardio training. They are also extremely easy to use, thus making them a winner with all age groups.

We would recommend the treadmill first because of the reasons mentioned above, also because there are few limiting factors for those wanting to use this machine. There is a lot less impact than walking or running on the road. There is little or no risk to joints, especially the knees. It is suitable for all levels of fitness and can be used in a rehabilitative situation if necessary.

cycles

OK, this is where the price tag makes a difference. If you are intending on spending a decent amount of time on your bike, buy something with a slightly higher price tag, it will be quieter and more comfortable. Cycles have changed a lot over the last ten years however and are now much more comfortable to use.

Resistance on low range bikes will be via a knob, which will either make pedalling harder or easier, the seats are a good size and comfortable and they are fully height adjustable. We recommend these machines for those who only want to spend 30 minutes max training. They are not great for interval work because the resistance adjustment can be fiddly when you are increasing and decreasing the load constantly.

Low range machines work off a heavy flywheel that is attached to the pedals. When you increase the resistance a strap tightens around the flywheel and restricts movement, thus making it harder to turn the pedals.

Mid range machines will be a little quieter because they work on magnetic resistance. They still have a flywheel, but they use magnets for resistance so that when the tension is increased, the magnets are moved closer to the flywheel, which again restricts movement and makes it harder to pedal. Because there is no physical contact between magnets and flywheel, the operation and movement is smoother.

These machines will be a little more comfortable to use, simply because of their size; they will be made from larger steel tubing and so be sturdier. Resistance settings are more responsive and so they will be better suited to interval or fitness training.

High range machines work on an electrical-powered magnetic force that provides the same smooth action as the mid range machines. This machine has a programmable computer that will automatically put you through few different programs including fitness and fat-burning regimes. There are several intensity levels designed to suit most people. High Range machines are comfortable and smooth and will be the ultimate machine for cardio training, designed to suit all forms of training.

Most York cycles come with a clip on ear lobe heart rate monitor, these things are pretty accurate and will do you fine if you don't want to spend the extra money to get a chest band style monitor. They simply clip on to your ear lobe and pick up a pulse that reads out on the computer screen of the cycle.

Cycles are safe for most people to use although if you have or have had a knee or hip injury, then take care with this one. If you suffer any pain or discomfort, give it a miss. If you haven't already bought your cardio machine, go and try them out. As we said earlier, don't feel embarrassed about spending some time on these machines in the showroom. We think it is imperative if you are to make a purchase that is completely right for you. It might also be a good idea to visit a physiotherapist for some advice if you are really worried. They will be able to check out your injury and hopefully let you know which movements will not be a good idea for you on an ongoing basis.

elliptical trainers

Most people know less about these machines than the standard cycles, treadmills and steppers. They basically work the same way as a cycle. The lower range models have a heavy-duty flywheel, the high range machine works on magnetic resistance.

The movement is totally different to that of a cycle though. It involves standing on foot-plates and rolling them around in an elliptical movement either forward or backwards. At the same time as your legs are moving, your upper body is working too. By holding on to the handles and pushing them to and from, your upper body muscles will be working to elevate your heart rate as well.

Base models have a relatively smooth movement and include a basic computer to keep track of time, speed and distance travelled. They have a manual tension that works the same way as the lower end cycles. This is well within your reach when training and so this machine could easily be used for a training regime that involves regular changes in the intensity.

The higher range machine has a smoother movement and better transition during tension adjustments because of its magnetic resistance. It also comes with an ear lobe heart rate monitor and has a telemetry pick up in built. So if you have a chest band monitor, the computer will pick up the beat while you are training. This is a handy feature to have if you have purchased a heart rate monitor to use during other forms of training. These machines also fold away for easy storage, something to consider if you are pushed for space.

This machine is great for elevating the heart rate because the upper body is brought into the equation as well. Your heart rate will come up quicker and you will be able to have a more intense workout simply because both ends of the body are working hard. Just about every muscle in the body is required for the proper operation of an elliptical trainer, and so the heart has to work hard to keep oxygenated blood flowing to those muscles, which in turn keeps them moving.

OK on to the limiting factors. As with the cycles if you currently have or have had in the past a knee injury of any kind, this machine is probably not for you. Shoulders are also required to work hard with this machine, so likewise with the upper body.

We recommend the elliptical trainer for those who have a core base of strength and no weaknesses in the major joints of the body with special emphasis placed on the knees, back and shoulders. If you have your heart set on this machine but are worried about the suitability, see a sports physiotherapist before making your final decision.

All types of training can be performed on this machine, no particular format stands out as the better or more effective. However if you do intend on using it for slow and steady fat burning or health training, be aware that you will be spending lengthy periods of time exercising, and because your arms and legs are both required for operation, you will be prone to muscle fatigue. This is not a huge problem - it may just be a matter of working yourself up to longer training periods.

steppers

At the time of publishing, York was currently carrying one stepper in their domestic stock range – The Big Foot Stepper. This stepper had been on the market for about seven years and was one of the first to emerge when steppers were introduced. As far as steppers go this one is fine, we would probably describe it as mid range. It comes with the usual computer console to keep track of time, step count, distance and tempo; it also has an earlobe heart rate monitor.

It uses spring-loaded shocks for resistance that work independently of each other, this is important as it allows for a smoother movement.

Steppers are a great machine for fitness training because, as the name suggests, they were invented to simulate stair climbing, and we all now how challenging that can be. As far as training formats go, they are fine for all, again be aware that spending lengthy periods of time on this machine will be hard work to start with but will become easier as your fitness and strength increases.

If you have any knee problems, this machine is not for you. There is a good deal of stress placed on the knees during this exercise, and so if you have an existing weakness, it will only serve to make the problem worse. If you really want to use a stepper, try doing some leg strengthening work first. Refer to our lower body strength routines that will build up some muscle in your legs and in turn support your knees. If after making your legs stronger you still experience pain when using the stepper, give it a miss and find something else, its not worth the constant pain and discomfort that a permanent injury will cause.

Over and above the machines already highlighted there is also a machine available which offers two exercises in one machine. It combines a rower with a cycle to allow versatility and efficient use of a small space.

This machine sounds like a bit of a gimmick but it is actually quite a good little set up. It works on magnetic resistance to power both the cycle and the rower, which means a quiet and more fluid movement. It is fully adjustable to suit people in the normal height range, the computer is detailed for both forms of exercise and it also includes a telemetry heart rate pick up for use with a chest band heart rate monitor.

Because it has the quality inclusions it comes in as a mid price range item that we believe is worth a go. We believe it would be fine with all training formats. The long haul stuff will be a bit difficult on the rower because you are basically stuck in one position for a long period of time without any room for wiggling around. We have always found the rower great for short intense bursts of exercise like those detailed in fitness or fast furious fat burning training. However this machine would be great to ease the boredom factor or to combine two different training formats such as health and fitness training.

SECTION TWELVE
getting started

what to wear

What you wear while you are exercising is important. You need to be comfortable and well supported. It can also help some people to look good, if you look good you feel good. So if you are one of these people then go and buy yourself some trendy training clothes, if it means you will feel more enthusiastic about your training – great, whatever works for you is fine by us!

The first thing to keep in mind here is comfort, remember that you will warm up. If it is winter, try layering, as you warm up you can take a layer off – a training top, a t-shirt and a light sweater will work well. In summer opt for something that is made of cotton. Singlets or training tops are a good idea as they allow the air to flow around your body, this keeps you cool. T-shirts are fine as long as they are loose fitting and again allow air to flow around the body. If you intend on doing a lot of running or walking, try on a pair of running shorts. These have high sides to allow freedom of movement through the legs and are made of lightweight fabric that is comfortable to wear.

Lycra looks great and feels good, but it can be hot while you are training. Choose good quality training clothes that incorporate a mix of cotton and lycra. This will breathe better and allow your body to perspire normally. Beware of tracksuit pants, they usually contain a large percentage of nylon and will be hot and uncomfortable to exercise in. Opt instead for shorts or cotton/lycra tights.

Good support is important for all females regardless of their bust size. Choose training tops that have a bra insert, or get yourself fitted for a decent sports bra, especially if you intend on doing some running.

Sport shoes are the next important consideration; how old are your current training shoes? If you answered six months or more, turn them over, are they showing signs of wear on the bottom? Sports shoes will wear quicker than most people realise, especially for those who exercise regularly. Don't wait until your shoes look really shabby or get a hole in the toe to replace them, chances are they should have been replaced long before.

Sports shoes are designed to offer you support and cushioning while you are exercising. The products that they are made from will compress over a period of time. When this happens, your shoe is not providing the cushioning and support that you require to avoid impact and foot and ankle injuries. Your shoe will be worn to the shape of your foot and the inner materials compressed well before it shows major signs of wear and tear on the outside.

Don't keep your training shoes for five years. We highly recommend you replace your trainers every twelve months, possibly sooner depending on your level of activity. When choosing new sports shoes, find a retail outlet that has informed and qualified staff, tell them exactly what you will be doing in your shoes and have the shoes fitted properly. Take your time wandering the shop with the shoes on and make sure that you choose the one that feels most supportive as well as comfortable.

Tip Try choosing a shoe based on its comfort and support rather than your physical attraction to it. The shoe that you think looks great may be totally wrong for your footfall and shape of foot.

Tip Keep your training shoes for when you are training. Get yourself a second pair of sports shoes to wear every day. This means that your training shoes won't wear out as quickly and so will offer you maximum support while you are exercising

choosing a program for you

Your program level should be based solely on your capabilities and goals. The programs have been split up into two categories:

1. strength/muscle size
2. fitness/fat loss

You must first decide whether your goals are to build muscle and gain some strength or burn off excess body fat and increase your fitness level. Most people will fall into either of these categories. Those wanting to gain some muscle size and increase their fitness as well will find that there is still a cardio component within the strength programs; and vice versa, if you want to burn body fat and build muscle you will find that there is a good deal of weight training involved in the fat loss programs.

Once you have completed the first 12-week cycle and gained some results you will be able to fine tune your training program and may even want to attempt writing your own program or trying a mix of the two categories. Whichever way you go, you will need to perform the fitness assessment first.

Once you have run through the fitness test and you have a result, follow the guidelines for your level of results. These guidelines will tell you which level you should start on – beginner, intermediate or advanced. Choose the relative program from chapter thirteen and make 12 copies (one for each week) and away you go!

organising your twelve week planner

Get on top of this before you start anything else. This is your training calendar, your map of where and what you will do each day for the 12 weeks.

Once you have chosen your program and level, you will also have the corresponding 12-week planner. You will only need to photocopy one of these because all 84 days are contained on one sheet.

Familiarise yourself with the details on the 12-week planner. Get a feel for what happens on what days and maybe even jot your training days down in your diary to make sure that you don't book something else in on a day and time that you should be training.

We suggest that you stick your 12-week planner on the wall in your training studio. Somewhere where you can easily see it and get to it to record your body weight reading for the week.

You will need to refer to this sheet on a daily basis to find out what you need to do that day for your training, or not do in the case of your days off!

The 12-week planner is designed to go hand-in-hand with your program card. The planner tells you what is on for the day and the program card will tell you how to do it.

filling in the forms

We have included detailed instructions with each form on how to fill in the appropriate areas. It is important that you take it on with enthusiasm and gusto. Follow the instructions to the tee and be enthusiastic about it. Take this stuff seriously, after all we are talking about your best asset here – your health and well being – the thing that so many of us take for granted.

Fill in these sheets each day if possible after/during each training session in the case of the program card and training diary. Evenings are the best time to fill in the food diary, once you have finished eating for the day. Pick a time that is quiet and sit down and go over everything you have eaten that day. If you want to carry the diary around with you during the day and write things down as you eat them, go ahead.

For most though it will be easier to do it once at the end of the day for ease of convenience. There are only four food diary sheets to fill in, we suggest one every three weeks to keep you on track and bring the bad habits to your attention.

It will be important for you to fill in your training program as you go so that you can record your increase in weight and intensity on cardio machines. Don't rely on your memory each time, there's a good chance that you will remember each weight and intensity level, but having everything recorded will make for a smoother a more effective workout. It will also help you down the track when you can refer back to starting weights on new exercises for renewed programs.

choosing a start date

Finding a date to start this lot will need some consideration as well. Don't go starting your 12-week program a week before your best friends wedding for instance, when you know you will have a big night out and then the wedding and the day after to contend with. Put it off until the following week.

Give some thought as to what is coming up in your life in the next few weeks that may effect your training, a holiday perhaps or a busy period at work. Work around this stuff. We aren't suggesting you put off starting your program for two months because of an event that far off.

Choose a time when you have no major events that may prevent you training for the first month of your program. This first month is the time when you are most likely to ditch a training day or go against your healthy eating habits. After the first month you will begin to see and feel results and will be more enthusiastic about the whole deal. You will also be well and truly entrenched in your routines and as a consequence will be more able to work other commitments around your training days/days off training and good eating.

your first training session

How exciting, you have made it to your first session. Your training studio is all set up and waiting for you, you have photocopied all your forms and you know just what to do and where to start and you have your favourite music playing.

What do you do now? Get into it! Knock yourself out. Have a great time. Enjoy the feeling that exercise gives you.

Congratulate yourself for making it. You have taken control of your life and you will change your health and fitness for the better. Well done. Do you know how many people never make it to this stage? Do you know how many people there are out there who have no energy to even think about doing regular exercise? There's a lot, so be proud of yourself and go out and sing the virtues of regular exercise and healthy eating.

Even if you only influence one of those people who has no inclination for exercise you will have made a positive difference to another life, you will have enhanced their life and made them realise what their bodies are capable of.

Expect to feel a high from your first session, it is a major achievement and should be treated as such. It could also be a while since you have done any amount of intense physical activity and so the increased blood flow to your muscles and organs will give you a heightened sense of healthiness and energy.

You may also expect to run out of energy fairly quickly during your first session, simply because your fitness level might be low. If you do start to experience fatigue throughout your first session, slow it down. Increase the rest times between sets or if you are doing cardio training try sipping cool water and concentrate on getting as much air as you can in through your nose and out through your mouth.

Try to stick to the program format if possible, you wouldn't expect anything else from these first couple of sessions and so this is no time to start being easy on yourself. Know that your tolerance level and your staying power will increase with every session.

Of course if you experience any unusual or particularly intense levels of pain, discomfort or difficulty with breathing stop exercising at once. Cool down and take it easy. Make sure that you have assessed your fitness level correctly and that you have started yourself on the program that is best suited to your capabilities. If you haven't, make the relevant adjustments. If you have, slow the pace down a little and decrease the intensity. If you continue to experience any difficulties with your training, get yourself to a medical practitioner for a check up.

Most of all, we encourage you to have fun. Enjoy your first session. Be proud of yourself for having the mental and physical strength to make such positive changes to your life, because we are proud of you too. Well done and good luck with it!

lifestyle questionnaire

1. What is your occupation? _____

2. Do you currently do any regular exercise? ☐ yes   ☐ no

If yes, what type of exercise? _____

Frequency? _____

Perceived Intensity   ☐ hard   ☐ medium   ☐ light   ☐ very light

How long have you been exercising regularly? _____

3. List in order from one to eight what you hope to achieve from your home training program.

- To reduce body fat ☐
- To improve aerobic capacity (heart/lung function) ☐
- To gain some muscle definition ☐
- To gain some muscle size ☐
- To gain overall fitness ☐
- To generally tone up ☐
- To reduce stress ☐
- Other _____ ☐

4. how many times a week are you prepared to commit to an exercise program?

_____

5. How would you describe your current physical condition?

☐ unwell   ☐ overweight   ☐ unfit   ☐ healthy   ☐ fit

the score

1. If your job has you in a sedentary position for the majority of the day, we recommend you do some regular cardio training for fitness purposes, even if your goal is to build muscle. Sitting down all day does little for heart/lung function and inhibits circulation. It also slows the metabolism. Try getting up from your desk every hour if possible. Allow yourself five minutes for walking and stretching before returning to your desk.

If your work requires you to be active, you have no problems here, move onto the next question.

2. If you answered no to this question, we suggest you take caution when beginning your exercise program. Start with the easier programs and be aware that you will suffer a degree of discomfort in the early days. We have also included this question to make you aware that you will find it mentally challenging to commit to your program and keep going if you haven't been doing any regularly physical activity. Take heart though, it isn't impossible and your rewards will be great.

If you have been doing some regular exercise, it is time to re-assess your training and structure your program specifically to suit your goals. Use the guidelines for frequency and intensity when deciding on how many times per week you will exercise and at what level of intensity.

If you have a long history of regular exercise, re-assess your training and your achievements. Look for areas that you would like to improve, perhaps in line with a particular sport that you play.

3. Listing what you hope to achieve from your program in order of importance will make it clear what sort of program you will need to follow. Once you have answered this question you will be able to set yourself some goals (if you haven't already done so).

4. By deciding how much time you are willing to devote to your training you will be able to make a self-affirmation for your program. You will also be able to compare what you wish to devote time-wise with what we suggest you should devote.

This question is important because it is a chance for you to be honest about the amount of time you really want to spend training each week. This is different to what we suggest. If the figures

GETTING STARTED

differ, find yourself a happy median somewhere in the middle.

5. If you are unwell, overweight or very unfit we suggest you take the necessary precautions when commencing an exercise program. Seek medical advice first and be aware if you are unwell that exercise is taxing on the immune system and so care should be taken with intensity levels. We also recommend against any heavy fitness or resistance training for the same reasons.

If you are overweight, heart rate monitoring is a must. Take it easy and don't pursue anything that feels uncomfortable of painful. Your range of movement will be restricted as will your stamina and you may find it difficult to sustain exercise for the length of time that your selected program suggests. If this is the case, keep going for as long as you feel you can and record on your program card where you stopped during that session. Aim to increase the duration of your sessions each time until you are getting through the prescribed program.

If you are fit and healthy, follow the standard guidelines for your age and ability.

Look at your lifestyle questionnaire as a whole now that you have completed it. It may be apparent from your answers that you need to make some serious changes in order to keep yourself healthy and avoid any unwanted injuries or illnesses in the future.

Maybe it will look the way you expected it to look, which isn't necessarily what you want. Take these questions seriously and come back to this questionnaire three to six months down the track and answer them again. By then you should be feeling a whole lot better about yourself both physically and mentally. It will be a reward to look back at the second lot of answers and see a person who is in control of they're health and well being.

medical questionnaire

1. When was your last medical check up? _____

2. Are you on prescription medication (some medicines may alter heart rate and blood pressure)?
_____

3. Have you been hospitalised recently? _____

4. Are you pregnant? _____

5. Have you given birth in the last six weeks? _____

6. Do you have or have you had?

☐ Stroke   ☐ Dizziness or fainting   ☐ Palpitations or chest pain

☐ Liver or kidney condition ☐ Glandular fever ☐ Diabetes

☐ Heart murmur   ☐ High blood pressure   ☐ Epilepsy

If you answered yes to ANY of the above questions, it is imperative that you see a medical practitioner before beginning any exercise program.

7. Do you have or have you had?

☐ Arthritis   ☐ Asthma   ☐ Cramps   ☐ Muscular pain

8. Do you have or have you had pain or major injuries in the following areas?

☐ Neck   ☐ Back   ☐ Knee   ☐ Ankles

9. Do you smoke?   ☐ YES   ☐ NO

10. Are you dieting or fasting?   ☐ YES   ☐ NO

If you answered yes to ANY of the above questions, we strongly recommend that you seek advice from a medical practitioner or the appropriate professional before beginning any form of exercise program.

page 214

fitness assessment

The series of tests below are designed to assess your endurance, strength, stamina and flexibility. The answers to these questions will enable you to evaluate your current level of fitness and identify areas that require work. The answers will also give you a starting point for your training and decide for you which program to begin with. Be honest and record true scores here, as it will give you an accurate starting block and reflect on future assessments. The tests have been specifically designed to be performed in their order, one to five. Record your result for each test, the scores follow

1. **Three-minute step test.** This test will evaluate your current cardiovascular fitness. Use a step that is 40cm in height. Step up and down at a rate of between 22 and 26 steps per minute (that's about 3 seconds per step). Make sure that you place your whole foot flat on the box when you step and step to a rhythm of 'up up down down' i.e. right foot up, left foot up, right foot down, left foot down and repeat. Keep your head up and your back straight. Perform step-ups for three minutes. Stop and take your pulse immediately. Count the beat for 15 seconds and then multiply that figure by four to get a number of beats per minute. Check your score and write it down.

   LEVEL I   - **Male 155bpm or more**
                 - **Female 160bpm or more**

   LEVEL II - **Male 141 - 155bpm**
                 - **Female 147 - 160pm**

   LEVEL III - **Male 125 – 140bpm**
                 - **Female 131 – 146bpm**

2. **One minute push-up test.** This test will evaluate your upper body strength. Position your hands directly under your shoulders with your fingers pointing forward and spread. Keep your torso straight and with ankles and knees together. Bend your arms and lower your body until your elbows reach a 90-degree angle i.e. nose almost to the carpet, making sure you keep your abdominal muscles tight. Try not to arch your back as you push yourself up, your body should remain on one straight plane. If you cannot do a full minute of push-ups, count the number of repetitions you can complete before your technique deteriorates. Note males should do push-ups on their toes, and females supported on their knees.

Male (toes)

LEVEL I	- 0 – 10
LEVEL II	- 11 – 30
LEVEL III	- 31+

Female (knees)

LEVEL I	- 0 – 20
LEVEL II	- 21 – 40
LEVEL III	- 41+

3. One minute crunch test. This test will evaluate your abdominal strength. Lie on the floor, on your back with your knees bent and feet flat on the floor about 12 inches from your bottom. Place your hands by your ears and keep your eyes up. Keep a gap between your chin and the top of your chest about the size of a tennis ball. Lift your shoulders, ensuring that you keep the tennis ball gap and your head stays in line with your spine. Keeping your lower back on the floor, bring your shoulders as high as you can, hold for a count of one and then return to the start position. As with the push-up test, if you cannot do a full minute of crunches, count the number of repetitions you can complete before your technique deteriorates.

LEVEL I	- Male and Female 0 – 25
LEVEL II	- Male and Female 26 – 35
LEVEL III	- Male and Female 36 – 50

4. Sit and reach test. This test will evaluate your lower back and hamstring flexibility. Sit on the floor with your legs extended in front of you and about shoulder width apart. Keep the backs of your knees and heels down and your toes up. Reach forward and measure how far down your legs your fingertips can touch without bending your knees.

LEVEL I	- Male and Female – Top of thighs
LEVEL II	- Male and female – Kneecap
LEVEL III	- Male and Female – Shins and beyond

body mass index (BMI) evaluation.

This test assesses your weight in relation to your height and provides an indication of how healthy your current body shape is. If you are carrying a greater amount of lean muscle tissue and little body fat, this test will not be accurate. Because the BMI only looks at a height and weight ratio and not body fat, lean muscle mass or bone structure it will not give an accurate indication for an individual whose body fat is low and muscle mass is high.

Because muscle is heavier than fat, overall bodyweight can be greater but not necessarily reflecting body fat. The BMI range is used to gauge the level of health in an individual of average body fat/muscle mass distribution. Therefore a very lean female carrying an above average percentage of muscle mass will be in an unhealthy BMI range when she is probably in actual fact at her optimum fitness level, the same applies to a male with similar percentages.

It is for these reasons we have decided not to include a BMI as part of your fitness assessment. Although it will be fairly accurate for most people, there is nothing concrete enough to base a fitness assessment on. However you may wish to review the chart on this page for working out your BMI for your own interest.

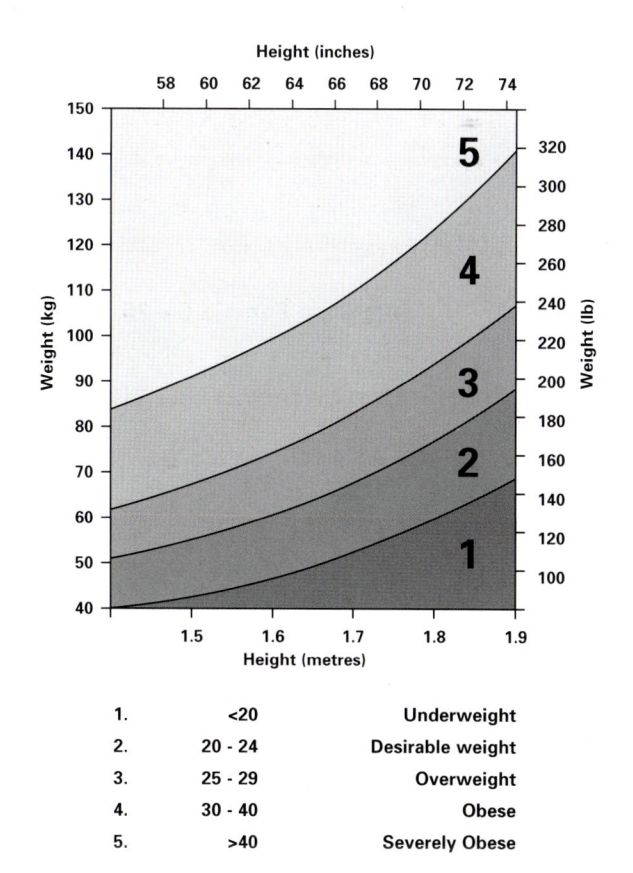

1.	<20	Underweight
2.	20 - 24	Desirable weight
3.	25 - 29	Overweight
4.	30 - 40	Obese
5.	>40	Severely Obese

body measurements

Body measurements are going to be the most accurate way to see your body shape change. For the same reasons as the BMI, the scales are not going to show you a true indication of what's going on. As you begin your training program, two things are going to happen. Your body fat levels will decrease and your muscle mass will increase. As well as this there may also be an increase in glycogen storage in the muscles and because glycogen attracts water (approx. 2.7grams to each gram of glycogen) this may also bump the scales up in the early stages of training.

A tape measure however cannot lie. And it is a good idea to make a few basic measurements before you start your program, whether you are looking to see your waist line decrease or your biceps increase and repeat the process each time you do a fitness assessment or at any regular interval.

Thigh (R) _____ cm   (L) _____ cm
Hip _____ cm
Waist _____ cm
Chest/bust _____ cm
Bicep (R) _____ cm   (L) _____ cm

Try to have someone else do the measurements for you, as it can be a little difficult, however it is not impossible to do it yourself. When you are measuring, try to stand as relaxed as possible with all muscles relaxed, not flexed, and in the case of torso measurements stand as tall as possible, take a full breath in, exhale half-way out and measure, again in a relaxed state. Make sure you measure the point at the greatest circumference of each area and make sure the tape measure stays flat. Follow the same procedure each time.

results

1.	level I	1 point	2.	level I	1 point
	level II	2 points		level II	2 points
	level III	3 points		level III	3 points
3.	level I	1 point	4.	level I	1 point
	level II	2 points		level II	2 points
	level III	3 points		level III	3 points

the score

Your test results will give you a good indication of your current fitness level. Workout your score and follow the instructions for the appropriate level.

LEVEL I – A score between 5 and 11 points indicates a lower level of fitness. It probably means that you have done little or no exercise for quite a while. Thus saying it will be important for you to start with the beginner programs to build up your level of fitness slowly and gently. Don't be discouraged by your score, use it as a benchmark for improvement, a turning point in your approach to your health and well being.

LEVEL II – A score of between 12 and 19 points indicates an average level of fitness. You are probably doing some regular exercise and maintaining your results. You should start on programs designed for intermediate training. These programs will provide you with a challenge and also the opportunity to increase your level of goal attainment.

LEVEL III – A score of 20 points or more indicates a high level of fitness. You have almost certainly been exercising regularly for a lengthy period of time and you will have an idea of how your body responds to exercise. Your results indicate that you are probably ready for an advanced level of training. However we recommend you start in the final four-week phase of the intermediate level as a prelude to launching into an advanced program. These programs have been designed for those who either need or want to train at a very high level and are keen to devote a lot of time to their training.

SECTION THIRTEEN programs

how to follow your 12-week program

In the following pages you will find a sample program card for your first week of training, a 12-week (84 day) planner, a training diary and a food diary for both strength/muscle size beginner, intermediate and advanced, and fitness/fat-loss beginner, intermediate and advanced. Please note that all of the chosen exercises for these programs can be substituted for any other similar exercise listed in this manual. Refer to the exercise listing.

before you start

Before you start your chosen training program, you will need to do a little preparation and planning. First you will need to make a few photocopies:

Instructions for progressing on your 12-week program	1 copy
12-week planner	1 copy
1-week program card	12 copies
Training diary	1 copy
Food diary	4 copies

Place these 19 pages in the order above and staple them together. This is now your complete operations manual for the next 12 weeks.

what are they for?

12-week planner

This is your complete 12-week training program at a glance. This sheet has been designed to show you what you should be doing everyday from day 1 to 84. Whether it be strength, cardio or both, whether your session is scheduled for the morning or the evening and where your days off will be. There is also provision for you to record your body weight at the start of every new week should you feel the urge to do so.

When you complete your training for a specific day, put a great big tick (✓) across the box. You will be amazed at the satisfaction this brings when you start to see row after row of ticks appearing down the page.

1-week program card

This is the one that tells you exactly what you should be doing on every scheduled training day for each individual week. It shows you what you do, for how long, how many sets and repetitions and which muscles to stretch. It relates directly to your 12-week (84 day) planner by showing you which day of 84 you are looking at.

How to fill in your program card: On your program card you will need to record a number of things:

1. The day number. Which number day it is of your scheduled 84. This includes days off.

2. Your chosen cardio activity for the day eg. running, swimming, stationery cycle, treadmill etc.

3. How long you did it for, recorded in minutes.

4. If you did a specific program on a cardio machine or a distance completed in an outdoor activity.

5. How intensely you work. If you use a scale of 1 – 10 whereby 1 would be barely moving and 10 would be an extremely high level you should be able to plan and gauge your intensity level or if you are using a heart rate monitor, what is your target heart rate zone.

6. The time your heart rate was within your specific heart rate training zone. If you have a heart rate monitor this is also a more accurate way of monitoring your intensity level.

7. How much weight you lifted for your programmed number of repetitions.

8. Which stretches were successfully completed at the end of each session marked by a tick (✓).

training diary

This sheet has been designed to show you any patterns that may emerge in regards to the time of day, your mood and your energy levels throughout your session. It is useful to help identify any changes that may be needed in your daily life, perhaps in your diet, your sleep patterns or how your training program is going to fit in around a working day eg are your sessions better before the phone starts ringing for the day or after the working day is done. These brief comments should be made at the completion of each session.

food diary

This one is used to keep you aware of everything that passes your lips from the time that you wake up to the time you retire. It is a good way to keep you on track because you become a lot more aware of what you are eating when you are writing everything down. We recommend you have four copies of the food diary in your program. This will give you one full week to record your food intake at three-week intervals.

Depending on how varied your diet is and how much discipline you need, you may only want to fill out a few days to get an idea of what is going on. Perhaps two weekdays and one day over the weekend, or you may need the full seven days to keep you tuned in.

The first thing to do is record the date below the day on your diary. There are then six meals for each day that can be recorded. Make sure you list everything you have eaten and record everything as closely as possible to its meal number.

Try to record quantities of food in cups and tablespoons and record things like; what sort of milk you had on your breakfast cereal and if you had butter on your toast or sandwiches. That way if you want to you can have a dietician or nutritionist analyse it for you.

By keeping a food diary you can start to see patterns forming for your potentially 'dangerous' periods of day. Maybe it's a sweet tooth at morning teatime, a few too many glasses of wine with dinner or that dessert that you probably didn't really need. It may also be that you are trying to gain weight and you might not be eating enough food throughout the day to aid sufficiently in muscle growth.

There are sample diets for you to have a look at in the nutrition section of this book. These will give you an idea of what you should be eating to reach your specific goal.

strength & muscle size - BEGINNERS

instructions for progressing on your 12-week program

- Follow your first weeks program card down the page from day 1 to 7 filling in the weight lifted (kgs or lbs) and the stretches completed.

- Follow the same routine until the end of week 4 making sure you also mark off every day on your 12-week (84 day) planner and fill out your training and food diary, if required.

- **At week 5 (day 29)** add a third full body strength session to your week on Wednesday (same session as Monday & Friday) and stretch at the completion of your workout. Thursday now becomes a P.M. stretch day, not a full day off. Don't forget to mark these on your program card over the top of any now-outdated information.

- Follow the same routine until the end of week 8 making sure you also mark off every day on your 12-week (84 day) planner and fill out your training and food diary, if required.

- **At week 9 (day 57)** add a second cardio session to your week on Saturday morning followed directly by your stretch (same as Tuesday).

Also add a fourth set of 15 repetitions to squats, pulldowns and bench press on your strength days. Don't forget to mark these on your program card over the top of any now-outdated information.

By the completion of week 12 you will need to re-assess your goals and decide whether you are to progress to the strength/muscle size intermediate level or if your fitness and body fat levels perhaps need to be addressed. We recommend you take a one week break between finishing one twelve week cycle and starting another.

Note: The weight you lift should be heavy enough to cause you some difficulty on the last three repetitions but not so heavy that you need to cheat to complete the movement. When the final repetitions become comfortably easy, it's time to increase the resistance. These increases will come randomly throughout your 12 weeks and will be different for everybody.

Photocopy this sheet at 140% on your photocopier to enlarge it to a full A4 working size

YORK Fitness
12 WEEK PLANNER

	monday	tuesday	wednesday	thursday	friday	saturday	sunday
WEEK 1 BODY WEIGHT kgs/lbs	Day 1 □ am ☒ pm — Full Body Strength	Day 2 □ am ☒ pm — Cardio	Day 3 □ am ☒ pm — Stretch	Day 4 □ am □ pm — Day off	Day 5 □ am ☒ pm — Full Body Strength	Day 6 □ am ☒ pm — Stretch	Day 7 □ am □ pm — Day off
WEEK 2 BODY WEIGHT kgs/lbs	Day 8 □ am ☒ pm — Full Body Strength	Day 9 □ am ☒ pm — Cardio	Day 10 □ am ☒ pm — Stretch	Day 11 □ am □ pm — Day off	Day 12 □ am ☒ pm — Full Body Strength	Day 13 □ am ☒ pm — Stretch	Day 14 □ am □ pm — Day off
WEEK 3 BODY WEIGHT kgs/lbs	Day 15 □ am ☒ pm — Full Body Strength	Day 16 □ am ☒ pm — Cardio	Day 17 □ am ☒ pm — Stretch	Day 18 □ am □ pm — Day off	Day 19 □ am ☒ pm — Full Body Strength	Day 20 □ am ☒ pm — Stretch	Day 21 □ am □ pm — Day off
WEEK 4 BODY WEIGHT kgs/lbs	Day 22 □ am ☒ pm — Full Body Strength	Day 23 □ am ☒ pm — Cardio	Day 24 □ am ☒ pm — Stretch	Day 25 □ am □ pm — Day off	Day 26 □ am ☒ pm — Full Body Strength	Day 27 □ am ☒ pm — Stretch	Day 28 □ am □ pm — Day off
WEEK 5 BODY WEIGHT kgs/lbs	Day 29 □ am ☒ pm — Full Body Strength	Day 30 □ am ☒ pm — Cardio	Day 31 □ am ☒ pm — Full Body Strength	Day 32 □ am ☒ pm — Stretch	Day 33 □ am ☒ pm — Full Body Strength	Day 34 □ am ☒ pm — Stretch	Day 35 □ am □ pm — Day off
WEEK 6 BODY WEIGHT kgs/lbs	Day 36 □ am ☒ pm — Full Body Strength	Day 37 □ am ☒ pm — Cardio	Day 38 □ am ☒ pm — Full Body Strength	Day 39 □ am ☒ pm — Stretch	Day 40 □ am ☒ pm — Full Body Strength	Day 41 □ am ☒ pm — Stretch	Day 42 □ am □ pm — Day off
WEEK 7 BODY WEIGHT kgs/lbs	Day 43 □ am ☒ pm — Full Body Strength	Day 44 □ am ☒ pm — Cardio	Day 45 □ am ☒ pm — Full Body Strength	Day 46 □ am ☒ pm — Stretch	Day 47 □ am ☒ pm — Full Body Strength	Day 48 □ am ☒ pm — Stretch	Day 49 □ am □ pm — Day off
WEEK 8 BODY WEIGHT kgs/lbs	Day 50 □ am ☒ pm — Full Body Strength	Day 51 □ am ☒ pm — Cardio	Day 52 □ am ☒ pm — Full Body Strength	Day 53 □ am ☒ pm — Stretch	Day 54 □ am ☒ pm — Full Body Strength	Day 55 □ am ☒ pm — Stretch	Day 56 □ am □ pm — Day off
WEEK 9 BODY WEIGHT kgs/lbs	Day 57 □ am ☒ pm — Full Body Strength	Day 58 □ am ☒ pm — Cardio	Day 59 □ am ☒ pm — Full Body Strength	Day 60 □ am ☒ pm — Stretch	Day 61 □ am ☒ pm — Full Body Strength	Day 62 ☒ am □ pm — Cardio + Stretch	Day 63 □ am □ pm — Day off
WEEK 10 BODY WEIGHT kgs/lbs	Day 64 □ am ☒ pm — Full Body Strength	Day 65 □ am ☒ pm — Cardio	Day 66 □ am ☒ pm — Full Body Strength	Day 67 □ am ☒ pm — Stretch	Day 68 □ am ☒ pm — Full Body Strength	Day 69 ☒ am □ pm — Cardio + Stretch	Day 70 □ am □ pm — Day off
WEEK 11 BODY WEIGHT kgs/lbs	Day 71 □ am ☒ pm — Full Body Strength	Day 72 □ am ☒ pm — Cardio	Day 73 □ am ☒ pm — Full Body Strength	Day 74 □ am ☒ pm — Stretch	Day 75 □ am ☒ pm — Full Body Strength	Day 76 ☒ am □ pm — Cardio + Stretch	Day 77 □ am □ pm — Day off
WEEK 12 BODY WEIGHT kgs/lbs	Day 78 □ am ☒ pm — Full Body Strength	Day 79 □ am ☒ pm — Cardio	Day 80 □ am ☒ pm — Full Body Strength	Day 81 □ am ☒ pm — Stretch	Day 82 □ am ☒ pm — Full Body Strength	Day 83 ☒ am □ pm — Cardio + Stretch	Day 84 □ am □ pm — Day off

YORK Fitness

Photocopy this sheet at 140% on your photocopier to enlarge it to a full A4 working size

CARDIO

activity	monday	tuesday	wednesday	thursday	friday	saturday	sunday
	day ___ of 84	day ___ of 84	day ___ of 84	day ___ of 84	day ___ of 84	day ___ of 84	day ___ of 84
duration	Cycle	Walk / Run			Cycle		
	5 mins	20 mins	mins	mins	5 mins	mins	mins
program / distance	manual				manual		
intensity level	5 out of 10	6-7 out of 10			5 out of 10		
time in training zone	N/A mins	N/A mins	mins	mins	N/A mins	mins	mins

STRENGTH

	wt / reps
Legs: barbell squats	15 / 15
leg extn.	15 / 15
leg curl	15 / 15
Back: pulldn v/hand close	15 / 15
low cable seated row	15 / 15
Chest: barbell bench press	15 / 15
flat bench flyes	15 / 15
Shoulder: db o'head press	15 / 15
Tricep: flat bench dips	15 / 15
Bicep: dumbell curl seated	15 / 15
Torso: crunches feet floor	15 / 15
Low Back hyper extn	15 / 15

FLEXIBILITY

hip bend	page 261
buttock	page 262
short groin	page 262
hamstring sit	page 263
calf stand	page 264
quadricep stand	page 263
tricep pull-down	page 258
shoulder pull-across	page 257
pecs standing	page 259
shoulder circles	page 257

strength & muscle size - INTERMEDIATE

instructions for progressing on your 12-week program

- Follow your first weeks split training program card down the page from day 1 to 7 filling in the weight lifted (kgs or lbs) and the stretches completed. Note that you will train half your body one day, and the other half the next.

- Follow the same routine until the end of week 4 making sure you also mark off every day on your 12-week (84 day) planner and fill out your training and food diary, if required.

- Make sure you do your torso exercises at every workout

- **At week 5 (day 29)** add a second cardio session to Wednesday evening followed directly by your stretch (same as Saturday). Don't forget to mark these on your program card over the top of any now-outdated information.

- Follow the same routine until the end of week 8 making sure you also mark off every day on your 12-week (84 day) planner and fill out your training and food diary, if required.

- **At week 9 (day 57)** reduce your last set on all exercises (except torso) to 6 repetitions (12 for lunges) and go as heavy as possible with good form. Record the weight. Don't forget to mark these on your program card over the top of any now-outdated information.

By the completion of week 12 you will need to re-assess your goals and decide whether you are to progress to the strength/muscle size advanced level or if your fitness and body fat levels perhaps need to be addressed. We recommend you take a one week break between finishing one twelve week cycle and starting another.

Note: The weight you lift should be heavy enough to cause you some difficulty on the last three repetitions but not so heavy that you need to cheat to complete the movement. When the final repetitions become comfortably easy, it's time to increase the resistance. These increases will come randomly throughout your 12 weeks and will be different for everybody.

YORK FITNESS 12 WEEK PLANNER

Photocopy this sheet at 140% on your photocopier to enlarge it to a full A4 working size

	monday	tuesday	wednesday	thursday	friday	saturday	sunday
WEEK 1 BODY WEIGHT kgs/lbs	☐ am ☒ pm Day 1 Leg, Back, Bicep	☐ am ☒ pm Day 2 Chest, Shoulder, Tricep	☐ am ☒ pm Day 3 Stretch	☐ am ☒ pm Day 4 Leg, Back, Bicep	☐ am ☒ pm Day 5 Chest, Shoulder, Tricep	☒ am ☐ pm Day 6 Cardio	☐ am ☐ pm Day 7 Day off
WEEK 2 BODY WEIGHT kgs/lbs	☐ am ☒ pm Day 8 Leg, Back, Bicep	☐ am ☒ pm Day 9 Chest, Shoulder, Tricep	☐ am ☒ pm Day 10 Stretch	☐ am ☒ pm Day 11 Leg, Back, Bicep	☐ am ☒ pm Day 12 Chest, Shoulder, Tricep	☒ am ☐ pm Day 13 Cardio	☐ am ☐ pm Day 14 Day off
WEEK 3 BODY WEIGHT kgs/lbs	☐ am ☒ pm Day 15 Leg, Back, Bicep	☐ am ☒ pm Day 16 Chest, Shoulder, Tricep	☐ am ☒ pm Day 17 Stretch	☐ am ☒ pm Day 18 Leg, Back, Bicep	☐ am ☒ pm Day 19 Chest, Shoulder, Tricep	☒ am ☐ pm Day 20 Cardio	☐ am ☐ pm Day 21 Day off
WEEK 4 BODY WEIGHT kgs/lbs	☐ am ☒ pm Day 22 Leg, Back, Bicep	☐ am ☒ pm Day 23 Chest, Shoulder, Tricep	☐ am ☒ pm Day 24 Stretch	☐ am ☒ pm Day 25 Leg, Back, Bicep	☐ am ☒ pm Day 26 Chest, Shoulder, Tricep	☒ am ☐ pm Day 27 Cardio	☐ am ☐ pm Day 28 Day off
WEEK 5 BODY WEIGHT kgs/lbs	☐ am ☒ pm Day 29 Leg, Back, Bicep	☐ am ☒ pm Day 30 Chest, Shoulder, Tricep	☐ am ☒ pm Day 31 Stretch	☐ am ☒ pm Day 32 Leg, Back, Bicep	☐ am ☒ pm Day 33 Chest, Shoulder, Tricep	☒ am ☐ pm Day 34 Cardio	☐ am ☐ pm Day 35 Day off
WEEK 6 BODY WEIGHT kgs/lbs	☐ am ☒ pm Day 36 Leg, Back, Bicep	☐ am ☒ pm Day 37 Chest, Shoulder, Tricep	☐ am ☒ pm Day 38 Stretch	☐ am ☒ pm Day 39 Leg, Back, Bicep	☐ am ☒ pm Day 40 Chest, Shoulder, Tricep	☒ am ☐ pm Day 41 Cardio	☐ am ☐ pm Day 42 Day off
WEEK 7 BODY WEIGHT kgs/lbs	☐ am ☒ pm Day 43 Leg, Back, Bicep	☐ am ☒ pm Day 44 Chest, Shoulder, Tricep	☐ am ☒ pm Day 45 Cardio Stretch	☐ am ☒ pm Day 46 Leg, Back, Bicep	☐ am ☒ pm Day 47 Chest, Shoulder, Tricep	☒ am ☐ pm Day 48 Cardio	☐ am ☐ pm Day 49 Day off
WEEK 8 BODY WEIGHT kgs/lbs	☐ am ☒ pm Day 50 Leg, Back, Bicep	☐ am ☒ pm Day 51 Chest, Shoulder, Tricep	☐ am ☒ pm Day 52 Cardio Stretch	☐ am ☒ pm Day 53 Leg, Back, Bicep	☐ am ☒ pm Day 54 Chest, Shoulder, Tricep	☒ am ☐ pm Day 55 Cardio	☐ am ☐ pm Day 56 Day off
WEEK 9 BODY WEIGHT kgs/lbs	☐ am ☒ pm Day 57 Leg, Back, Bicep	☐ am ☒ pm Day 58 Chest, Shoulder, Tricep	☐ am ☒ pm Day 59 Cardio Stretch	☐ am ☒ pm Day 60 Leg, Back, Bicep	☐ am ☒ pm Day 61 Chest, Shoulder, Tricep	☒ am ☐ pm Day 62 Cardio	☐ am ☐ pm Day 63 Day off
WEEK 10 BODY WEIGHT kgs/lbs	☐ am ☒ pm Day 64 Leg, Back, Bicep	☐ am ☒ pm Day 65 Chest, Shoulder, Tricep	☐ am ☒ pm Day 66 Cardio Stretch	☐ am ☒ pm Day 67 Leg, Back, Bicep	☐ am ☒ pm Day 68 Chest, Shoulder, Tricep	☒ am ☐ pm Day 69 Cardio	☐ am ☐ pm Day 70 Day off
WEEK 11 BODY WEIGHT kgs/lbs	☐ am ☒ pm Day 71 Leg, Back, Bicep	☐ am ☒ pm Day 72 Chest, Shoulder, Tricep	☐ am ☒ pm Day 73 Cardio Stretch	☐ am ☒ pm Day 74 Leg, Back, Bicep	☐ am ☒ pm Day 75 Chest, Shoulder, Tricep	☒ am ☐ pm Day 76 Cardio	☐ am ☐ pm Day 77 Day off
WEEK 12 BODY WEIGHT kgs/lbs	☐ am ☒ pm Day 78 Leg, Back, Bicep	☐ am ☒ pm Day 79 Chest, Shoulder, Tricep	☐ am ☒ pm Day 80 Cardio Stretch	☐ am ☒ pm Day 81 Leg, Back, Bicep	☐ am ☒ pm Day 82 Chest, Shoulder, Tricep	☒ am ☐ pm Day 83 Cardio	☐ am ☐ pm Day 84 Day off

Photocopy this sheet at 140% on your photocopier to enlarge it to a full A4 working size

YORK fitness

CARDIO

	monday	tuesday	wednesday	thursday	friday	saturday	sunday
	day ___ of 84	day ___ of 84	day ___ of 84	day ___ of 84	day ___ of 84	day ___ of 84	day ___ of 84
activity	treadmill	treadmill		treadmill	treadmill	walk / run	
duration	5 mins	5 mins	mins	5 mins	5 mins	30 mins	mins
program / distance	manual	manual		manual	manual	manual	
intensity level	5 out of 10	5 out of 10		5 out of 10	5 out of 10	6-7 out of 10	
time in training zone	N/A mins	N/A mins	mins	N/A mins	N/A mins	N/A mins	mins

STRENGTH

	monday	tuesday	wednesday	thursday	friday	saturday	sunday
Legs: barbell squats	wt/reps 10 10 10			10 10 10 10			
forward lunges	wt/reps 20 20 20			20 20 20			
leg curl	wt/reps 10 10 10			10 10 10			
Back: pulldn o/hand wide	wt/reps 10 10 10			10 10 10			
single arm db row	wt/reps 10 10 10			10 10 10			
Bicep: dumbell hammer curl	wt/reps 10 10 10			10 10 10			
Chest: machine bench press	wt/reps	10 10 10			10 10 10		
Pec Dec	wt/reps	10 10 10			10 10 10		
Shoulder: db o/head press	wt/reps	10 10 10			10 10 10		
dumbell raise side	wt/reps	10 10 10			10 10 10		
Tricep: high cable pushdn	wt/reps	10 10 10			10 10 10		
Torso: crunches feet bench	wt/reps 15 15 15	15 15 15		15 15 15	15 15 15		
Low Back hyper extn	wt/reps 15 15 15	15 15 15		15 15 15	15 15 15		

FLEXIBILITY

		monday	tuesday	wednesday	thursday	friday	saturday	sunday
hip bend	page 261	✓						
buttock	page 262	✓						
short groin	page 262	✓						
hamstring sit	page 263	✓						
calf stand	page 264	✓						
quadricep stand	page 263	✓						
tricep pull-down	page 258	✓						
shoulder pull-across	page 257	✓						
pecs standing	page 259	✓						
shoulder circles	page 257	✓						

strength & muscle size - ADVANCED

instructions for progressing on your 12-week program

- View your training program card and note that you will be training 6 days per week with weights, splitting your body into 3 training parts. These sessions will be shorter in time (approx. 30 mins) than the intermediate level, but far more intense. These sessions are designed to be 'short and sharp' and avoid you pushing weights for an hour, 6 times a week.
- Follow the first week of your 3-way split training program card down the page from day 1 to 7 filling out the weights lifted (kgs or lbs) and the stretches completed.
- Your routine for most exercises will work in a pyramiding fashion where you will begin with a lighter weight for the highest number of repetitions (12) and gradually add weight to each set as you reduce the repetitions, finally finishing with an all out set of 6.
- You will notice the word fail in the repetition section of some exercises. This means complete as many repetitions as possible until you can do no more. Record the number and try to beat this number every session.
- Make sure you do your abdominal work at every session.
- Follow the same routine with Thursday being your day off, until week 4 making sure you also mark off every day on your 12-week (84 day) planner and fill out your training and food diary, if required.
- **At week 5 (day 29)** add a 30-minute cardio session to Tuesday and Saturday mornings and return for your weight session in the evening. There is no provision for recording these sessions, however your session can be anything you choose for 30 minutes with an intensity of 6–7 out of 10.
- Follow the same routine until the end of week 8 making sure you also mark off every day on your 12-week (84 day) planner and fill out your training and food diary, if required.
- **At week 9 (day 57)** add one more 'drop set' to every exercise that finishes with 6 repetitions. The drop set should be done as soon as you finish your 6th repetition with no rest between these 2 sets. Reduce the weight you are lifting back to the same weight you previously lifted for 10 repetitions and blast out a further 10-15 reps or muscle failure, whichever comes first. There is no provision for recording this on your program card, mark it down wherever you can next to your ' 6 rep' weight.

Note: We recommend you take a one week break between finishing one twelve week cycle and starting another. The weight you lift should be heavy enough to cause you some difficulty on the last three repetitions but not so heavy that you need to cheat to complete the movement.

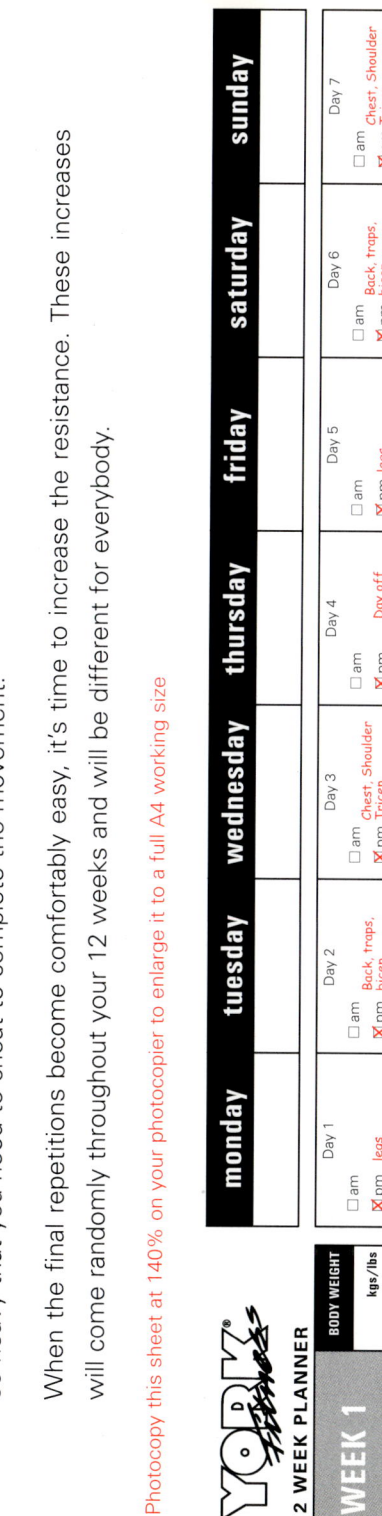

When the final repetitions become comfortably easy, it's time to increase the resistance. These increases will come randomly throughout your 12 weeks and will be different for everybody.

Photocopy this sheet at 140% on your photocopier to enlarge it to a full A4 working size

YORK Fitness — 12 WEEK PLANNER

		monday	tuesday	wednesday	thursday	friday	saturday	sunday
WEEK 1	BODY WEIGHT ___ kgs/lbs	Day 1 ☐ am ☒ pm legs	Day 2 ☐ am ☒ pm Back, traps, bicep	Day 3 ☐ am ☒ pm Chest, Shoulder Tricep	Day 4 ☐ am ☒ pm Day off	Day 5 ☐ am ☒ pm legs	Day 6 ☐ am ☒ pm Back, traps, bicep	Day 7 ☐ am ☒ pm Chest, Shoulder Tricep
WEEK 2	BODY WEIGHT ___ kgs/lbs	Day 8 ☐ am ☒ pm legs	Day 9 ☐ am ☒ pm Back, traps, bicep	Day 10 ☐ am ☒ pm Chest, Shoulder Tricep	Day 11 ☐ am ☒ pm Day off	Day 12 ☐ am ☒ pm legs	Day 13 ☐ am ☒ pm Back, traps, bicep	Day 14 ☐ am ☒ pm Chest, Shoulder Tricep
WEEK 3	BODY WEIGHT ___ kgs/lbs	Day 15 ☐ am ☒ pm legs	Day 16 ☐ am ☒ pm Back, traps, bicep	Day 17 ☐ am ☒ pm Chest, Shoulder Tricep	Day 18 ☐ am ☒ pm Day off	Day 19 ☐ am ☒ pm legs	Day 20 ☐ am ☒ pm Back, traps, bicep	Day 21 ☐ am ☒ pm Chest, Shoulder Tricep
WEEK 4	BODY WEIGHT ___ kgs/lbs	Day 22 ☐ am ☒ pm legs	Day 23 ☐ am ☒ pm Back, traps, bicep	Day 24 ☐ am ☒ pm Chest, Shoulder Tricep	Day 25 ☐ am ☒ pm Day off	Day 26 ☐ am ☒ pm legs	Day 27 ☐ am ☒ pm Back, traps, bicep	Day 28 ☐ am ☒ pm Chest, Shoulder Tricep
WEEK 5	BODY WEIGHT ___ kgs/lbs	Day 29 ☐ am ☒ pm legs	Day 30 ☒ am 30 min Cardio ☒ pm Back, traps, bicep	Day 31 ☐ am ☒ pm Chest, Shoulder Tricep	Day 32 ☐ am ☒ pm Day off	Day 33 ☐ am ☒ pm legs	Day 34 ☒ am 30 min Cardio ☒ pm Back, traps, bicep	Day 35 ☐ am ☒ pm Chest, Shoulder Tricep
WEEK 6	BODY WEIGHT ___ kgs/lbs	Day 36 ☐ am ☒ pm legs	Day 37 ☒ am 30 min Cardio ☒ pm Back, traps, bicep	Day 38 ☐ am ☒ pm Chest, Shoulder Tricep	Day 39 ☐ am ☒ pm Day off	Day 40 ☐ am ☒ pm legs	Day 41 ☒ am 30 min Cardio ☒ pm Back, traps, bicep	Day 42 ☐ am ☒ pm Chest, Shoulder Tricep
WEEK 7	BODY WEIGHT ___ kgs/lbs	Day 43 ☐ am ☒ pm legs	Day 44 ☒ am 30 min Cardio ☒ pm Back, traps, bicep	Day 45 ☐ am ☒ pm Chest, Shoulder Tricep	Day 46 ☐ am ☒ pm Day off	Day 47 ☐ am ☒ pm legs	Day 48 ☒ am 30 min Cardio ☒ pm Back, traps, bicep	Day 49 ☐ am ☒ pm Chest, Shoulder Tricep
WEEK 8	BODY WEIGHT ___ kgs/lbs	Day 50 ☐ am ☒ pm legs	Day 51 ☒ am 30 min Cardio ☒ pm Back, traps, bicep	Day 52 ☐ am ☒ pm Chest, Shoulder Tricep	Day 53 ☐ am ☒ pm Day off	Day 54 ☐ am ☒ pm legs	Day 55 ☒ am 30 min Cardio ☒ pm Back, traps, bicep	Day 56 ☐ am ☒ pm Chest, Shoulder Tricep
WEEK 9	BODY WEIGHT ___ kgs/lbs	Day 57 ☒ am ☒ pm Legs + drop sets	Day 58 ☒ am 30 min Cardio ☒ pm Back, traps, bicep + drop sets	Day 59 ☐ am ☒ pm Chest, Shoulder Tricep + drop sets	Day 60 ☐ am ☒ pm Day off	Day 61 ☐ am ☒ pm Legs + drop sets	Day 62 ☒ am 30 min Cardio ☒ pm Back, traps, bicep + drop sets	Day 63 ☐ am ☒ pm Chest, Shoulder Tricep + drop sets
WEEK 10	BODY WEIGHT ___ kgs/lbs	Day 64 ☒ am ☒ pm Legs + drop sets	Day 65 ☒ am 30 min Cardio ☒ pm Back, traps, bicep + drop sets	Day 66 ☐ am ☒ pm Chest, Shoulder Tricep + drop sets	Day 67 ☐ am ☒ pm Day off	Day 68 ☐ am ☒ pm Legs + drop sets	Day 69 ☒ am 30 min Cardio ☒ pm Back, traps, bicep + drop sets	Day 70 ☒ am Chest, Shoulder ☒ pm Tricep + drop sets
WEEK 11	BODY WEIGHT ___ kgs/lbs	Day 71 ☒ am ☒ pm Legs + drop sets	Day 72 ☒ am 30 min Cardio ☒ pm Back, traps, bicep + drop sets	Day 73 ☒ am Chest, Shoulder ☒ pm Tricep + drop sets	Day 74 ☐ am ☒ pm Day off	Day 75 ☐ am ☒ pm Legs + drop sets	Day 76 ☒ am 30 min Cardio ☒ pm Back, traps, bicep + drop sets	Day 77 ☐ am ☒ pm Chest, Shoulder Tricep + drop sets
WEEK 12	BODY WEIGHT ___ kgs/lbs	Day 78 ☒ am ☒ pm Legs + drop sets	Day 79 ☒ am 30 min Cardio ☒ pm Back, traps, bicep + drop sets	Day 80 ☒ am Chest, Shoulder ☒ pm Tricep + drop sets	Day 81 ☐ am ☐ pm Day off	Day 82 ☐ am ☒ pm Legs + drop sets	Day 83 ☒ am 30 min Cardio ☒ pm Back, traps, bicep + drop sets	Day 84 ☐ am ☒ pm Chest, Shoulder Tricep + drop sets

YORK Fitness

Photocopy this sheet at 140% on your photocopier to enlarge it to a full A4 working size

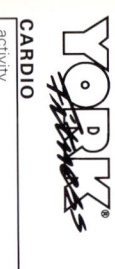

CARDIO

	monday	tuesday	wednesday	thursday	friday	saturday	sunday
activity	day ___ of 84	day ___ of 84	day ___ of 84	day ___ of 84	day ___ of 84	day ___ of 84	day ___ of 84
duration	cycle	cycle	cycle	cycle	cycle	cycle	cycle
program / distance	5 mins	5 mins	5 mins	5 mins	5 mins	5 mins	5 mins
intensity level	manual	manual	manual	manual	manual	manual	manual
time in training zone	5 out of 10	5 out of 10	5 out of 10	5 out of 10	5 out of 10	5 out of 10	5 out of 10
	N/A mins	N/A mins	N/A mins	N/A mins	N/A mins	N/A mins	N/A mins

STRENGTH

		mon	tue	wed	thu	fri	sat	sun
Legs: barbell squats	wt/reps	12 10 8 6			12 10 8 6		12 10 8 6	12 10 8 6
single leg squats	wt/reps				10 8 6		10 8 6	10 8 6
straight leg dead lift	wt/reps	12 10 8 6			12 10 8 6		12 10 8 6	12 10 8 6
calves: stand single leg db	wt/reps	15 15 15 15			15 15 15 15		15 15 15 15	15 15 15 15
Back: chin up w/hand close	wt/reps		fail fail fail fail			fail fail fail fail	fail fail fail fail	fail fail fail fail
bent over barbell row	wt/reps		10 8 6			10 8 6	10 8 6	10 8 6
Traps: barbell upright row	wt/reps		12 10 8 6			12 10 8 6	12 10 8 6	12 10 8 6
Bicep: barbell curl	wt/reps		10 8 6			10 8 6	10 8 6	10 8 6
chest: barbell bench press	wt/reps			12 10 8 6			12 10 8 6	12 10 8 6
incline db flyes	wt/reps			10 8 6			10 8 6	10 8 6
should: barbell o/head press	wt/reps			12 10 8 6			12 10 8 6	12 10 8 6
Tricep: parallel bar dips	wt/reps			fail fail fail			fail fail fail	fail fail fail
abdominals: decline situps	wt/reps	20 20 20 20	20 20 20 20	20 20 20 20	20 20 20 20	20 20 20 20	20 20 20 20	20 20 20 20

FLEXIBILITY

hip bend	page 261	✓
buttock	page 262	✓
short groin	page 262	✓
hamstring sit	page 263	✓
calf stand	page 264	✓
quadricep stand	page 263	✓
tricep pull-down	page 258	✓
shoulder pull-across	page 257	✓
pecs standing	page 259	✓
shoulder circles	page 257	✓

additional advanced strength training techniques

There are many different techniques you can use to stimulate muscle growth once you have reached the advanced level. These are more demanding and challenging than the normal lifting of a weight from point A to point B and back to point A again. Some of these techniques will require a training partner and all of them will require a definite focus and strong mind-set to work through the discomfort and force the muscles to grow bigger and stronger.

1. **Super sets** – This is when you perform two exercises together with no rest between sets. You can either train two opposing muscles in a push/pull super set eg bicep curls and tricep extension or two exercises for the same muscle group eg tricep dips and tricep pushdowns.

2. **Tri sets** – The same as a super set, using the same muscle group, but with a third exercise added and still without rest between sets.

3. **Giant sets** – This is an extension of the tri set but adding another 'same set' exercise to make four sets in a row for the same muscle group.

4. **Multi exercise sets** – For this technique you would need to perform your total number of sets for one muscle group all at once, making every exercise different eg ten different exercises for biceps completed without rest.

5. **Forced reps** – Have your training partner assist you when you reach the point of muscle failure by taking just enough weight on the lift to enable you to complete the repetition and force out a few more reps beyond muscle failure. Also known as 'spotting'.

6. **Negatives** – When you reach the point of muscle failure on the lifting phase, have your training partner assist you through the lifting phase and then let you control the weight through the negative or lowering phase. This is possible because you will almost always be able to lower a weight with control that you can't necessarily lift.

7. **Forced negatives** – Have your training partner place additional force on the 'negative' or lowering phase by pushing against the weight you are trying to control to provide a heavier resistance on the way down than on the way up.

8. **Drop set** – When you have finished your last repetition for your last set, decrease the weight you are lifting to 75% of that weight, and without rest finish off one more set to failure.

9. **Descending sets** – Use this one for your last set of an exercise. As soon as you complete your last repetition, reduce the weight by 75% and push out as many more reps as possible. Repeat this process as many times as required to reach total muscle failure.

10. **Pre-exhaust** – Begin training a major muscle group with an isolation exercise to pre-fatigue the muscle, then move on to a compound exercise to totally fatigue the muscle eg peck dec before bench press.

11. **Pyramids** – Start your first set of an exercise with a moderate weight for higher repetitions and as the sets progress, add weight to each set whilst decreasing the reps of that set eg reps of 12, 10, 8, 6.

12. **Reverse pyramids** – Start with a moderate weight for the first set to warm up, then go to maximum weight for minimum reps and decrease the weight and increase the reps for every additional set eg reps 6, 8, 10, 12.

13. **One and a halfs** – These involve one full repetition followed by a half rep, and then alternating between full and half reps until the set is finished.

14. **21's** – These are a more advanced version of one and a halfs in that you cover the upper and lower range in your half reps. Start with seven reps in the lower range, seven reps in the upper range and then seven full reps, performing 21 reps in total for each set.

15. **Partial reps** – This is a good way to continue to shock the muscle at the completion of a set when no more full reps can be done. Push out as many partial reps as you possibly can to finish off the set.

16. **Compounding** – Compounding is most easily described as a combination of super setting and pre-exhausts. You choose an isolation exercise first eg dumbell flyes and then move straight to the compound eg bench press in a superset fashion, then rest.

17. **Cheating** – These are done to enable you to lift a heavy weight through the weakest point in the range by using a gentle body motion to 'cheat' the weight up and therefore providing an overload to the muscles through the strongest points eg standing barbell curl.

18. **Catches** – These can be done on machines that require both limbs to work together eg leg extension. Lift the weight to the top with both limbs and then lower it back to the start with only one.

fitness & fat loss - BEGINNERS

instructions for progressing on your 12-week program

- Follow your first weeks training program card down the page from day 1 to 7 filling in the weight lifted (kgs or lbs) and the stretches completed.

- Follow the same routine until the end of week 4 making sure you also mark off every day on your 12-week (84 day) planner and fill out your training and food diary, if required.

- **At week 5 (day 29)** add a third cardio and strength session to your week on a Wednesday (same as Monday and Friday) and stretch at the completion of your workout.

Also add 10 additional minutes to the duration of your cardio sessions making them all 40 minutes duration, with 30 minutes at 50-60% Max HR and increase your torso reps from 10 to 20. Thursday will now become a pm stretch day, not a full day off. Don't forget to mark these on your program card over the top of any now-outdated information.

- Follow the same routine until the end of week 8 making sure you also mark off every day on your 12-week (84 day) planner and fill out your training and food diary, if required.

- **At week 9 (day 57)** increase the intensity of Monday, Wednesday and Friday's sessions to a level of 60-70% Max HR and reduce the duration of your session to 30 minutes. Saturday's cardio session and all else remains the same. Don't forget to mark these on your program card over the top of any now-outdated information.

By the completion of week 12 you will need to re-assess your goals and decide whether you are to progress to the fitness/fat loss intermediate level or if your muscle size/strength levels perhaps need to be addressed.

We recommend you take a one week break between finishing one 12 week cycle and starting another.

YORK FITNESS – 12 WEEK PLANNER

Note: The cardio activity that has been selected is not necessarily the activity that you must do. The cardio activity that you choose is up to you, so long as you work at the appropriate intensity level. Keep the intensity of your strength component high by moving quickly between exercises with little rest and increase your weights as the final 5 repetitions become too easy.

Photocopy this sheet at 140% on your photocopier to enlarge it to a full A4 working size

	monday	tuesday	wednesday	thursday	friday	saturday	sunday
WEEK 1 BODY WEIGHT kgs/lbs	Day 1 ☐ am ☒ pm 30 mins Cardio + Strength	Day 2 ☐ am ☐ pm	Day 3 ☐ am ☐ pm	Day 4 ☐ am ☐ pm	Day 5 ☐ am ☒ pm 30 mins Cardio + Strength	Day 6 ☒ am ☐ pm 30 mins Cardio	Day 7 ☐ am ☐ pm Day off
WEEK 2 BODY WEIGHT kgs/lbs	Day 8 ☐ am ☒ pm 30 mins Cardio + Strength	Day 9 ☐ am ☐ pm Stretch	Day 10 ☐ am ☐ pm Day off	Day 11 ☐ am ☒ pm 30 mins Cardio + Strength	Day 12 ☐ am ☒ pm 30 mins Cardio + Strength	Day 13 ☒ am ☐ pm 30 mins Cardio	Day 14 ☐ am ☐ pm Day off
WEEK 3 BODY WEIGHT kgs/lbs	Day 15 ☐ am ☒ pm 30 mins Cardio + Strength	Day 16 ☐ am ☒ pm Stretch	Day 17 ☐ am ☐ pm Day off	Day 18 ☐ am ☒ pm 30 mins Cardio + Strength	Day 19 ☐ am ☒ pm 30 mins Cardio + Strength	Day 20 ☒ am ☐ pm 30 mins Cardio	Day 21 ☐ am ☐ pm Day off
WEEK 4 BODY WEIGHT kgs/lbs	Day 22 ☐ am ☒ pm 30 mins Cardio + Strength	Day 23 ☐ am ☒ pm Stretch	Day 24 ☐ am ☐ pm Day off	Day 25 ☐ am ☒ pm 30 mins Cardio + Strength	Day 26 ☐ am ☒ pm 30 mins Cardio + Strength	Day 27 ☒ am ☐ pm 30 mins Cardio	Day 28 ☐ am ☐ pm Day off
WEEK 5 BODY WEIGHT kgs/lbs	Day 29 ☐ am ☒ pm 40 mins Cardio + Strength	Day 30 ☐ am ☒ pm Stretch	Day 31 ☐ am ☒ pm Day off	Day 32 ☐ am ☐ pm Day off	Day 33 ☐ am ☒ pm 30 mins Cardio + Strength	Day 34 ☒ am ☐ pm 40 mins Cardio	Day 35 ☐ am ☐ pm Day off
WEEK 6 BODY WEIGHT kgs/lbs	Day 36 ☐ am ☒ pm 40 mins Cardio + Strength	Day 37 ☐ am ☒ pm Stretch	Day 38 ☐ am ☒ pm 40 mins Cardio + Strength	Day 39 ☐ am ☒ pm Stretch	Day 40 ☐ am ☒ pm 40 mins Cardio + Strength	Day 41 ☒ am ☐ pm 40 mins Cardio	Day 42 ☐ am ☐ pm Day off
WEEK 7 BODY WEIGHT kgs/lbs	Day 43 ☐ am ☒ pm 40 mins Cardio + Strength	Day 44 ☐ am ☒ pm Stretch	Day 45 ☐ am ☒ pm 40 mins Cardio + Strength	Day 46 ☐ am ☒ pm Stretch	Day 47 ☐ am ☒ pm 40 mins Cardio + Strength	Day 48 ☒ am ☐ pm 40 mins Cardio	Day 49 ☐ am ☐ pm Day off
WEEK 8 BODY WEIGHT kgs/lbs	Day 50 ☐ am ☒ pm 40 mins Cardio + Strength	Day 51 ☐ am ☒ pm Stretch	Day 52 ☐ am ☒ pm 40 mins Cardio + Strength	Day 53 ☐ am ☒ pm Stretch	Day 54 ☐ am ☒ pm 40 mins Cardio + Strength	Day 55 ☒ am ☐ pm 40 mins Cardio	Day 56 ☐ am ☐ pm Day off
WEEK 9 BODY WEIGHT kgs/lbs	Day 57 ☐ am ☒ pm 40 mins Cardio + Strength	Day 58 ☐ am ☒ pm Stretch	Day 59 ☐ am ☒ pm 40 mins Cardio + Strength	Day 60 ☐ am ☒ pm Stretch	Day 61 ☐ am ☒ pm 40 mins Cardio + Strength	Day 62 ☒ am ☐ pm 40 mins Cardio	Day 63 ☐ am ☐ pm Day off
WEEK 10 BODY WEIGHT kgs/lbs	Day 64 ☐ am ☒ pm 40 mins Cardio + Strength	Day 65 ☐ am ☒ pm Stretch	Day 66 ☐ am ☒ pm 30 mins Cardio + Strength	Day 67 ☐ am ☒ pm Stretch	Day 68 ☐ am ☒ pm 30 mins Cardio + Strength	Day 69 ☒ am ☐ pm 40 mins Cardio	Day 70 ☐ am ☐ pm Day off
WEEK 11 BODY WEIGHT kgs/lbs	Day 71 ☐ am ☒ pm 30 mins Cardio + Strength	Day 72 ☐ am ☒ pm Stretch	Day 73 ☐ am ☒ pm 30 mins Cardio + Strength	Day 74 ☐ am ☒ pm Stretch	Day 75 ☐ am ☒ pm 30 mins Cardio + Strength	Day 76 ☒ am ☐ pm 40 mins Cardio	Day 77 ☐ am ☐ pm Day off
WEEK 12 BODY WEIGHT kgs/lbs	Day 78 ☐ am ☒ pm 30 mins Cardio + Strength	Day 79 ☐ am ☒ pm Stretch	Day 80 ☐ am ☒ pm 30 mins Cardio + Strength	Day 81 ☐ am ☒ pm Stretch	Day 82 ☐ am ☒ pm 30 mins Cardio + Strength	Day 83 ☒ am ☐ pm 40 mins Cardio	Day 84 ☐ am ☐ pm Day off

Photocopy this sheet at 140% on your photocopier to enlarge it to a full A4 working size

YORK fitness

CARDIO

	monday	tuesday	wednesday	thursday	friday	saturday	sunday
day	___ of 84	___ of 84	___ of 84	___ of 84	___ of 84	___ of 84	___ of 84
activity	Treadmill				Treadmill	Outdoor walk	
duration	30 mins	mins	mins	mins	30 mins	30 mins	mins
program / distance	manual				manual		
intensity level	50–60% max HR				50–60% max HR	50–60% max HR	
time in training zone	20 mins	mins	mins	mins	20 mins	20 mins	mins

STRENGTH

	monday		tuesday		wednesday		thursday		friday		saturday		sunday	
	wt	reps	wt	reps	wt	reps	wt	reps	wt	reps	wt	reps	wt	reps
Legs: Pulsing Lunges	–	20							–	20				
Back: Low Cable Seat Row	20	20							20	20				
Chest: Machine Bench Press	20	20							20	20				
Torso: Crunches feet floor	10	10							10	10				
Low Back hyper ext	10	10							10	10				

FLEXIBILITY

		monday	tuesday	wednesday	thursday	friday	saturday	sunday
hip bend	page xxx	✓						
buttock	page xxx	✓						
short groin	page xxx	✓						
hamstring sit	page xxx	✓						
calf stand	page xxx	✓						
quadricep stand	page xxx	✓						
tricep pull-down	page xxx	✓						
shoulder pull-across	page xxx	✓						
pecs standing	page xxx	✓						
shoulder circles	page xxx	✓						

fitness & fat loss - INTERMEDIATE

- Follow your first weeks training program card down the page from day 1 to 7 filling in the weight lifted (kgs or lbs) and the stretches completed.

- Follow the same routine until the end of week 4 making sure you also mark off every day on your 12-week (84 day) planner and fill out your training and food diary, if required.

- **At week 5 (day 29)** increase your Monday, Wednesday and Friday cardio sessions to 40 minutes at an intensity of 70-80% Max HR for 30 minutes. Increase your Saturday session to an intensity level of 60-70% Max HR for 40 minutes and make Thursday a strength day, the same as Tuesday. Stretch at the completion of every workout and don't forget to mark these on your program card over the top of any now-outdated information.

- Follow the same routine until the end of week 8 making sure you also mark off every day on your 12-week (84 day) planner and fill out your training and food diary, if required.

- **At week 9 (day 57)** increase your intensity only on Wednesdays session to an intensity level of 80-90% Max HR and reduce your session to 30 minutes total with only 20 minutes at the new higher heart rate level.

Also add another 5 minutes to the cardio component of your strength days, making these now 20 minutes in total. Everything else should remain the same. Stretch at the completion of every workout and don't forget to mark these on your program card over the top of any now-outdated information.

By the completion of week 12 you will need to re-assess your goals and decide whether you are to progress to the fitness/fat loss advanced level or if your muscle size/strength levels perhaps need to be addressed. We recommend you take a one week break between finishing one twelve week cycle and starting another.

Note: The cardio activity that has been selected is not necessarily the activity that you must do. The cardio activity that you choose is up to you, so long as you work at the appropriate intensity level. Keep the intensity of your strength component high by moving quickly between exercises with little rest and increase your weights as the final 5 repetitions become too easy.

Photocopy this sheet at 140% on your photocopier to enlarge it to a full A4 working size

YORK Fitness WORLDWIDE

12 WEEK PLANNER

	monday	tuesday	wednesday	thursday	friday	saturday	sunday
WEEK 1 BODY WEIGHT ___ kgs/lbs	Day 1 — 30 mins Cardio — ☐ am ☒ pm	Day 2 — Strength — ☐ am ☒ pm	Day 3 — 30 mins Cardio — ☐ am ☒ pm	Day 4 — Day off — ☐ am ☐ pm	Day 5 — 30 mins Cardio — ☐ am ☒ pm	Day 6 — 40 mins Cardio — ☒ am ☐ pm	Day 7 — Day off — ☐ am ☐ pm
WEEK 2 BODY WEIGHT ___ kgs/lbs	Day 8 — 30 mins Cardio — ☐ am ☒ pm	Day 9 — Strength — ☐ am ☒ pm	Day 10 — 30 mins Cardio — ☐ am ☒ pm	Day 11 — Day off — ☐ am ☐ pm	Day 12 — 30 mins Cardio — ☐ am ☒ pm	Day 13 — 40 mins Cardio — ☒ am ☐ pm	Day 14 — Day off — ☐ am ☐ pm
WEEK 3 BODY WEIGHT ___ kgs/lbs	Day 15 — 30 mins Cardio — ☐ am ☒ pm	Day 16 — Strength — ☐ am ☒ pm	Day 17 — 30 mins Cardio — ☐ am ☒ pm	Day 18 — Day off — ☐ am ☐ pm	Day 19 — 30 mins Cardio — ☐ am ☒ pm	Day 20 — 40 mins Cardio — ☒ am ☐ pm	Day 21 — Day off — ☐ am ☐ pm
WEEK 4 BODY WEIGHT ___ kgs/lbs	Day 22 — 30 mins Cardio — ☐ am ☒ pm	Day 23 — Strength — ☐ am ☒ pm	Day 24 — 30 mins Cardio — ☐ am ☒ pm	Day 25 — Day off — ☐ am ☐ pm	Day 26 — 30 mins Cardio — ☐ am ☒ pm	Day 27 — 40 mins Cardio — ☒ am ☐ pm	Day 28 — Day off — ☐ am ☐ pm
WEEK 5 BODY WEIGHT ___ kgs/lbs	Day 29 — 40 mins Cardio — ☐ am ☒ pm	Day 30 — Strength — ☐ am ☒ pm	Day 31 — 40 mins Cardio — ☐ am ☒ pm	Day 32 — Strength — ☐ am ☒ pm	Day 33 — 40 mins Cardio — ☐ am ☒ pm	Day 34 — 40 mins Cardio — ☒ am ☐ pm	Day 35 — Day off — ☐ am ☐ pm
WEEK 6 BODY WEIGHT ___ kgs/lbs	Day 36 — 40 mins Cardio — ☐ am ☒ pm	Day 37 — Strength — ☐ am ☒ pm	Day 38 — 40 mins Cardio — ☐ am ☒ pm	Day 39 — Strength — ☐ am ☒ pm	Day 40 — 40 mins Cardio — ☐ am ☒ pm	Day 41 — 40 mins Cardio — ☒ am ☐ pm	Day 42 — Day off — ☐ am ☐ pm
WEEK 7 BODY WEIGHT ___ kgs/lbs	Day 43 — 40 mins Cardio — ☐ am ☒ pm	Day 44 — Strength — ☐ am ☒ pm	Day 45 — 40 mins Cardio — ☐ am ☒ pm	Day 46 — Strength — ☐ am ☒ pm	Day 47 — 40 mins Cardio — ☐ am ☒ pm	Day 48 — 40 mins Cardio — ☒ am ☐ pm	Day 49 — Day off — ☐ am ☐ pm
WEEK 8 BODY WEIGHT ___ kgs/lbs	Day 50 — 40 mins Cardio — ☐ am ☒ pm	Day 51 — Strength — ☐ am ☒ pm	Day 52 — 40 mins Cardio — ☐ am ☒ pm	Day 53 — Strength — ☐ am ☒ pm	Day 54 — 40 mins Cardio — ☐ am ☒ pm	Day 55 — 40 mins Cardio — ☒ am ☐ pm	Day 56 — Day off — ☐ am ☐ pm
WEEK 9 BODY WEIGHT ___ kgs/lbs	Day 57 — 40 mins Cardio — ☐ am ☒ pm	Day 58 — Strength — ☐ am ☒ pm	Day 59 — 30 mins Cardio — ☐ am ☒ pm	Day 60 — Strength — ☐ am ☒ pm	Day 61 — 40 mins Cardio — ☐ am ☒ pm	Day 62 — 40 mins Cardio — ☒ am ☐ pm	Day 63 — Day off — ☐ am ☐ pm
WEEK 10 BODY WEIGHT ___ kgs/lbs	Day 64 — 40 mins Cardio — ☐ am ☒ pm	Day 65 — Strength — ☐ am ☒ pm	Day 66 — 30 mins Cardio — ☐ am ☒ pm	Day 67 — Strength — ☐ am ☒ pm	Day 68 — 40 mins Cardio — ☐ am ☒ pm	Day 69 — 40 mins Cardio — ☒ am ☐ pm	Day 70 — Day off — ☐ am ☐ pm
WEEK 11 BODY WEIGHT ___ kgs/lbs	Day 71 — 40 mins Cardio — ☐ am ☒ pm	Day 72 — Strength — ☐ am ☒ pm	Day 73 — 30 mins Cardio — ☐ am ☒ pm	Day 74 — Strength — ☐ am ☒ pm	Day 75 — 40 mins Cardio — ☐ am ☒ pm	Day 76 — 40 mins Cardio — ☒ am ☐ pm	Day 77 — Day off — ☐ am ☐ pm
WEEK 12 BODY WEIGHT ___ kgs/lbs	Day 78 — 40 mins Cardio — ☐ am ☒ pm	Day 79 — Strength — ☐ am ☒ pm	Day 80 — 30 mins Cardio — ☐ am ☒ pm	Day 81 — Strength — ☐ am ☒ pm	Day 82 — 40 mins Cardio — ☐ am ☒ pm	Day 83 — 40 mins Cardio — ☒ am ☐ pm	Day 84 — Day off — ☐ am ☐ pm

Photocopy this sheet at 140% on your photocopier to enlarge it to a full A4 working size

YORK Fitness WORLDWIDE

CARDIO

activity		monday	tuesday	wednesday	thursday	friday	saturday	sunday
		day ___ of 84	day ___ of 84	day ___ of 84	day ___ of 84	day ___ of 84	day ___ of 84	day ___ of 84
duration		Cycle	Treadmill	Cycle		Cycle	Outdoor walk	
		40 mins	15 mins	40 mins		40 mins	40 mins	mins
program / distance		manual	manual	manual		manual		
intensity level		60-70% max HR	70-80% max HR	60-70% max HR		60-70% max HR	50-60% max HR	
time in training zone		30 mins	10 mins	30 mins		30 mins	30 mins	mins

STRENGTH

		wt / reps
Legs: Walking Lunges		20 / 20
Dumbell Squats		20 / 20
Back: Single Arm db Row		20 / 20
Pulldn u/hand c/grip		20 / 20
Chest: Machine Bench Press		20 / 20
Pec deck		20 / 20
Torso: Crunches feet bench		20 / 20
Crunches feet elev.		20 / 20
Low Back hyper ext		

FLEXIBILITY

hip bend	page xxx	✓
buttock	page xxx	✓
short groin	page xxx	✓
hamstring sit	page xxx	✓
calf stand	page xxx	✓
quadricep stand	page xxx	✓
tricep pull-down	page xxx	✓
shoulder pull-across	page xxx	✓
pecs standing	page xxx	✓
shoulder circles	page xxx	✓

fitness & fat loss - ADVANCED

instructions for progressing on your 12-week program

- Follow your first weeks training program card down the page from day 1 to 7 filling in the weight lifted (kgs or lbs) and the stretches completed.

- Follow the same routine until the end of week 4 making sure you also mark off every day on your 12-week (84 day) planner and fill out your training and food diary, if required.

- **At week 5 (day 29)** make Fridays session a high intensity session for the week (same as Monday and Wednesday) and move it to the A.M. timeslot. This should now give you 3 x 30 minute sessions at 80-90% Max HR

Also add 10 repetitions to all torso exercises making them sets of 30. Stretch at the completion of every workout and don't forget to mark these on your program card over the top of any now-outdated information.

- Follow the same routine until the end of week 8 making sure you also mark off every day on your 12-week (84 day) planner and fill out your training and food diary, if required.

- **At week 9 (day 57)** add a 30 minute walk to Tuesday and Thursday in the A.M. timeslot at the same intensity level as Saturday (60-70% Max HR), this should be a reasonably easy session. You should still come back for your P.M. strength session. There is no provision for marking this on your program card, you will need to mark it down wherever you can in the cardio section next to your 20-minute session for the afternoon.

Stretch at the completion of every workout and don't forget to mark these on your program card over the top of any now-outdated information. We recommend you take a one week break between finishing one twelve week cycle and starting another.

YORK Fitness 12 WEEK PLANNER

Advanced tips: You will notice that most of your cardio sessions are scheduled for the A.M. timeslot. There are 2 reasons for this. One is that as your sessions for an advanced exerciser are shorter, they can be completed before the start of a busy work-day. Two and more importantly, your body will use fat stores more efficiently for energy first thing in the morning before eating anything. The only thing that should pass your lips before you exercise is a glass of water. If you can put off having breakfast until after you have showered and dressed, your body will keep burning up calories due to a revved up metabolism.

Photocopy this sheet at 140% on your photocopier to enlarge it to a full A4 working size

	monday	tuesday	wednesday	thursday	friday	saturday	sunday
WEEK 1 BODY WEIGHT kgs/lbs	Day 1 — ☒am ☐pm — 30 min Cardio	Day 2 — ☐am ☒pm — Strenght	Day 3 — ☐am ☒pm — 30 min Cardio	Day 4 — ☐am ☒pm — Strenght	Day 5 — ☒am ☐pm — 40 min Cardio	Day 6 — ☒am ☐pm — 40 min Cardio	Day 7 — ☐am ☐pm — Day off
WEEK 2 BODY WEIGHT kgs/lbs	Day 8 — ☒am ☐pm — 30 min Cardio	Day 9 — ☐am ☒pm — Strenght	Day 10 — ☐am ☒pm — 30 min Cardio	Day 11 — ☐am ☒pm — Strenght	Day 12 — ☒am ☐pm — 40 min Cardio	Day 13 — ☒am ☐pm — 40 min Cardio	Day 14 — ☐am ☐pm — Day off
WEEK 3 BODY WEIGHT kgs/lbs	Day 15 — ☒am ☐pm — 30 min Cardio	Day 16 — ☐am ☒pm — Strenght	Day 17 — ☐am ☒pm — 30 min Cardio	Day 18 — ☐am ☒pm — Strenght	Day 19 — ☒am ☐pm — 40 min Cardio	Day 20 — ☒am ☐pm — 40 min Cardio	Day 21 — ☐am ☐pm — Day off
WEEK 4 BODY WEIGHT kgs/lbs	Day 22 — ☒am ☐pm — 30 min Cardio	Day 23 — ☐am ☒pm — Strenght	Day 24 — ☐am ☒pm — 30 min Cardio	Day 25 — ☐am ☒pm — Strenght	Day 26 — ☒am ☐pm — 40 min Cardio	Day 27 — ☒am ☐pm — 40 min Cardio	Day 28 — ☐am ☐pm — Day off
WEEK 5 BODY WEIGHT kgs/lbs	Day 29 — ☒am ☐pm — 30 min Cardio	Day 30 — ☐am ☒pm — Strenght	Day 31 — ☐am ☒pm — 30 min Cardio	Day 32 — ☐am ☒pm — Strenght	Day 33 — ☒am ☐pm — 40 min Cardio	Day 34 — ☒am ☐pm — 40 min Cardio	Day 35 — ☐am ☐pm — Day off
WEEK 6 BODY WEIGHT kgs/lbs	Day 36 — ☒am ☐pm — 30 min Cardio	Day 37 — ☐am ☒pm — Strenght	Day 38 — ☒am ☐pm — 30 min Cardio	Day 39 — ☐am ☒pm — Strenght	Day 40 — ☒am ☐pm — 30 min Cardio	Day 41 — ☒am ☐pm — 40 min Cardio	Day 42 — ☐am ☐pm — Day off
WEEK 7 BODY WEIGHT kgs/lbs	Day 43 — ☒am ☐pm — 30 min Cardio	Day 44 — ☐am ☒pm — Strenght	Day 45 — ☒am ☐pm — 30 min Cardio	Day 46 — ☐am ☒pm — Strenght	Day 47 — ☒am ☐pm — 30 min Cardio	Day 48 — ☒am ☐pm — 40 min Cardio	Day 49 — ☐am ☐pm — Day off
WEEK 8 BODY WEIGHT kgs/lbs	Day 50 — ☒am ☐pm — 30 min Cardio	Day 51 — ☐am ☒pm — Strenght	Day 52 — ☒am ☐pm — 30 min Cardio	Day 53 — ☐am ☒pm — Strenght	Day 54 — ☒am ☐pm — 30 min Cardio	Day 55 — ☒am ☐pm — 40 min Cardio	Day 56 — ☐am ☐pm — Day off
WEEK 9 BODY WEIGHT kgs/lbs	Day 57 — ☒am ☐pm — 30 min Cardio	Day 58 — ☐am ☒pm — Strenght	Day 59 — ☒am ☐pm — 30 min Cardio	Day 60 — ☐am ☒pm — Strenght	Day 61 — ☒am ☐pm — 30 min Cardio	Day 62 — ☒am ☐pm — 40 min Cardio	Day 63 — ☐am ☐pm — Day off
WEEK 10 BODY WEIGHT kgs/lbs	Day 64 — ☒am ☐pm — 30 min Cardio	Day 65 — ☐am ☒pm — Strenght	Day 66 — ☒am ☐pm — 30 min Cardio	Day 67 — ☐am ☒pm — Strenght	Day 68 — ☒am ☐pm — 30 min Cardio	Day 69 — ☒am ☐pm — 40 min Cardio	Day 70 — ☐am ☐pm — Day off
WEEK 11 BODY WEIGHT kgs/lbs	Day 71 — ☒am ☐pm — 30 min Cardio	Day 72 — ☐am ☒pm — Strenght	Day 73 — ☒am ☐pm — 30 min Cardio	Day 74 — ☐am ☒pm — Strenght	Day 75 — ☒am ☐pm — 30 min Cardio	Day 76 — ☒am ☐pm — 40 min Cardio	Day 77 — ☐am ☐pm — Day off
WEEK 12 BODY WEIGHT kgs/lbs	Day 78 — ☒am ☐pm — 30 min Cardio	Day 79 — ☒am ☐pm — Strenght	Day 80 — ☒am ☐pm — 30 min Cardio	Day 81 — ☒am ☐pm — Strenght	Day 82 — ☒am ☐pm — 30 min Cardio	Day 83 — ☒am ☐pm — 40 min Cardio	Day 84 — ☐am ☐pm — Day off

Note: The cardio activity that has been selected is not necessarily the activity that you must do. The cardio activity that you choose is up to you, so long as you work at the appropriate intensity level. Keep the intensity of your strength component high by moving quickly between exercises with little rest and increase your weights as the final 5 repetitions become too easy.

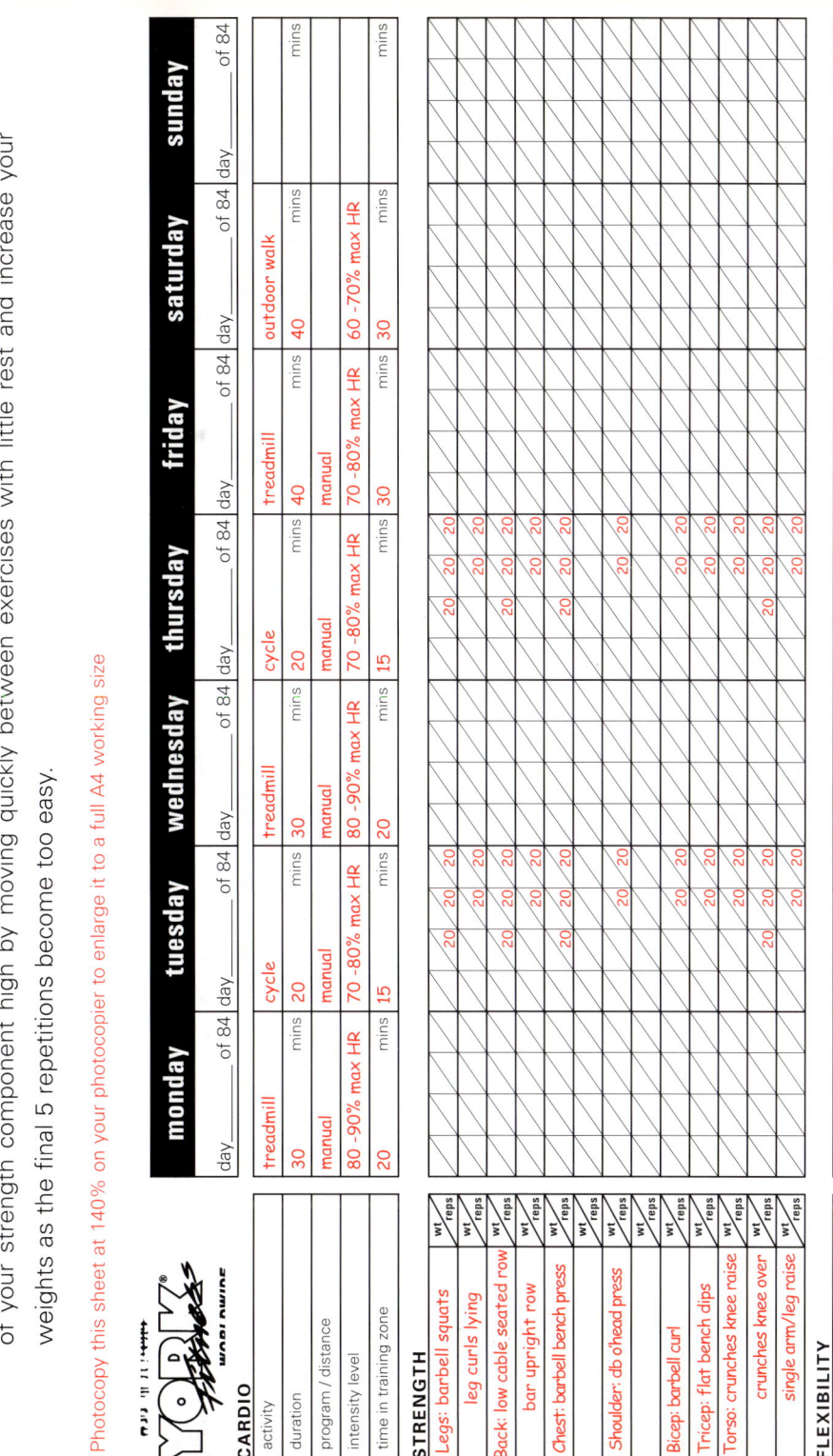

Photocopy this sheet at 140% on your photocopier to enlarge it to a full A4 working size

YORK FITNESS WORLDWIDE

CARDIO

	monday	tuesday	wednesday	thursday	friday	saturday	sunday
	day ___ of 84	day ___ of 84	day ___ of 84	day ___ of 84	day ___ of 84	day ___ of 84	day ___ of 84
activity	treadmill	cycle	treadmill	cycle	treadmill	outdoor walk	
duration	30 mins	20 mins	30 mins	20 mins	40 mins	40 mins	mins
program / distance	manual	manual	manual	manual	manual		
intensity level	80 -90% max HR	70 -80% max HR	80 -90% max HR	70 -80% max HR	70 -80% max HR	60 -70% max HR	
time in training zone	20 mins	15 mins	20 mins	15 mins	30 mins	30 mins	mins

STRENGTH

	monday wt/reps	tuesday wt/reps	wednesday wt/reps	thursday wt/reps	friday wt/reps	saturday wt/reps	sunday wt/reps
Legs: barbell squats		20		20			
leg curls lying		20		20			
Back: low cable seated row		20		20			
bar upright row		20		20			
Chest: barbell bench press		20		20			
		20		20			
Shoulder: db o'head press		20		20			
Bicep: barbell curl		20		20			
Tricep: flat bench dips		20		20			
Torso: crunches knee raise		20		20			
crunches knee over		20		20			
single arm/leg raise		20		20			

FLEXIBILITY

hip bend	page xxx	✓					
buttock	page xxx	✓					
short groin	page xxx	✓					
hamstring sit	page xxx	✓					
calf stand	page xxx	✓					
quadricep stand	page xxx	✓					
tricep pull-down	page xxx	✓					
shoulder pull-across	page xxx	✓					
pecs standing	page xxx	✓					
shoulder circles	page xxx						

THE 30 MINUTE EXPRESS WORKOUT

The phrase we most always hear from potential new exercisers is 'I'd really like to but I just can't find the time'. The secret is obviously not in waiting around and trying to find the time, but rather in making the time in your lifestyle. Most people involved in a fitness program are not doing it because they have nothing else to do, they are in control of their time.

With a home gym set-up, you will never have the time excuse again. Your gym is always open, never crowded, you won't get wet when it's raining travelling between the lounge room and your training room and the only thing you have to worry about parking is your bottom on the equipment!

Understandably some people's lifestyles are a little fuller than others. It is for this reason that we have put together the 30-minute express workout. There should be no one out there who cannot find 30 minutes, three times per week for this general health and fitness program.

Perhaps you could cut out some TV time (try keeping a 'TV diary' one week to see what you really didn't need to watch), or maybe you could set your alarm clock for half an hour earlier in the morning or go to bed half an hour later at night. If your problem is household chores then try delegating some of the work to others living under your roof. The time is there, and how badly you want to see your results will be determined by how hard you look to 'find the time'.

This session will also be useful for those already involved in a training program who unavoidably have a day when nothing has gone to plan and time has got away. It's the all too familiar situation of 'I've only got half an hour, I won't get anything done in that time, it's probably not worth starting now. I'll start again tomorrow'

WRONG! Get into the 30-minute express and you will be amazed at how good you feel afterward.

- Begin with 15 minutes cardio of your choice. Allow a five minute warm-up and then 10 minutes at 70-80% of your maximum heart rate.

- Go straight to the strength component of the workout without rest and complete one set of each exercise for 15 repetitions (20 in total for lunges) making sure each set is taken to complete exhaustion and every repetition is done slowly and smoothly.

- Complete all 13 exercises one after the other and finish with a quick full body stretch.

Photocopy this sheet at 140% on your photocopier to enlarge it to a full A4 working size

YORK Fitness

CARDIO

activity	monday date:___	tuesday date:___	wednesday date:___	thursday date:___	friday date:___	saturday date:___	sunday date:___
activity	treadmill	treadmill	treadmill	treadmill	treadmill	treadmill	treadmill
duration	15 mins	15 mins	15 mins	15 mins	15 mins	15 mins	15 mins
program / distance	manual	manual	manual	manual	manual	manual	manual
intensity level	70-80% max HR	70-80% max HR	70-80% max HR	70-80% max HR	70-80% max HR	70-80% max HR	70-80% max HR
time in training zone	10 mins	10 mins	10 mins	10 mins	10 mins	10 mins	10 mins

STRENGTH

	wt/reps	wt/reps	wt/reps	wt/reps	wt/reps	wt/reps	wt/reps
forward lunges	20	20	20	20	20	20	20
leg extension	15	15	15	15	15	15	15
leg curl lying	15	15	15	15	15	15	15
pulldown u/hand close	15	15	15	15	15	15	15
machine bench press	15	15	15	15	15	15	15
low cable seated row	15	15	15	15	15	15	15
pec deck	15	15	15	15	15	15	15
upright row (bar or dumbell)	15	15	15	15	15	15	15
dumbell o/head shoulder press	15	15	15	15	15	15	15
bicep dumbell curl seated	15	15	15	15	15	15	15
tricep flat bench dips	15	15	15	15	15	15	15
torso crunches feet bench	15	15	15	15	15	15	15
lower back hyperextention	15	15	15	15	15	15	15

FLEXIBILITY

hip bend	page 261	✓
buttock	page 262	✓
short groin	page 262	✓
hamstring sit	page 263	✓
calf stand	page 264	✓
quadricep stand	page 263	✓
tricep pull-down	page 258	✓
shoulder pull-across	page 257	✓
pecs standing	page 259	✓
shoulder circles	page 257	✓

tips for writing your own program

There will come a time, hopefully sooner rather than later, when you will want and need to start writing your own custom designed strength programs. You may find certain body parts need more or less work than others, you want to train for a specific reason or you may just be getting a little bored with the programs provided and want to experiment with something different, thus finding out what works well for you.

All these things are a natural progression on any strength program and varying the stimulation you place on your body will help to keep you progressing as well as keeping your mind active. With so many different exercises to choose from, boredom should not be an issue.

There is however one important thing that you will need to clearly understand, and that is how to differentiate between a compound exercise and an isolation exercise:

Compound – Compound exercises are those that involve the use of a number of muscles working together creating movement through a number of joints eg bench press or squats.

Isolation – Isolation exercises are those that usually isolate one single muscle and create movement through only one single joint eg pec dec/flyes or leg extension.

Once you have grasped this, the following tips will further assist you in designing an effective custom program.

- If you are doing a full-body session, try to work from the largest muscles to the smallest i.e. legs, back, chest, shoulders, triceps, biceps and abdominals. The main reason for this is that you will find it difficult to work the muscles of your back if your biceps are fatigued. The same goes for chest if you have already worked triceps and shoulders.

- Always allow at least 48 hours recovery time between working the same muscle group.

- If you are writing a split-routine, try not to schedule chest work the day after a heavy tricep workout as the triceps will not have recovered and will be forced to work while in recovery mode, consequently the muscle will have no power. This is similar to that of the full body biggest to smallest idea.

- As a rule, try to perform a compound exercise before you do an isolation exercise as you will lift more weight and use more muscles in your compound exercise and then finish off with isolation. There are of course exceptions to every rule and for this one, have a look at the pre-exhaust technique in the additional advanced strength training techniques section.

- When writing your custom program, try to always include at least one compound exercise for each muscle group and then an isolation exercise. For example, when training the muscles of the chest, always include one compound pressing movement, then an isolation flye movement. Rather than doing something like pec deck and flyes together and no press movement as you will miss the benefits of good, heavy compound lifting which is where the major gains will be made for strength and muscle size.

- Where repetitions are concerned, the general, broad-based theory is that a heavier weight lifted for fewer repetitions (6-12) will stimulate muscle size and strength. While a lighter weight lifted for a greater number of repetitions (15-20) will be more beneficial for muscle endurance and can be used for higher heart rate training like circuits and cross training.

- Before you include advanced exercises on your program, make sure that you have a good feeling for how the weights move through space and a definite feel for where the exercise is working as well as a good base level of strength. For some this may come after only a matter of weeks. If so there is no reason why you shouldn't give them a go and include them in your program.

YORK Fitness 12 WEEK PLANNER

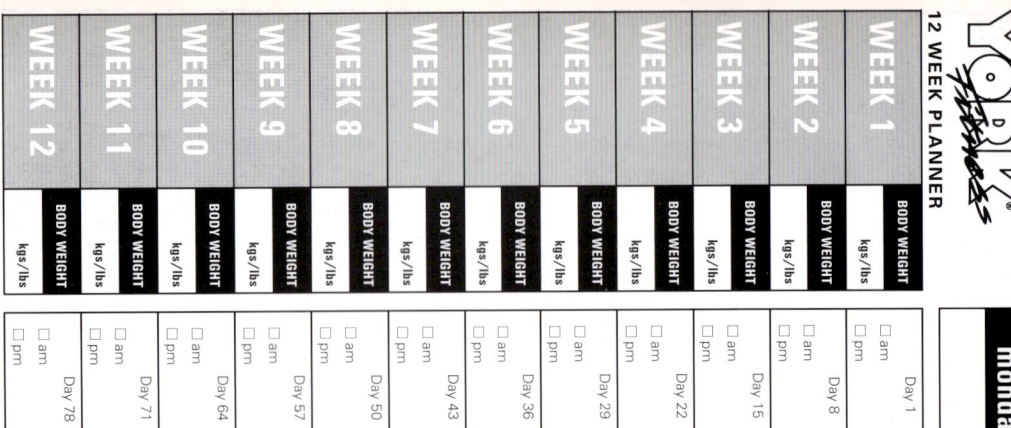

Photocopy this sheet at 140% on your photocopier to enlarge it to a full A4 working size

	monday	tuesday	wednesday	thursday	friday	saturday	sunday
WEEK 1 BODY WEIGHT ___ kgs/lbs	Day 1 □am □pm	Day 2 □am □pm	Day 3 □am □pm	Day 4 □am □pm	Day 5 □am □pm	Day 6 □am □pm	Day 7 □am □pm
WEEK 2 BODY WEIGHT ___ kgs/lbs	Day 8 □am □pm	Day 9 □am □pm	Day 10 □am □pm	Day 11 □am □pm	Day 12 □am □pm	Day 13 □am □pm	Day 14 □am □pm
WEEK 3 BODY WEIGHT ___ kgs/lbs	Day 15 □am □pm	Day 16 □am □pm	Day 17 □am □pm	Day 18 □am □pm	Day 19 □am □pm	Day 20 □am □pm	Day 21 □am □pm
WEEK 4 BODY WEIGHT ___ kgs/lbs	Day 22 □am □pm	Day 23 □am □pm	Day 24 □am □pm	Day 25 □am □pm	Day 26 □am □pm	Day 27 □am □pm	Day 28 □am □pm
WEEK 5 BODY WEIGHT ___ kgs/lbs	Day 29 □am □pm	Day 30 □am □pm	Day 31 □am □pm	Day 32 □am □pm	Day 33 □am □pm	Day 34 □am □pm	Day 35 □am □pm
WEEK 6 BODY WEIGHT ___ kgs/lbs	Day 36 □am □pm	Day 37 □am □pm	Day 38 □am □pm	Day 39 □am □pm	Day 40 □am □pm	Day 41 □am □pm	Day 42 □am □pm
WEEK 7 BODY WEIGHT ___ kgs/lbs	Day 43 □am □pm	Day 44 □am □pm	Day 45 □am □pm	Day 46 □am □pm	Day 47 □am □pm	Day 48 □am □pm	Day 49 □am □pm
WEEK 8 BODY WEIGHT ___ kgs/lbs	Day 50 □am □pm	Day 51 □am □pm	Day 52 □am □pm	Day 53 □am □pm	Day 54 □am □pm	Day 55 □am □pm	Day 56 □am □pm
WEEK 9 BODY WEIGHT ___ kgs/lbs	Day 57 □am □pm	Day 58 □am □pm	Day 59 □am □pm	Day 60 □am □pm	Day 61 □am □pm	Day 62 □am □pm	Day 63 □am □pm
WEEK 10 BODY WEIGHT ___ kgs/lbs	Day 64 □am □pm	Day 65 □am □pm	Day 66 □am □pm	Day 67 □am □pm	Day 68 □am □pm	Day 69 □am □pm	Day 70 □am □pm
WEEK 11 BODY WEIGHT ___ kgs/lbs	Day 71 □am □pm	Day 72 □am □pm	Day 73 □am □pm	Day 74 □am □pm	Day 75 □am □pm	Day 76 □am □pm	Day 77 □am □pm
WEEK 12 BODY WEIGHT ___ kgs/lbs	Day 78 □am □pm	Day 79 □am □pm	Day 80 □am □pm	Day 81 □am □pm	Day 82 □am □pm	Day 83 □am □pm	Day 84 □am □pm

Photocopy this sheet at 140% on your photocopier to enlarge it to a full A4 working size

YORK FITNESS

	monday	tuesday	wednesday	thursday	friday	saturday	sunday
CARDIO	day ___ of 84	day ___ of 84	day ___ of 84	day ___ of 84	day ___ of 84	day ___ of 84	day ___ of 84
activity							
duration	___ mins	___ mins	___ mins	___ mins	___ mins	___ mins	___ mins
program / distance							
intensity level							
time in training zone	___ mins	___ mins	___ mins	___ mins	___ mins	___ mins	___ mins

STRENGTH

	wt/reps	wt/reps	wt/reps	wt/reps	wt/reps	wt/reps	wt/reps

FLEXIBILITY

hip bend	page 261
buttock	page 262
short groin	page 262
hamstring sit	page 263
calf stand	page 264
quadricep stand	page 263
tricep pull-down	page 258
shoulder pull-across	page 257
pecs standing	page 259
shoulder circles	page 257

YORK Fitness
TRAINING DIARY

Photocopy this sheet at 140% on your photocopier to enlarge it to a full A4 working size

	monday	tuesday	wednesday	thursday	friday	saturday	sunday
WEEK 1 — time of day / mood / energy level							
WEEK 2 — time of day / mood / energy level							
WEEK 3 — time of day / mood / energy level							
WEEK 4 — time of day / mood / energy level							
WEEK 5 — time of day / mood / energy level							
WEEK 6 — time of day / mood / energy level							
WEEK 7 — time of day / mood / energy level							
WEEK 8 — time of day / mood / energy level							
WEEK 9 — time of day / mood / energy level							
WEEK 10 — time of day / mood / energy level							
WEEK 11 — time of day / mood / energy level							
WEEK 12 — time of day / mood / energy level							

YORK Fitness FOOD DIARY

Photocopy this sheet at 140% on your photocopier to enlarge it to a full A4 working size

	monday	tuesday	wednesday	thursday	friday	saturday	sunday
	date:	date:	date:	date:	date:	date:	date:
1 MEAL 1 BREAKFAST							
2 MEAL 2 AM SNACK							
3 MEAL 3 LUNCH							
4 MEAL 4 PM SNACK							
5 MEAL 5 DINNER							
6 MEAL 6 SUPPER							

our ten favourite exercises and why you should do them

Below we have listed ten exercises that are favourites of ours for the reasons outlined in section two. There is one exercise per major muscle group and we suggest where possible you add these to your training program.

1. **front thigh** – barbell squats. Page 76 This one will often be described as the best exercise you can do. It not only works all the muscles of the lower body but also brings into play the abdominal and lower back muscles for stability, the strength of the upper body for balance and heart rate elevation.

2. **back thigh** – leg curls lying. Page 87 When it comes to isolating the hamstrings, you can't go wrong with this one. Because you can keep both legs and hips square against the bench, you can really pull in hard and direct all the work to the hamstrings with little risk of twisting and moving.

3. **lower leg** – calf raise standing single leg. Page 93 This exercise is a favourite because of ease of performance. All you need is a dumbell and an elevated surface and both legs can be worked quickly and effectively. You don't need to use a lot of weight either as you are already lifting your own body weight on only one leg.

4. **back** – low cable seated row. Page 99 Of all the back exercises to choose from, cable and free weight, we have chosen this one because it gives the greatest feeling of the back muscles contracting as you squeeze your shoulder blades together and push your chest out. It also provides a good forward stretch.

5. **upper back** – barbell upright row. Page 107 The barbell upright row appeals to us because it is a relatively fluent movement with the barbell tracking in front of you whilst giving a good squeeze on the trapezius.

6. **chest** – bench press. Pages 115, 117, 120 A bench press where you are pushing weight away from you at a 90degree angle eg flat bench press with barbell or a machine press is almost always going to be the best chest exercise. This is your most powerful exercise for this muscle group and will also work the deltoids and triceps. It is one of the best overall strength developers.

7. **shoulders** – dumbell overhead press seated. Page 130 As the bench press is for the chest, so to is the overhead press for the shoulders. Our preference here would be for dumbells for two reasons. One is the ease of getting into a pressing position with dumbells, and two is the greater range of motion you get from using dumbells.

8. **front arms** – standing barbell curls. Page 142 This is your most basic curling movement and it is for this reason that it is our pick. There should be minimal risk of twisting as you curl and you should be able to feel a strong, even load against the biceps.

9. **back arms** – dips. Pages 158, 162 Dips can be done just about anywhere – on a bench, coffee table, chair or if you are out walking, a park bench. Dips are a very versatile exercise and very effective. When completed with good form, dips will give you a good 'worked' sensation.

10. **torso** – crunches feet on bench. Page 169 Of all the gadgets and gizmos available on the television shopping shows, nothing will ever replace a well-executed abdominal crunch. With this crunch, your lower back is supported hard against the floor and your abdominals squeeze hard through a perfect crunching range. If you do this correctly, you won't need many repetitions to get that 'burning' feeling.

SECTION FOURTEEN flexibility

Flexibility is most easily described as the measure of how our bodies move, determined by our muscles and joints.

The more we stretch our muscles and joints, the more we can increase the range of motion available throughout our bodies.

When building a stretching routine into your fitness/strength training program, the most important thing to remember is that if you are going to work a specific muscle or muscle group in any way you should also be stretching that same muscle. Also remember that a muscle that is worked must also be stretched. Stretching immediately after working a muscle will help to restore length and decrease the level of post exercise muscle soreness.

Flexibility levels will differ with everybody so it is therefore important to work at your own level and concern yourself only with improvements to your own range of motion and not everyone else's.

When you do stretch it is imperative that you only stretch when your muscles are warm. The best way to prepare your muscles for stretching is by performing a brief period of aerobic activity, ten minutes of brisk walking for instance. If you are exercising in colder conditions, make sure that you allow a little extra time to fully warm up and take extra care when you start your stretch routine.

As you follow your training program card, you will find that your flexibility routine is done at the end of your workout, after you have completed your cardio and strength component. However we also recommend you stretch throughout your session especially if you are following a strength routine. You should also run through the list of stretches on days when you may have nothing else scheduled training-wise. It is on those non-training days that a pre-stretch warm up is a must.

There are many limiting factors with everybody as far as flexibility is concerned. Genetics, joint structure, body mass and any current injuries are all specific areas that will enhance or inhibit an individual's level of flexibility.

However the one common factor with us all is age. The older we get the less flexible we become and the longer it takes to see improvements. Although increased flexibility may not be able to be achieved at the same rate as we get older, due to changes in our connective tissue, it should still be developed at all ages and should go hand in hand with our strength and fitness program from today through the rest of your life.

benefits of stretching

Increased suppleness
Improved posture
Reduced risk of injury

Increased mental and physical relaxation
Reduced muscle soreness/tension
Greater physical fitness

How to stretch

- Only stretch when your body is warm
- stretch only to a mild discomfort, never pain
- hold each stretch for 10 – 20 seconds
- rest and repeat

Tip Stretch gently and slowly and relax into each stretch

We have selected 20 of what we believe to be the most effective stretches for full body flexibility and range of motion to be used in conjunction with your training program.

Included on your program card are ten selected stretches to be completed at the end of each training session. We also recommend you do a brief version of the same ten after your cardio and prior to starting your strength routine to prepare your muscles for the weight they are about to lift. For example, do each stretch only once and hold for about ten seconds.

You may also find the remaining ten stretches useful to include in your own routine that will aid in improving your total overall flexibility and may be done at some stage every day if desired. It should only take around 15 minutes to complete all 20 stretches as a daily routine.

This basic guide to flexibility is a fairly general covering of what is a rather complex topic. There are of course many more stretches and stretching techniques that we have not covered in this home exercise guide. For a more comprehensive insight into the subject of flexibility, we suggest taking a look at one of the many publications dealing specifically with the topic of stretching and flexibility.

1. pull behind

muscles stretching: **Trapezius (upper back)**

Middle deltoids (shoulders)

Biceps (front arms)

The action: Stand upright with your feet about shoulder width apart keeping your chest high and your eyes focused straight ahead. Bring your right hand across behind your back and grasp your right wrist with your left hand. Gently pull down and across while at the same time dropping your left ear towards your left shoulder. Hold the stretch and repeat for the left side.

Tip Try not to allow your head to drop forward or your body to twist as you stretch.

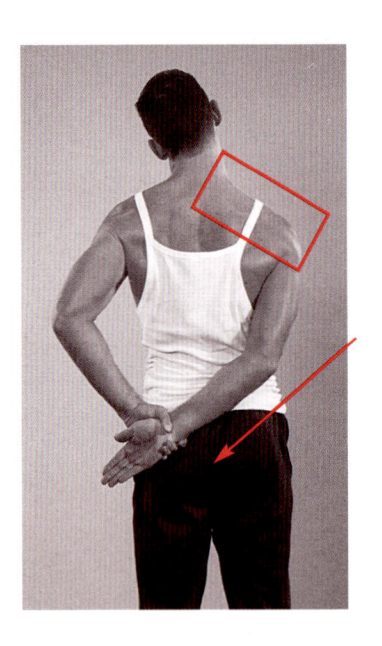

2. shoulder circles

muscles stretching:	**Trapezius (upper back)**
	Deltoids (shoulders)
	Rhomboids (mid back)
areas released:	**neck, shoulders, chest**

The action: Stand upright with your feet about shoulder width apart keeping your chest high and your eyes focused straight ahead. Lift both shoulders up towards your ears and gently roll them backwards and down. Pause for a moment and then reverse the direction. Roll in circles

Tip Try to feel every circle rather than just rolling around.

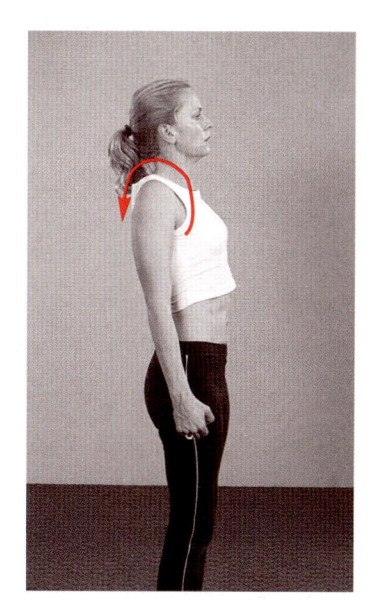

3. shoulder pull across

muscles stretching:	**Rear deltoids (shoulders)**
	Middle deltoids (shoulders)

The action: Stand upright with your feet about shoulder-width apart keeping your chest high and your eyes focused straight ahead. Bring your right arm across in front of your upper chest and gently pull the elbow further across. Hold the stretch and repeat for the left side.

Tip Try not to allow your head to drop forward or your body to twist as you stretch.

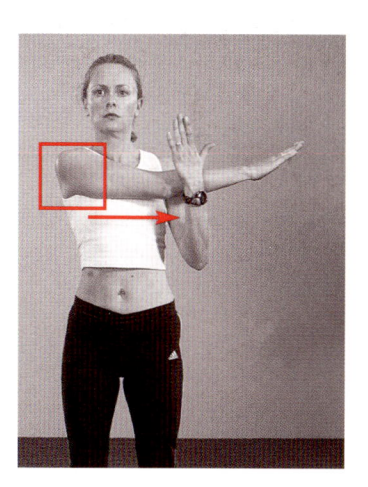

4. tricep pull down

muscles stretching   Triceps (back arms)

The action: Stand upright with your feet about shoulder width apart keeping your chest high and your eyes focused straight ahead. Bring your right arm down behind your head so your fingertips touch your spine. Gently pull your right elbow down behind your head. Hold the stretch and repeat for the left side.

Tip Try not to allow your head to drop forward or your body to twist as you stretch.

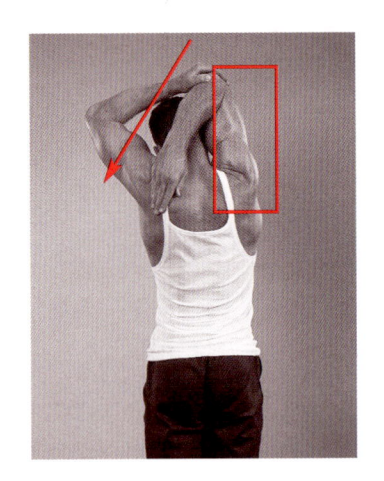

5. high reach

muscles stretching: Latissimus dorsi (back)

areas released: shoulder, elbow, wrist

The action: Stand upright with your feet about shoulder width apart keeping your chest high and your eyes focused straight ahead. Bring your arms together out in front and clasp your hands, interlocking your fingers. Turn your palms inside out and stretch your arms out in front. Gently lift your arms overhead and reach up as high as you can. Hold the stretch.

Tip Try to have your hands finish as close to directly above your head as possible.

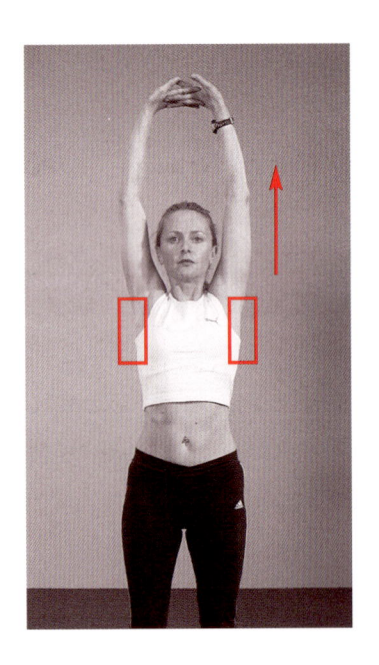

6. pecs supported

muscles stretching: **Pectorals (chest)**

Front deltoids (shoulders)

The action: Stand upright close to a vertical piece on your home gym or use a door frame. Place your right forearm against the vertical section to form a 90-degree angle at your elbow. Step your right foot forward to lean into the stretch and at the same time turn your chest away from your right arm. Hold the stretch and repeat for the left side.

Tip Try to stand tall and keep your shoulders back to avoid twisting through the upper body.

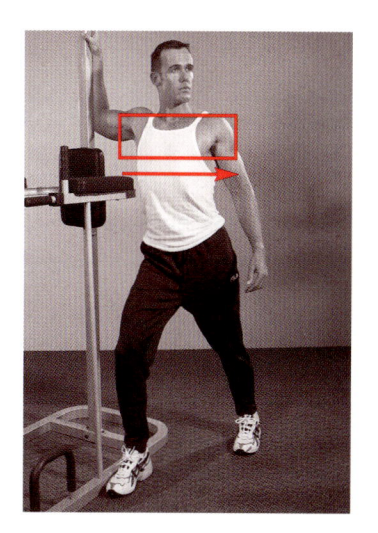

7. pecs standing

muscles stretching: **Pectorals (chest)**

Front deltoids (shoulders)

The action: Stand upright with your head up and shoulders back. Clasp your hands together behind your back and interlock your fingers. Straighten your arms and roll your shoulders back until you feel a stretch across the chest and shoulders. To intensify the stretch, begin to lift your arms. Hold the stretch.

Tip Try to stand tall and keep your shoulders back and avoid arching your lower back.

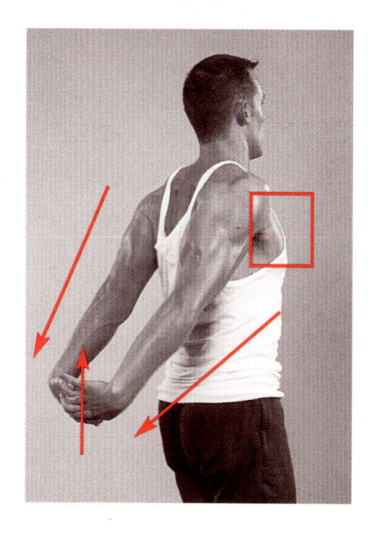

8. forearm flexors

muscles stretching: Forearm flexors (wrists)

The action: Stand upright with your head up and shoulders back. Outstretch your right arm, palms up and grasp your right hand fingers with your left hand. Bend your wrist and fingers down so your fingers point towards the floor. Try to keep your stretching arm straight as you stretch. Hold the stretch and repeat for the left side.

Tip Try to stand tall and keep your shoulders back and avoid arching your lower back.

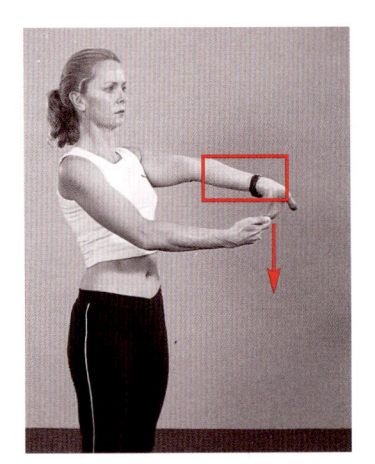

9. cat stretch

muscles stretching Abdominals (tummy)

Erectors (lower back)

area released spine

The action: Drop down to the floor supported by your hands and knees with your hands directly below your shoulders and your knees at the same width. Relax your belly button down towards the floor as you slightly lift your head and stick your backside out. You should feel a stretch in your abdominal muscles. Begin then to tuck your belly button in towards your spine as you round your back upwards while tucking your bottom and head under. You should feel a stretch in the muscles of your back and shoulders and through your spine. Hold the stretch at the top and the bottom

Tip Remember to stretch slowly and gently to avoid any sharp back and neck pain.

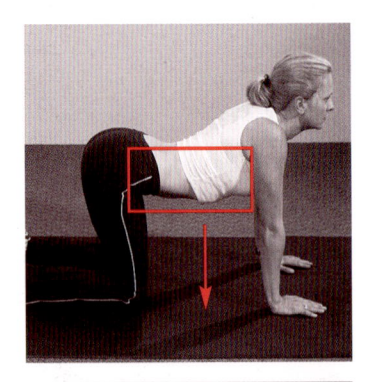

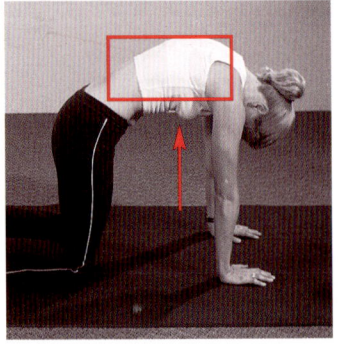

10. front hip

muscles stretching: Rectus femoris (high front thigh)

The action: Kneel down on the floor with your right knee and place your left foot flat on the floor well forward in front. Place your right hand at the back of your right hip and gently rock your pelvis forward while your left hand is supported on your left knee. Keep your chest up, shoulders back and your eyes focused straight ahead. Begin to lean your hips forward as you take your body weight on your left foot while your right hand supports your right hip. Hold the stretch and repeat for the left side.

Tip Remember to set your hips up with the pelvic rock before you commence the stretch and hold that hip position.

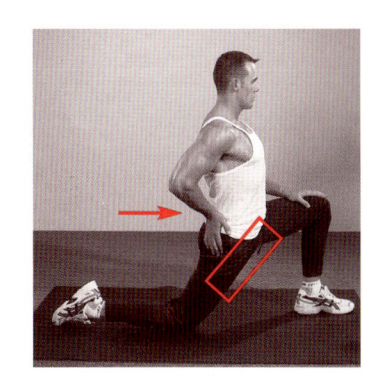

11. hip bend

muscles stretching: Gluteals (backside)

Hamstrings upper (back thigh)

The action: Lie down on the floor on your back with both legs outstretched. Raise your left knee in towards your chest and grasp your knee with both hands. Gently pull your left knee in and across towards your right shoulder while keeping your right leg straight. Hold the stretch and repeat for the left side.

Tip Try to avoid hunching your shoulders as you pull your knee in to the stretch.

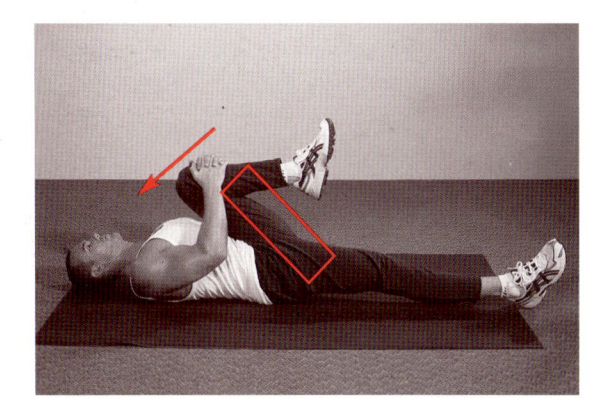

12. buttock

muscles stretching: Gluteals (backside)

Hamstrings upper (back thigh)

Deep hip rotators

The action: Lie down on the floor on your back with both feet flat against the floor about 12 inches away from your bottom. Raise your right leg up and lay your right ankle across your left knee. Reach your right hand forward to go beneath your right calf and your left hand forward to go past the outside of your left leg and clasp both hands together in front of your knee. Gently start to pull your left knee towards you, drawing your right ankle closer to your chest. You should feel this stretch mostly in the outside of your hips. Hold the stretch and repeat for the left side.

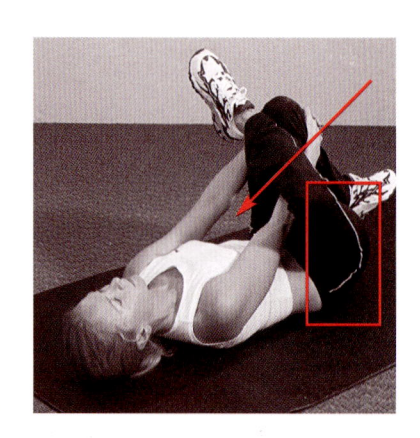

Tip Try to relax your head and shoulders against the floor and if you can't reach your hands to the front of your knee, grab both hands behind your knee.

13. short groin

muscles stretching: Short hip adductors (groin inner thigh)

Lateral hip

The action: Sit down on the floor with the bottoms of your feet pushed flat against each other. Draw your heels in as close to you as is comfortable. Grasp both ankles with your hands and sit as straight and tall as possible. As you gently start to lean forward with your back straight, begin pushing your knees towards the floor with your elbows. Hold the stretch.

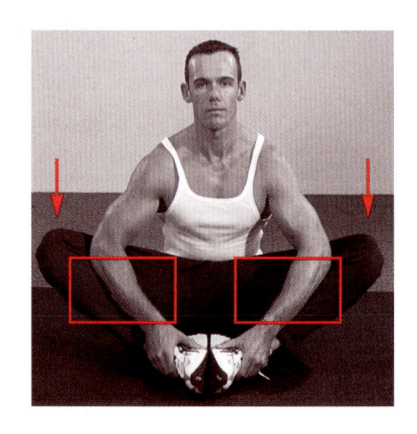

Tip Try not to let your head drop and your back to round as you lean forward.

14. quadricep stand

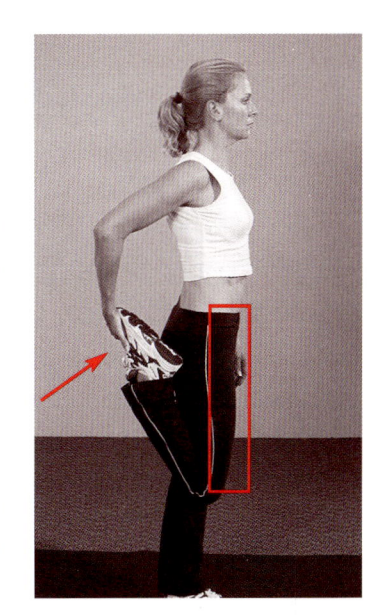

muscles stretching: Quadriceps (front thigh)

Rectus femoris (high front thigh)

The action: Stand upright with your eyes focused straight ahead. Bend your right knee to bring your right ankle toward your bottom and grasp your right ankle with your right hand. At the same time as you pull your right knee backwards try to push your right hip forward. It is important that you stand as straight as you can. Hold the stretch and repeat for the left side.

Tip You may need to hold onto a support if you are not comfortable with your balance. This stretch can also be done by grabbing your ankle with the opposite hand to give a slightly different stretch across the muscle.

15. hamstring sit

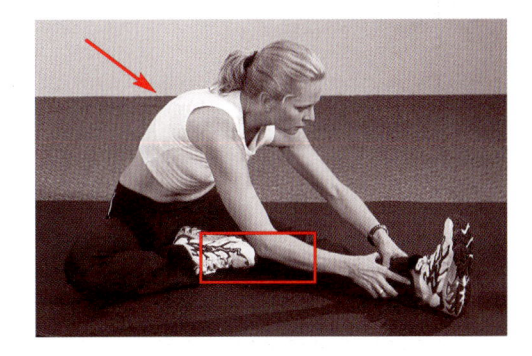

muscles stretching Hamstrings (back thigh)

Gluteus maximus (backside)

Gastrocnemius (lower leg calf)

The action: Sit down on the floor with your right leg outstretched and your toes pointing towards the ceiling. Bring your left foot in so the bottom of your left foot is supported against the inner thigh of your right leg. With your head up and shoulders back, gently start to lean forward from the hips pushing your chest out towards your right knee. Be sure to keep your back and your right leg straight as you reach out towards your right toe. Hold the stretch and repeat for the left side.

Tip You may also do this stretch by using a rolled up towel to place around your foot and hold each end like a rope. This will reduce the temptation to round your back if you can't quite reach your outstretched toe.

16. front shin

muscles stretching: Tibialis (lower leg front)

areas released: anterior knee and ankle joints

The action: Kneel down on the floor leaning your body weight forward onto your hands. Point your toes out directly behind you and gently sit back towards your heels. Try to sit as upright and straight as your flexibility will allow you. Hold the stretch.

Tip You will need to pay extra care and attention to your ankles and knees in this stretch, especially if you have any pre existing problems in these areas.

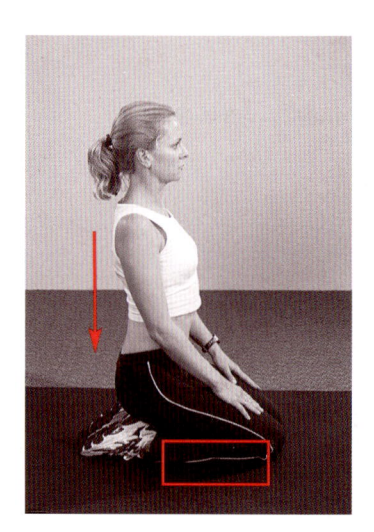

17. calf stand

muscles stretching: Gastrocnemius (lower leg calf)

The action: Start in a feet together, upright position. Place both hands on your left knee and raise your right foot and place it back on the floor well behind your front left foot with the toes from both feet pointing straight ahead. Keep your right leg straight and begin to lean forward onto your left leg as you push your right heel down into the floor. Hold the stretch and repeat for the left side.

Tip Make sure you keep both feet pointing straight ahead.

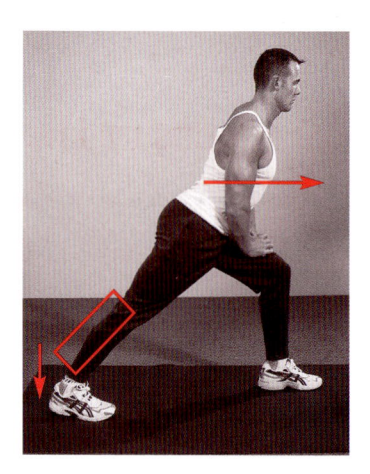

18. two hand lat stretch

muscles stretching: Latissimus dorsi (back)
Pectorals (chest)
Intercostals (rib area)

The action: Approach a vertical part of your home gym and grasp with a double hand grip at about chest height with your feet positioned at shoulder width. Begin to bend from your knees and hips in a partial squat action and place your head between your biceps as you keep both arms straight. You should feel a good stretch from under your arms down towards your waist. Hold the stretch.

Tip Try to imagine you are trying to drag your machine across the floor as you stretch, but without actually moving it.

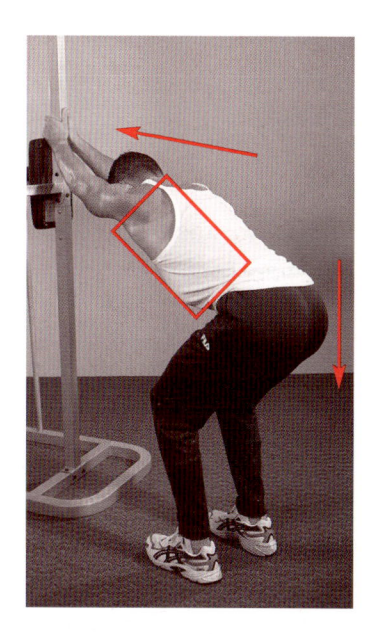

19. hamstring stand

muscles stretching: Hamstrings (back thigh)
Gluteus maximus (backside)
Gastrocnemius (lower leg calf)

The action: From an upright standing position, place your right heel down on the floor with your right leg straight and focus on pulling your right toes back towards your right shin. Place both hands on your left knee for balance and while keeping your head and shoulders back, gently start to lean forward from the hips pushing your chest out towards your right knee. Be sure to keep your back and your right leg straight as you lean out towards your right toe. Hold the stretch and repeat for the left side.

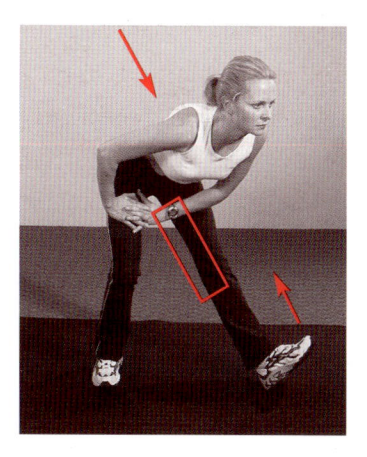

Tip Try not to let your back round as you lean out towards your knee.

20. gym ball stretch over

muscles stretching: Abdominals (tummy)
Rectus femoris (high front thigh)

areas released vertebral column, shoulder, chest

The action: Sit on top of your gym ball with both feet flat on the floor. Gently begin to walk both feet away from the ball while at the same time lie back onto the ball until your body is fully supported lying over the ball. With your hands placed beside your head, gently drop your head back towards the floor behind you until you feel a comfortable stretch in the abdominals and vertebral column. You may feel a slight stretching discomfort at the beginning of this stretch. Hold the stretch.

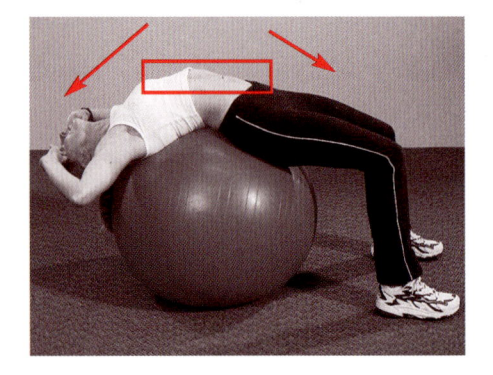

Tip To advance on this stretch, when you are comfortable with your balance, try extending your arms straight out above your head and straightening your legs.

FLEXIBILITY

SECTION FIFTEEN

good nutrition

Your nutrition will be no harder to conquer than your fitness, in fact it will probably be easier – there is less physical effort involved – it's all will power. We all know that we are not supposed to eat anything deep-fried and that most sweet things are bad for you. But how many of us know exactly why they are bad, other than the fact that they make you 'fat'?

Good nutrition is made so much easier by knowing what your body does with food once it goes into your mouth. What does your body need on a daily basis to keep it going? What happens to all that fish and chips, chocolate and ice cream once you eat it? Do you think that if you knew the answers to these questions it would be easier to stay on track? The answer is yes. Think of food as fuel for your body, not something that you just do out of habit a few times a day.

Enjoy what you eat and try as many different flavours as you can. Take an interest in the contents of the food that you consume. Read labels before you buy food in the supermarket. Learn about organic produce and how good it is for your body and the environment. Look for treats that are also healthy for you to eat, like all natural ice cream, raw nuts and preservative-free breads.

If you take the same interest in your diet as you do in your training, you should have no problems. Your body will also crave healthy food once you are doing some regular exercise. Try to listen to the signals that your body sends you. If you find yourself craving a particular food there is probably a good reason (even if it's chocolate!). Interpret what your body tells you and follow those instincts.

We suggest that you don't follow fat grams and calories too closely, this can easily become an obsession. Rather aim to get most of your nutrition each day from food that has gone through the least amount of processes as possible.

It is a good idea to check how many grams of fat you are consuming on a daily basis occasionally though. The biggest trap with most people's diets is still the amount of saturated fat they are consuming. By checking your overall fat intake on your food diary every three weeks you will be able to gauge whether or not you are on track. Follow the guidelines below for how many grams of fat you should be consuming on a daily basis.

For those who are wishing to reduce body fat:	30 – 40g per day
For most women and children:	30 – 50g per day
For most men:	40 – 60g per day
For active teenagers & very active adults:	70g per day

where are you now

If you are well and truly entrenched in bad eating habits, it will be hard to change. There are so many foods that taste great but aren't that great for you. Not just from a fat content point of view either. These foods are usually enhanced to make them taste so good. They can be high in sugar, salt and artificial enhancers, all of which our bodies have no use for. But our taste buds love them, and that's why companies produce the stuff. Your goal is to understand that these things, although they taste great are not good for you in abundance. Exercise your will power and enjoy them in moderation on your day off each week.

There is a little more to it than just how much fat and sugar you are consuming though. Most people we have encountered over the years are actually not eating enough food on a daily basis. Many miss breakfast, skip lunch altogether or grab a coffee because they are too busy to stop and eat and then overcompensate at dinner. Sound familiar?

Not consuming enough fruit and vegetables is another trap that many people fall into. Fresh produce doesn't last that long, is time consuming to prepare and expensive to buy in bulk. Many fridges tend to be full of foodstuffs that are quick and easy to prepare; and that certainly doesn't mean fruit and vegetables.

Sit down now and have a good honest think about your diet and what you consume on average on a daily basis. Do you eat breakfast lunch and dinner most days with the odd snack between meals to keep you going? Do you eat too much take away food? Do you drink too much alcohol? Read on and we will give you the answers and the guidelines.

popular myths

We hear stuff all the time about our diets and what is good or bad for us. Some of this information is accurate and based on current technical research. The rest is rumours and innuendos, the type of thing that has been said for years without any scientific back up for whether it is true or not. Here we aim to dispel some of those myths.

Potatoes, pasta and bread are fattening.

This one comes from a time when calorie counting was popular. These foods are carbohydrates. They are an excellent source of sustainable energy and tend to be high in calories because of their density. If consumed in large quantities carbohydrates are unsuitable for those wishing to reduce their body fat levels, but we would not deem them 'fattening'. Carbohydrates are less of a threat to a lean body than saturated fat and refined sugar.

Any fat in your diet is bad.

Wrong. Fat is an essential ingredient for the body. It is our long stay energy supply and is vital if our bodies are to function properly and remain healthy. Fat comes in good and bad varieties. Bad fats (saturated) are not essential for our bodies to function, they will have adverse effects for us such as heart disease and unhealthy weight gain. Good fats (mono/poly-unsaturated) on the other hand provide healthy energy.

If you want to lose weight, don't eat.

Wrong again. Eat more to lose more. If you restrict your food intake your body will go into survival mode. It will decrease the rate at which it burns fat and rather than burning it your body will store it.

If you exercise, it doesn't matter what you eat.

Spending an hour on the treadmill to work off that piece of chocolate cake isn't going to work. One doesn't cancel out the other, and in fact once you are exercising regularly it is even more important for you to eat healthily. Your body will require plenty of nutrient dense food to prevent illness and deficiencies.

starting the day

OK, so you've heard the saying that breakfast is the most important meal of the day. Guess what? It's true. Consider the fact that you haven't eaten anything in around eight or nine hours. How could you then expect your body to function efficiently for another few hours while you burn off energy reserves?

Your metabolism is fired up by food, that's why it is important to break-the-fast by eating something healthy in the morning. Think of your metabolism as a fire and food is the wood to fuel that fire. When the fire is burning bright, the body is working efficiently and burning off fuel instead of storing it for later. When the fire burns low, the body goes into survival mode, slows down the burning process and stores whatever comes in for later, just in case.

This is the main reason why fitness professionals and nutrition experts recommend you eat six smaller meals per day rather than three big ones – to help keep the fire burning bright. It makes sense then that a hearty and healthy start to the day is important because this is the time when your metabolism burns low and your body feels sluggish.

If you do not feel comfortable with eating in the morning, train yourself slowly and gently. Start with something small like a piece of wholemeal toast topped with a low fat spread or some fresh tomato and avocado. Try to avoid butter, margarine or stodgy high fat spreads, your body will have trouble digesting them first thing in the morning and they will induce feelings of lethargy by lunchtime. If the toast doesn't sound too appealing try a piece of fruit and maybe some low fat fruit yoghurt.

There are also some good breakfast bars on the market today. So if you find that you can't face eating first thing in the morning, try taking a fruit or breakfast bar and a piece of fruit with you and eat it on the way to work. If you are not working, shower and wake yourself up first, maybe go out for a walk, and then try nibbling little by little.

Avoid the temptation to start the day with tea or coffee. This will put something in your stomach and give your body the false impression of nourishment. Make your tea or coffee after you have eaten breakfast.

Ultimately we suggest you start the day with a good quality cereal, fruit and low fat yoghurt. This will provide all the good stuff that you need to kick-start yourself into the day and should keep you going until lunchtime or close to it.

Start the day with a stretch in bed before you get up, then rise grab a tall glass of water and maybe head out for a walk or run. When you come back, hit the shower, dress ready for the day and then sit down to your healthy breakfast. We absolutely guarantee that you will not regret getting up half an hour earlier to do it. You will feel alive and firing on all cylinders, ready to tackle the day. You will probably find that you will be more productive throughout the day as well

eating on the run

The perfect scenario above sounds great but how do you achieve it if you pack as much as possible into your day and get little or no time to yourself anyway. The only meal of the day you stop for is dinner, and even that you skip sometimes because you're too tired to be bothered.

It is possible to eat healthy food, and enough of it, on the run. It will just take a little more preparation time and some imagination.

Breakfast on the run has already been covered above. The alternative to a breakfast bar and piece of fruit on the way to work is to keep some cereal at work. We have both done this in the past, mostly because we are not morning people, but still have to eat. Have your cereal and fruit over the morning paper or while replying to yesterday's emails. Plan your day while eating, that way you are not rushing around trying to fit things in, you are sitting at your desk and accomplishing two tasks at once, quietly and comfortably.

Lunch is a tricky one. We have encountered so many people over the years that just find it impossible to stop for lunch, and if they do it's a boozy business lunch that tends to defeat the purpose. Our advice here is to have food in the top drawer of your desk, in your bag or the glove box of your car and eat while you work. Although it is much preferable for both the mind and the body to rest during the day for at least 15 minutes, we also understand that busy people can be stressed more by finding time to stop than eating on the go.

Aim to stop for lunch every other day. Your work and colleagues will benefit in the afternoon because you will be refreshed and refuelled and ready to go for a few more hours. Keep a store of muesli bars on hand, throw a piece of fruit in your briefcase before you leave for work or buy a slab of protein drinks – they taste better refrigerated but it isn't essential.

Next time you visit the supermarket check the shelves for foods that store well and are easy to eat on the run. Beware though that these foods quite often contain artificial ingredients, so read the back of the pack before you go loading up the trolley.

We highly recommend you stop for dinner most nights. Fast food dinners can be a major fat trap, and lets face it, by that time of night who wants to still be racing around? Do yourself a favour and slow down in preparation for bed and a good nights sleep.

If you must eat dinner on the run, try to prepare something yourself that can be easily re-heated. Avoid frozen meals, even though they claim to be low in fat, they still are not a great alternative to lean meat and fresh vegetables, and a quick stir-fry won't take long to whip up. Buy the meat and veggie's pre-chopped to save time.

cooking dinner

That brings us to cooking dinner. How often do you have take away or eat out for dinner each week? If you answered more than three times per week, you are consuming too much commercially prepared food. You probably think that you are making healthy choices, and some fast foods are better than others. But the bottom line is that you have no real idea of exactly what has gone into what you are eating. How much oil did they cook your pasta in? Did they trim excess fat from your chicken? If you are serious about healthy eating and more importantly reducing body fat, make the extra effort to cook at home.

Buy yourself a good low-fat cookbook that lists fat, carbohydrate and protein in grams, and calories or kilojoules. They are not that hard to find and the recipes contained within these books are usually easy to follow and quick to prepare.

As a rule, include a good-sized serve of vegetables for each person and a portion of lean meat. We suggest you limit your starchy carbohydrates (rice, pasta, potatoes) at dinner. These foods are more difficult to digest and are also a powerhouse of energy which is more likely to be stored overnight than burnt off because of the bodies extremely low level of activity during sleep.

Be prepared when cooking meals at home. Do a big shop every week and have a well- stocked pantry. Keep a week or two's worth of meat in your freezer and when cooking food like spaghetti bolognese, cook double and freeze half for an emergency dinner somewhere down the track. Buy frozen vegetables as well, these contain the same nutrient value as fresh ones believe it or not and are a good alternative to not eating a serve of veggies at all! Foods that can be easily prepared and put in the oven to cook are also good. This frees up your time to do something else while your meal is cooking.

When it comes to entertaining, use your imagination. Low fat meals don't only come in the standard family meal variety and if you're thinking decadent desert, then go ahead. If it is the weekend and you have worked hard at your diet and exercise plan all week then you deserve it!

pantry survival list

Keeping your pantry stocked full of the kinds of foodstuffs that can quickly and easily constitute a tasty, low-fat, nutritious meal is a must. Below we have listed our favourite staple food supplies that will never leave you short of a tasty meal!

in the pantry

Tinned low-salt tomatoes	Lentils
Tinned potatoes	Organic tinned soup
Tins of tuna in spring water	Low-salt tomato paste
Tins of low-salt salmon	Wholemeal Pasta
Red kidney beans	Rice, brown and Arborio
Baked beans, low-salt	Couscous
Good quality olive oil	Tinned fruit in natural juice
Long life heat-treated skim milk	Natural unsalted nuts
Wheat germ	Dried fruit
Rolled oats	Honey

in the freezer

lean cuts of red and white meat	organic bread
assorted pre-packed vegetables	filo pastry
strawberries, raspberries & blueberries	fresh pasta
home pre-cooked meals	fresh pasta sauce
low-fat ice cream	

in the fridge

fresh vegetables in assorted colours	fresh fruit in assorted colours
cottage cheese	low-fat yoghurt
fresh eggs	fresh salad leaves
low-fat cheese	

the importance of drinking water

Did you know that your body is made up of around 80 percent water? Water is responsible for transporting vitamins and minerals around the body. It flushes toxins from the kidneys and keeps the brain functioning in a healthy fashion. It will also aid in the reduction of fluid retention by flushing out retained fluids.

Drinking water is essential for those exercising, by the time you start to feel thirsty through training and sweating you are already on the road to dehydration. Sip water before during and after your training session. The same goes for people in hot and humid or windy and warm conditions where your body will lose a lot of fluid without you being completely aware of it.

Tea, coffee, fizzy drinks, cordials and sweetened juices do not count as re-hydration fluids. These drinks have only a small water content and also contain substances which the body identifies as food, therefore digesting them through a different process and not absorbing the fluid efficiently. Tea and coffee also contain a diuretic which has the opposite effect to hydration of the bodies systems.

Herbal teas and unsweetened juices can contribute to your fluid intake for the day. But we suggest that you get the majority of the recommended 1.5 to 2 litres per day from still water.

what about alcohol

Alcohol is fine to consume in small amounts. If you enjoy a glass or two of wine each night with dinner, continue to do so. There are many proven healthy qualities contained in wine especially red wine. Red wine tends to contain antioxidants which are the good guys for our bodies, so if you do drink wine with dinner, try sticking with red.

All varieties of beer are high in kilojoules, something that a lot of people don't realise. That classically named 'beer belly' is an apt description for something that happens to people who tend to drink a lot of beer – excess unhealthy body fat around the mid section. There is unfortunately nothing good about beer at all, other than the obvious fact that it tastes so good after a long day!

GOOD NUTRITION

Try to limit your beer intake to one or two a day and have at least two totally beer-free days per week. If you are trying to reduce your body fat, we suggest that you reduce your intake of beer even further.

Spirits are very low in kilojoules. That's the good news. However the soft drinks that most people mix with them are packed full of sugar, have you ever heard someone ask for a scotch and diet coke? Now you know why!

We highly recommend that you have two alcohol free days each week. Alcohol is still identified by the body as a toxin, it has no real use for our systems. Drink equal amounts of water with alcohol and remember that if it is only taken in moderation, alcohol has no real adverse effects on the body.

Beer 1 can, 375ml	555kj
White wine, 1 glass, 150ml	465kj
Red wine 1 glass, 150ml	425kj
Champagne 1 glass, 150ml	405kj
Spirits 1 nip, 30ml	270kj (average)

time out

Just as we suggest you take regular time out from your training, we also suggest time out from your healthy eating program. Your day off training should be your day to relax your diet too. If you have been good all week, eating the right food avoiding the bad, then relax and have the things you like and enjoy.

Most people will take a day off from their program on the weekend. As we have said previously, this is the time when most of us socialise, eat out, and drink more alcohol.

It is important that you take time out with your diet. Food serves a purpose, but it is also meant to be enjoyed. There are a lot of foods that are not all that good for us but that taste fantastic. Everyone has a weakness that should be indulged. If you don't enjoy these indulgences on a regular basis, sticking to a strict eating regime mid week will be hard, and downright boring.

Try to relax on your day off and not feel guilty. You will not sabotage your results by taking time out and in the long run can only do yourself benefit. Most days you will be good, eating the right foods and feeling great. On your day off you will have the things you love but that you know you can't eat in abundance all week long if you are to reduce your body fat levels and maintain or increase your lean muscle mass.

Your approach and enthusiasm for your training will not wane, neither will your enthusiasm for reaching your goals. Because you will not feel deprived.

eating out

Eating out is something that we all enjoy doing. Having somebody else prepare, cook and serve your meal is a great treat, especially when you can get up and leave without cleaning the kitchen afterwards!

Commercially prepared food is a trap for poor nutrition and high fat though. If you are eating in top restaurants every night you won't be suffering from poor nutrition because (hopefully!) they are using the best quality meat and produce. You will however also find that there will probably be a good deal more fat in the meals than what you would otherwise use at home. And anyway, how many of us eat out at top restaurants every night?

We're not suggesting you refrain from eating out altogether, just that you limit the amount of times you do so each week and be aware that eating out, even if you make a healthy selection, won't be the same as a home cooked meal.

We urge you to eat out once or twice a week, preferably on your 'day off'. It will be good for your motivation levels, and it doesn't have to be dinner; perhaps you like to have breakfast out on the weekends or lunch with a friend. Do whatever you enjoy doing and know that it won't do your program any harm if done in moderation.

We also suggest you eat whatever it is that you enjoy. Remember, this is your day off and your chance to have the kinds of food that you shouldn't mid-week when you are training hard and eating well.

good and bad fast foods

Some take away foods are definitely a better choice that others, for their high level of nutritional value and for their lower levels of saturated fat we suggest:

Beef burger with salad	18g total fat,	1640kj (average)
Chicken burger with salad	15g total fat,	1785kj (average)
Kebab – chicken	25g total fat,	2815kj (average)
– lamb	37g total fat,	3210kj (average)
BBQ or rotisserie chicken (breast qtr with skin)	13g total fat,	900kj (average)
Sandwiches or rolls (lean meat and salad)	6g total fat,	840kj (average)

Pizzas aren't a bad choice either; stick with the gourmet variety though. They tend to contain less fat because the amount of cheeses and oils are less than traditional pizzas.

Now we come to the baddies, we advise against these because they will contain the opposite to those above: higher levels of saturated fat and low nutritional value.

Pie	24g total fat,	1660kj (average)
Sausage roll	23g total fat,	1560kj (average)
Hot dog	24g total fat,	1850kj (average)
Fish and chips	44g total fat,	3130kj (average)
Fried chicken	15g total fat,	900kj (average)

fat grams in popular snack foods

cheese crackers, 4, 16g	4g total fat,	315kj
chocolate biscuits, 2, 20g	3.5g total fat,	365kj
cheddar cheese, 30g	10g total fat,	505kj
milk chocolate, 10 squares, 50g	13.5g total fat,	1080kj
doughnut-iced, 1, 80g	19.5g total fat,	1425kj
peanuts, 50g	26g total fat,	1285kj
pate, 50g	12g total fat,	620kj
popcorn, 1 cup, 10g	2.5g total fat,	195kj
potato crisps, 50g packet	16g total fat,	1050kj
pretzels, 30g	1g total fat,	470kj

good fats, bad fats

You have probably heard that there are some fats that are OK to eat or that are even good for you. It's true, despite popular belief that all fats are bad, some are fine for you to eat but still in moderation.

Saturated fat, which we have already mentioned, is the one to stay away from. Bad fats include butter, margarine, shortening or lard and fat on meat products. Check nutritional details on foods in the supermarket, most will list saturated fat separately. Processed foods will usually be high in saturated fat as well.

Unsaturated fats are the good guys, most contain essential fatty acids. These are the ones that our body requires on a regular basis to maintain a whole host of normal functions. These include olive, sesame and canola oils, fish, nuts, seeds and of course avocados.

Good fats should not be eaten in abundance though, they still contain high levels of fat that isn't great for anyone in bulk amounts long term. One small portion of any good fat each day will be enough to supply your body with the essential fatty acids that it needs .

healthy alternatives

Below we have listed some healthy alternatives to those high fat/processed foods that are popular at all meal times.

Breakfast	**substitute with**
Sugary processed cereals	whole wheat cereals
Buttered toast	mashed avocado/cottage cheese
Fried eggs	poached eggs

Lunch	**substitute with**
Fish and chips	grilled fish and salad
Burgers	sandwiches
Creamy pasta	soup and toast

Dinner	**substitute with**
Roast leg of lamb	roasted fillet of beef
Spaghetti Bolognese	wholemeal pasta & tomato-based sauce
Creamy curries	Stir fry's

what is a diet

What does the word diet mean to you? Unfortunately over the years the word 'diet' has been used to describe an eating format for someone who is trying to lose weight. For most when the word diet is mentioned the thought of celery sticks and low-fat cottage cheese springs to mind!

But it shouldn't be that way. Ever heard of a dietician? This isn't someone who restricts your eating in order to lose weight, it is someone who analyses what people eat in order to assess and fix all kinds of different ailments from skin diseases to food allergies to hormone imbalances.

Diet is a word used to describe what a person eats, any person, not just those who are looking to reduce their body fat levels.

Of those who have followed a fad diet in the past, most will see immediate results and then a plateau, usually followed by weight gain, hence the term 'yo yo dieting'. Another popular one that most of us are familiar with.

Weight levels go up and down as you restrict your food intake to a lower nutrient level than your body requires. This slows the metabolism.

Our bodies were never designed for nutrient or calorific restriction. We are designed to eat a whole range of different foods on a regular basis and take regular bouts of exercise. Both of which have been mixed up over the centuries. We now tend to do a whole lot less exercise and to counteract the effect we restrict our food intake.

Restricting what you eat in order to lose weight will get you little or no results. Initially your body weight will reduce, owing to your metabolism slowing down through loss of fuel (food). When you lose weight you will not only be losing body fat but healthy lean muscle mass.

Lean muscle mass is the good stuff, you don't want to lose that, it helps to keep your metabolism firing which in turn keeps you burning body fat. The overall effect of constantly going on fad diets to lose weight is that you fluctuate between healthy weight ranges and reduce your overall metabolic rate.

People who fad diet regularly find it impossible to maintain a healthy and normal weight range and will rarely be at a stage where their body is physically healthy and functioning normally. This is not a healthy or permanent way to lose weight.

Your diet or eating plan should be something that easily fits in with your lifestyle. You should try to include a large range of foods that will provide you with the vitamins and nutrients that you need to function normally while effectively fighting against disease.

Variety in your diet will not only provide you with essential requirements, it will also give you variety of taste, smell and colour. This is important to stimulate your senses and keep you interested in food. Eating good quality food is really enjoyable and once you start eating healthily you will realise that contrary to what most people believe, good food actually tastes much better than bad food.

GOOD NUTRITION

Our diet should provide us with a constant source of energy throughout the day, starting with a wholesome breakfast and following through the right sources of carbohydrates protein and fats for lunch, dinner and snacks in between.

Most importantly of all though, it should be enjoyable. Food isn't something to be avoided; it is something to be enjoyed in both quality and quantity. Stop placing emphasis on your diet as a means to losing weight and start looking at it as a way of fuelling your body and allowing you to get the results from your training that you are after.

sample fitnes fat-loss eating plan

Meal 1.
cereal and non-fat milk
1 piece of fruit
500ml of water

Meal 2.
1-2 slices of wholemeal toast or;
2 crispbread crackers
$1/2$ cup low-fat cottage cheese with celery

Meal 3.
wholemeal sandwich – no butter – with;
chicken/tuna/lean beef and salad
500ml of water

Meal 4.
low-fat yoghurt
1 piece of fruit

Meal 5.
chicken (no skin)/lean beef/fish and;
steamed vegetables or salad to fill
500ml of water

Meal 6.
$1/2$ cup of low-fat cottage cheese with;
celery and/or carrot

THIS IS NOT A DIET!

This is a sample eating plan designed to show you the sorts of foods you could include to achieve your fitness and fat-loss results. Feel free to substitute any of the above foods for a similar food type. For example if you are training for a higher level of fitness, you may need to add a few more energy foods to your lunch or pre-training snack. You may also wish to contact a dietician who can set a diet plan tailored specifically for you.

Foods that may be eaten anytime

carbohydrates: most fruit and vegetables

protein: lean meat, fish, egg-whites, tofu, low-fat cottage cheese, low-fat/non-fat milk, low-fat yoghurt

fats: good fats in small amounts such as avocado, nuts, olive and canola oil

Foods best eaten before meal 4

*carbohydrates: starch-based carbohydrates such as pasta, rice, potatoes, pumpkin, bread

*The reason for this is that too many high-energy foods eaten later in the day will not be utilised whilst sleeping and tend to be stored as fat, not to mention messing with your blood-sugar levels.

The most important thing about following any relatively strict eating plan is that you must never tell yourself "I am not allowed to eat that". Our belief is that you can eat anything you want, it's really the amounts that do the damage. It is for this reason that one day of your seven-day eating plan should be a 'free-day' (usually over the weekend). This means you may enjoy things like alcohol, ice cream, pizza etc. but obviously in moderation and only once a week.

Use this day as your weekly goal to work towards and live a little. Know that you have earned it when it comes around and use it to keep you from feeling deprived.

GOOD NUTRITION

sample strengthmuscle size eating plan

Meal 1. cereal and non-fat milk
1 piece of fruit
low-fat yoghurt
2 slices of wholemeal toast with jam/honey/peanut butter
500ml of water

Meal 2. 3 boiled eggs (discard 2 yolks)
2 crispbread crackers
1 cup of water

Meal 3. 1/4 or 1/2 chicken (no skin)
wholemeal bread roll – no butter
cold rice salad or pasta salad
1 cup of fruit salad
500ml of water

Meal 4. low-fat muesli bar
low-fat yoghurt
1 piece of fruit
1 cup of water

Meal 5. chicken (no skin)/lean beef/fish and;
1/2 cup legumes (beans, peas, lentils etc) and;
steamed vegetables or salad and;
a small serve of pasta/rice or 1 baked/boiled potato
500ml of water

Meal 6. 1/2 cup low-fat cottage cheese with;
celery and/or carrot
1 cup of tinned or fresh fruit

THIS IS NOT A DIET!

This is a sample eating plan designed to show you the sorts of foods you could include to achieve your strength and muscle size gains. Feel free to substitute any of the above foods for a similar food type as this is only one example of a healthy eating plan to help achieve strength and muscle size without gaining excess body fat. It is appropriate for a person of approximately 70kg in weight who is training regularly. You may wish also to contact a dietician who can set up a diet plan specifically for you.

Foods that may be eaten anytime

carbohydrates: most fruit and vegetables

protein: lean meat, fish, egg whites, tofu, low-fat cottage cheese, low-fat/non-fat milk, low-fat yoghurt

fats: good fats in small amounts such as avocado, nuts, olive and canola oil

Foods best eaten before meal 4

*carbohydrates: starch-based carbohydrates such as pasta, rice, potatoes, pumpkin, bread

*The reason for this is that too many high-energy foods eaten later in the day will not be utilised whilst sleeping and tend to be stored as fat, not to mention messing with your blood-sugar levels.

On a strength/muscle size eating plan, a small amount of starch-based carbohydrates is not going to make a significant difference to your overall body fat levels but will however be beneficial in the muscle building process.

The most important thing about following any relatively strict eating plan is that you must never tell yourself "I am not allowed to eat that". Our belief is that you can eat anything you want, it's really the amounts that do the damage. It is for this reason that one day of your seven-day eating plan should be a 'free-day' (usually over the weekend). This means you may enjoy things like alcohol, ice cream, pizza etc. but obviously in moderation and only once a week.

Use this day as your weekly goal to work towards and live a little. Know that you have earned it when it comes around and use it to keep you from feeling deprived.

sample eating for health plan

Meal 1. cereal and non-fat milk
1 piece of fruit
500ml of water

Meal 2. 2 slices of raisin toast
low-fat flavoured milk

Meal 3. wholemeal sandwich – no butter – with;
chicken/tuna/lean beef and;
cheese or avocado and salad
500ml of water

Meal 4. 1 low-fat muffin
1 piece of fruit
1 cup of tea or coffee

Meal 5. chicken (no skin)/lean beef/fish and;
steamed vegetables or salad and;
small serve of pasta/rice or 1 baked/boiled potato
500ml of water

Meal 6. 1 cup of fruit salad
1 scoop low-fat ice cream

THIS IS NOT A DIET!

This is a sample eating plan designed to show you the sorts of foods you could include to maintain a healthy eating lifestyle. Feel free to substitute any of the above foods for a similar food type.

Foods that may be eaten anytime

carbohydrates:	most fruit and vegetables
protein:	lean meat, fish, egg-whites, tofu, low-fat cottage cheese, low-fat/non-fat milk, low-fat yoghurt
fats:	good fats in small amounts such as avocado, nuts, olive and canola oil

Foods best eaten before meal 4

*carbohydrates:	starch-based carbohydrates such as pasta, rice, potatoes, pumpkin, bread

*The reason for this is that too many high-energy foods eaten later in the day will not be utilised whilst sleeping and tend to be stored as fat, not to mention messing with your blood-sugar levels.

On a healthy eating or body maintenance plan, a small amount of starch-based carbohydrates is not going to make a significant difference to your overall body fat levels.

The most important thing about following any relatively strict eating plan is that you must never tell yourself "I am not allowed to eat that". Our belief is that you can eat anything you want, it's really the amounts that do the damage. It is for this reason that one day of your seven-day eating plan should be a 'free-day' (usually over the weekend). This means you may enjoy things like alcohol, ice cream, pizza etc. but obviously in moderation and only once a week.

Use this day as your weekly goal to work towards and live a little. Know that you have earned it when it comes around and use it to keep you from feeling deprived.

Glossary

Aerobic – This means exercising 'with oxygen'. Aerobic exercises are those involving low-level intensity eg walking or jogging.

Anaerobic – This means exercising 'without oxygen'. Anaerobic exercise is fast, explosive work that cannot be sustained for long periods of time eg sprinting or weight lifting.

Antioxidants – Necessary nutrients for the body to help fight the build up of free radicals and disease.

Cardio training – Aerobic or anaerobic exercise designed to improve health and fitness of the heart, lungs and body composition of fat and muscle.

Circulation – The flow of blood around the body.

Circuit training – A training method where a series of exercises are performed in succession for short periods of time with a timed rest between each exercise.

Compound exercises - Compound exercises are those that involve the use of a number of muscles working together creating movement through a number of joints.

Connective tissue – Tendons that connect bones and muscles together.

Essential fatty acids – Fats that our bodies can't produce. We must obtain them through our diet, they are essential for keeping out bodies healthy and fighting off disease.

Flexibility – The measure of how our bodies move, determined by our muscles and joints.

Form – The style in which a repetition is performed - properly and safely or loose and unsafely.

Glycogen – This form of energy otherwise known as glucose is stored in the muscles.

Isolation exercises – Isolation exercises are those that usually isolate one single muscle and create movement through only one single joint.

Lean muscle mass – A measure of muscle excluding fat.

Maximum heart rate (MHR) – The maximum level to which a person should raise their heart rate. Determined by age.

Metabolism – The process by which food comes into the body and the rate at which it is used.

Multi-gym – A machine that offers the opportunity to perform a number of exercises, usually with a cabling system.

Muscle failure – The point at which the muscles are no longer capable of lifting a weight.

Opposing muscles – Using opposite muscles eg back and chest or quadriceps and hamstrings.

Post exercise muscle soreness – The level of discomfort felt in the muscles following a training session. Caused by unfamiliar or overly strenuous exercise.

Range of movement – The distance that your muscles and joints are capable of moving through.

Repetitions – The number of times a resistance exercise is performed.

Resistance training – Training with weights or using your body to resist some other force eg push ups or chin ups.

Saturated fat – The bad fats. Fat that is solid at room temperature. Has been linked to high blood pressure and heart disease.

Sets – A group of repetitions.

Training zone – A calculated upper and lower heart rate zone in which you would attempt to keep your heart rate. Zones vary depending on your goals.

Unsaturated fat – The good fats. Fat that is liquid at room temperature. It is essential for many of the functions of the body.

Bibliography

The following books have been consulted in compiling this book.

Jeffrey Hodges – Sports Mind – Hawk Personal Excellence, 1993

Dennis Waitley – The Psychology of Winning – Business Education Institute Pty Ltd

Gary Egger & Nigel Champion – The Fitness Leaders Handbook, Third Edition – Kangaroo Press Pty Ltd, 1990

Matt Roberts – 90-day Fitness Plan – Dorling Kindersley Ltd, 2001-10-19

Bill Phillips & Michael D'Orso – Body for Life – Harper Collins Publishers, 1999

Rosemary Stanton – Fat & Fibre Counter – Wilkinson Books, 1993

Kate Grenville – Writing from Start to Finish – Allen & Unwin, 2001

Acknowledgments

We would firstly like to thank Paul Boyle from York Fitness Australia, for his support and constructive advice during this whole process. Without Paul this book would look totally different! He was always on hand to provide us with anything we needed, from product information to the use of the York Fitness Sydney showroom for our photo shoot. Thanks Paul we really appreciate it.

Thanks also to Dad for giving up so much of his time to organise the lighting and photography equipment for our photo shoot. Not to mention the years of support he has given us during Phyne Physique's successful lifespan. Thanks Dad.

A special thank you to Callum, Bev and Sean for putting up with us during the final three months of our project in Wellington, New Zealand. We know there were times when you just wanted your house and attic back, free of computers, printers and paperwork!

A big thank you also to our book designer Sam Auger. He took on our project without fully realising what he was in for, but stuck it out to the end and did a brilliant job. We really appreciate all those late nights you spent in your home office pumping out chapter after chapter.

We would also like to thank Alex Cramb for planting the seed. We vividly remember that morning sitting at a café in Balmain when Alex pointed out in no uncertain terms just which of our projects should be given priority! Alex also gave us his time on many occasions to help us with great ideas and advice on how things are done in the publishing world. Thanks also to Paul Gosney for doing our portrait shots in his Balmain studio at a very reasonable rate!

Last of all a very big thank you to all of our clients whom we have worked with during the years at Phyne Physique. You guys have given us the experience that we needed to write this book. Without that experience we wouldn't have a good 'feel' for what people really need from home training. We would especially like to thank all of you who we used to bounce ideas off once this project was underway. Your thoughts and ideas have been invaluable.

Index

A

Abdominals (torso) 74, 167-178

Accessories 43

Advanced machines 37

Advantages and disadvantages of free weights 61

Advantages and disadvantages of machines 60

Alcohol 276-277

Ankle/wrist weights 46

B

Back arms (triceps) 73, 152-163

Back (latissimus dorsi) 71,

Back thigh (hamstrings) 70, 85-89

Beer 276, 277

Blank program cards 248-251

BMI (body mass index) 217

Body measurements 217-218

Boxing equipment 42-43

Breakfast 270

C

Cardio equipment 38-39, 198

Cardio for fitness 191-194

Cardio for good health 183-185

Cardio for weight loss 186-191

Chest (pectorals) 72, 115-127

Clothing, what to wear 204-205

Commitment 6

Compound exercises 246

D

Diet myths 270-271

Diet, what is a 281-283

Dinner 274

E

Eating plan, sample fitness/fat loss 283-284

Sample strength/muscle size 285-287

Sample for health 287-288

Eating out 278

Education 5

Elliptical trainers 42, 200-201

Equipment for your studio 26-48

Exercise bikes 39-40, 199-200

Exercise mats 46

F

Fast foods 279

Fat grams, required 269

In fast foods 279

In snack foods 280

Fats, good and bad 280

Favourite Exercises 18-19, 252-253

Fitness assessment 215-216, results 218, the score 218-219

Fitness/fat loss programs,

    Beginners 235-237

    Intermediate 238-240

    Advanced 241-243

Flexibility 254-255

Food diary 222

Forearms (wrists) 73, 164-166

Front arms (biceps) 73, 141-151

Front thigh (quadriceps) 70, 75-84

G

Goals, goal setting 19-23,

H

Heart rate, monitors 47-48

    Target 195-196

    Chart 196

    Maximum 195, 196

    Checking pulse 185

I

Injury prevention 12

Isolation exercises 246

L

Lifestyle questionnaire 211, results 212-213

Lower back (torso) 74, 179-180

Lower leg (gastrocnemius) 70, 91-94

Lunch 272, 273

M

Medical questionnaire 214

Metabolism 271

Motivation 4, 14-15

Multigyms 35-37,

Muscle soreness 67

O

One-minute crunch test 216

One minute push up test 215

P

Perceived rate of exertion 197

R

Repetitions 62-63,

Resistance training – see strength training

Rest and recovery 8

S

Section of an existing room 50-52

Sets 63

Shoulder circles 257

Shoulders (deltoids) 72, 128-140

Sit and reach test 216

Skipping ropes 46-47,

Spirits 277

Stepping machines 41, 202-203

Strength training 58

Strength training programs,

    Beginners 224-226

    Intermediate 227-229

    Advanced 230-232

Strength training techniques 233-234

Stretches, Buttock 262

    Calf stand 264

    Cat stretch 260

    Forearm flexors 260

    Front hip 261

    Front shin 264

    Gym ball stretch over 266

    Hamstring sit 263

    Hamstring stand 265

    High reach 258

    Hip bend 261

    Pecs standing 259

    Pecs supported 259

    Pull behind 256

    Quadriceps stand 263

    Short groin 262

    Shoulder circles 257

    Shoulder pull across 257

    Tricep pull down 258

    Two hand lat stretch 265

Stretching, benefits of 255-256

    How to 255

T

The garage 54-56

The spare room 52-54

Thirty-minute express workout 244-245

Three-minute step test 215

Training diary 23-25, 222

Treadmills 40, 198-199

Twelve week planner 207, 221

U

Upper back (trapezius) 71, 95-113

W

Water intake 276

Weight training belts 44

Weight training gloves 45

Wine 276, 277

Writing your own program 246-247

notes:

notes: